T0401374

PROGRESS IN CELL GROWTH PROCESS RESEARCH

PROGRESS IN CELL GROWTH PROCESS RESEARCH

TAKUMI HAYASHI
EDITOR

Nova Biomedical Books
New York

LIBRARY OF CONGRESS CATALOGING-IN-PUBLICATION DATA

Progress in cell growth process research / Takumi Hayashi (editor).
        p. ;cm.
Includes bibliographical references and index.
ISBN 978-1-60456-325-2(hardcover)
1. Cells—Growth. I. Hayashi,Takumi.
[DNLM: 1. Cell Growth. Processes—physiology. QU 375 P964 2008]
QH604.7.P76 2008
571.8'49—dc22
                        2008002845

Published by Nova Science Publishers, Inc. ✦ New York

CONTENTS

PREFACE

When used in the context of reproduction of living cells the phrase "cell growth" is shorthand for the idea of "growth in cell populations by means of cell reproduction." During cell reproduction one cell (the "mother" cell) divides to produce two daughter cells.

Cell proliferation, which depends on the intimately linked processes of growth and division, is a fundamental systems-level attribute of all life forms. The precise regulation of proliferation in response to internal and external cues is critical for development, tissue renewal and evolutionary fitness, while in the disregulation of cell proliferation underlies a variety of human diseases, most notably cancer and aging. Historically, breakthroughs in our understanding of cell growth and division have derived from cross-fertilization results and ideas from researchers studying a wide range of model organisms, from yeast to humans. The basis for cell proliferation entails the control of key signaling and cell cycle regulators through transcriptional, translational, post-translational, genetic, and epigenetic mechanisms. Indeed, many conceptual breakthroughs in cell regulation have been derived from analysis of basic cell cycle mechanisms. This book is dedicated to new research from around the globe in this field.

Chapter 1 - The endothelium can no longer be regarded as an inert layer of cells lining the inside surface of the vascular system. It is now becoming clear that endothelial cells (EC) actively and reactively participate in multifaceted reactions and can mount anti- and pro-inflammatory and protective responses depending on environmental conditions. Endothelial cell dysfunction or activation also contributes to a variety of disease states. Considering the role of the endothelium in the initiation and propagation of vascular wall injury, there is a need for the discovery of validated biomarkers to serve as predictors for activation of inflammatory cascades in the development of vascular injury. Among the laboratory methods available for the detection of endothelial dysfunction, the use of species- and disease-specific endothelial cell culture models enables the presentation of heterogenous endothelial phenotypes and the assessment of environmental conditions on endothelial cell function. This review describes various in vitro EC culture systems with respect to developing therapeutic interventions in cardiovascular diseases. Understanding the mechanisms of EC dysfunction is a prerequisite for EC-targeted therapy to reduce the incidence of cardiovascular diseases.

Chapter 2 - Intracellular redox balance, i.e. the ratio between oxidizing and reducing species within the cell, plays a significant role in the regulation of cellular processes. Redox balance results from the activities of enzymatic systems that produce or neutralize oxidizing species. Aerobic metabolism significantly affects intracellular redox balance through the formation of reactive oxygen species. ROS. ROS, including superoxide anion, singlet oxygen, hydrogen peroxide and hydroxyl radical, are potent oxidizing agents that largely alter redox balance and target a variety of cellular components. Mitochondrial respiration as well as cytosolic and membrane oxidases contribute largely to the regulation of intracellular redox balance.

In the past, intracellular accumulation of ROS was thought to lead exclusively to an unspecific damage to cellular components. Nowadays, the physiological relevance of redox balance regulation by ROS has been reevaluated. In fact, emerging data suggest that ROS function as signaling molecules that regulate cellular processes such as angiogenesis, fat development, stem cell renewal, and apoptosis. Furthermore, ROS were shown to regulate stem cell pools maintenance and proliferation and to adjust their differentiation program.

Here the authors review the current knowledge about ROS control of cellular growth and differentiation, discuss the critical and context specific role of ROS in regulating cell processes and finally hypothesize that integration of the different tissue specific regulatory circuits with the alteration of redox balance induced by ROS accumulation determines cell fate.

Chapter 3 - Generally, normal diploid somatic cells cultivated in standard growth media supplemented with ordinary fetal bovine serum do not replicate indefinitely. However, under similar culture conditions transformed cells with abnormal chromosome complements replicate indefinitely. Interestingly, embryonic stem cells contain diploid karyotype yet they have unlimited proliferation potential if maintained in appropriate culture conditions. Although normal somatic stem cells also contain diploid chromosomes, they are unable to proliferate indefinitely in vitro. In contrast to embryonic stem cells, somatic stem cells can potentially be used in autologous cell transplantation but their restricted proliferation limits their successful application in clinical settings. Therefore, improvement of proliferation of somatic stem cells is not only desirable for clinical, but also for research applications. The authors have recently developed a two-step cell culture protocol to improve the proliferation of various types of normal somatic cells derived from diverse mammalian species. In the first step of the method, immortal hybrid cells are generated containing polyploid chromosomes derived from normal cells by fusing normal somatic cells with a hypo-diploid immortal murine cell line GM05267 using polyethylene glycol. In the second step, conditioned media are collected from the proliferating hybrid cells and subsequent cultivation of normal parental somatic cells in the presence of this conditioned media to generate long-term growing somatic cell lines containing diploid chromosomes. In the present article, the background of the discovery of a two-step cell culture protocol will be presented along with an update of recent findings to demonstrate that this method has general applicability. The generation of hybrid cells using the specific murine cell line can be used in the generation of hybrids with tissue specific cell types and can be used to produce tissue specific growth-factors to improve the proliferation of tissue specific somatic cells, including adult stem cells.

Chapter 4 - Embryonic stem cells that derive from the inner cell mass of the blastocyst induce a variety of tissues and form the central nervous system. The cells that differentiate into neural progenitor cells exist on the ventricular zone of the embryonic brain and produce neuronal and glial cells during the developmental period. Although neurogenesis—the generation of new neuronal cells—has been thought to terminate after the embryonic stage, it has recently been found that neural progenitor cells exist in parts of the adult brain, namely the subventricular zone and the dentate gyrus of the hippocampus. Furthermore, it has been suggested that glial fibrillary acidic protein (GFAP)-positive cells are capable of trans-differentiating to give rise to neural progenitor cells in the adult brain. In the processes of cell growth, neural progenitor cells derived from GFAP-positive cells express a variety of cell-specific markers such as nestin, polysialylated neural cell adhesion molecule (PSA-NCAM), and others. In addition, the proliferation rate of neural progenitor cells and expression level of cell markers during cell growth is altered by various conditions such as increases in mitotic activity related to exercise, environmental enrichment, and ischemic insult, whereas decreases in cell proliferation are related to aging and stress. This chapter describes recent research on the function of neural plasticity–related molecules and discusses their role in adult neurogenesis.

Chapter 5 - Manipulation of the cell cycle is an important strategy used by viruses to cope with the changing environments in virally infected cells. Viral infection may lead to inhibition or promotion of cell growth processes and may, in some cases, result in the arrest of the host cell cycle so as to promote viral replication. Cell growth may be slowed by inhibition of cellular DNA or RNA synthesis, inhibition of cell cycle progression by interaction with host cell proteins, and progression of apoptosis. These changes are thought to provide favorable conditions for the replication of viruses before elimination by the host immune system. After viral replication, apoptosis is often induced, resulting in lysis and the release of viruses. On the other hand, oncoproteins of DNA viruses are known to interact with proteins in the retinoblastoma family, which are tumor suppressors. These viruses have the potential to induce transformation of host cells. Such observations have led to experimental concepts regarding, for example, the culturing of cells from primary cells by expression of oncogenes. Signaling pathways, which may be activated or inactivated by viral infection, also play important roles in cell growth. In this review, the authors highlight molecular mechanisms of host cell growth regulation by the interactions of viral proteins and host proteins.

Chapter 6 - Lung carcinoma is one of the most common malignant tumors in the world, and is the leading cause of carcinoma death in the United States. Despite recent advances in understanding the molecular biology of lung carcinoma and the introduction of multiple new chemotherapeutic agents for its treatment, its dismal 5-year survival rate (< 15%) has not changed substantially. It is well known that tobacco use is the most important risk factor for the development of lung carcinoma in the United States. In particular, non-small cell lung cancer (NSCLC), the most common lung malignancy, demonstrates a strong etiologic association with smoking. Smoking susceptibility is influenced by both genetic and environmental factors. Although nicotine, the major pharmacologically active substance in cigarette smoke, has been shown to be involved in lung cancer, the mechanisms by which this agent affects human lung cancer occurrence and progression remain incompletely elucidated. Recent work suggests that multiple factors and pro-oncogenic signaling pathways are involved in this process. In this review, the authors summarize the extensive network of co-mediators and cellular mechanisms that have implicated nicotine in lung tumorigenesis with the hope of improving understanding in this field. Our intention is to foster the development of new strategies to successfully break the cycle of nicotine-mediated lung carcinogenesis. Further work in this area is likely to lead to the identification of novel targets for early detection and treatment.

Chapter 7 - The monitoring of cell growth *in vitro* is used not only for the investigation of cultivation processes but also for medical diagnosis, cytotoxicity testing, and drug development. The *in vitro* characterization of cells without any labelling is increasingly required to guarantee the cell culture environment during the experiments. As one of those non-invasive methods, electrical impedance spectroscopy has been investigated over the last decades. Impedance spectroscopy is a reliable and quantifiable technique to measure the ratio of alternating potential to current. Since the bi-lipid layer of cell membrane has low conductivity, the behaviour of cells (e.g. movement, adhesion, spreading, or detachment) affects current flow or potential distribution across the cell layer. The electrical properties of thin cell monolayer and even single cell related with morphological changes have been measured by micro systems with impedance spectroscopy. Under various environments (e.g. during the cell cultivation, toxification, or infection), the impedances dependent on the minute changes in the cell/substrate and cell/cell gap have been monitored. In this chapter, a technical and applicative review of impedance spectroscopy for *in vitro* monitoring of cell monolayer growth is presented.

Chapter 8 - Oxidative stress caused by reactive oxygen species (ROS) is capable of disturbing the integrity of cell membranes via peroxidation of membrane lipids and alteration of the structure and function of macromolecules. Reactive aldehydes, in particular 4-hydroxynonenal (HNE), are endogenous end products resulting from the lipid peroxidation of polyunsaturated fatty acids of membrane lipids. For a long time, HNE has been considered as a mainly toxic product of lipid peroxidation, implicated in the pathophysiology of several diseases such as neurodegenerative diseases, ischemia/reperfusion states, atherosclerosis, diabetes, and cancer. However, HNE is permanently formed also under physiological conditions, and has signaling activities in regulation of cell cycle, proliferation, differentiation and apoptosis. A complex network of signal cascades involving HNE is intensively studied. Various signaling pathways are directly or indirectly affected by HNE, because HNE is able to react with a number of cellular elements. Due to the strong affinity to bind to bioactive macromolecules, in particular proteins and peptides, HNE could modify their structure and consequently their function. Formation of HNE-cell surface protein adducts could mimic ligand-cell surface receptor binding, and induce activation of receptor-triggered signal transduction. Thus, HNE is considered also as a growth regulating factor, interfering with the cytokine activities. Interaction of HNE with other growth factors and their influence on cell proliferation will be topic of this article.

Chapter 9 - Glutamate is not only the major excitatory neurotransmitter in the central nervous system (CNS), glutamate receptors have also been found in peripheral non-excitable cells. In addition to eliciting excitatory currents, glutamate can also regulate a broad range of other biological responses. Of particular interest is the discovery that peripheral glutamatergic signalling differentially modifies the proliferation of tumor cells, depending on ingredients in the external milieu (e.g. the external glutamate content). Furthermore, glutamate antagonists effectively suppress cancer growth, inhibit cell division and migration, enhance cell death, and alter the morphology of tumor cells. The authors results indicate that glutamate, the receptor agonists kainate and AMPA (alpha-amino-3-hydroxy-5-methyl-4-isoxsazolepropionic acid), but also the antagonist CNQX (6-cyano-7-nitroquinoxaline-2,3-dione) significantly modified the proliferation of human promonocytic lymphoma (U937) cells. Furthermore, the authors could show that CPCCOEt (7-hydroxyiminocyclopropan[b]chromen-1a-carboxylic acid ethyl ester), a subtype-specific, non-competitive metabotropic glutamate receptor-1 antagonist, significantly, dose-dependently, and reversibly attenuated cell proliferation of both HBMC (human Bowes melanoma) and n15006 melanoma cells. In addition, they observed a synergistic effect of CPCCOEt and docetaxel, a commonly used cytostatic agent. Recent data now indicate that the same glutamate receptor antagonist can also inhibit the growth of multidrug resistant medullary thyroid carcinoma (MTC) cells. In conclusion, this data supplies evidence that glutamate is far more than an excitatory neurotransmitter; glutamate has an important impact on cell growth as well, and glutamate receptor antagonists may augment existing cancer therapies either alone or through synergies with other chemotherapeutic drugs.

In: Progress in Cell Growth Process Research
Editor: Takumi Hayashi, pp. 1-4

ISBN 978-1-60456-325-2
© 2008 Nova Science Publishers, Inc.

Expert Commentary

DEPOLARIZING ACTIVITY OF GABA DURING ADULT NEUROGENESIS: A DEVELOPMENTAL PROCESS?

Philippe Taupin[1, 2, 3]*

[1] National Neuroscience Institute, Singapore
[2] National University of Singapore
[3] Nanyang Technological University, Singapore

In the mammalian nervous system, nerve cells are born during the prenatal phase of development, with the exception of the granule cells of the dentate gyrus (DG) of the hippocampus [1]. The granule cells of the DG are mostly born during the first two weeks postnatal. In the adult nervous system, contrary to a long-held dogma, neurogenesis, the generation of new neuronal cells, occurs throughout adulthood, in discrete regions of the brain, primarily the DG and the subventricular zone (SVZ) [2, 3]. Neuronal cells born during adulthood that become integrated into circuits and survive to maturity are very stable. They may permanently replace granule cells born during development. The mechanism of integration of newly generated neuronal cells in the preexisting network remains poorly understood [4]

In the early 60s, Altman published the first report related to the generation of new neuronal cells in discrete areas of the adult mammalian brain, the hippocampal DG and SVZ, along the ventricles, in rodents [5]. These studies were substantiated and confirmed in the 70s and 80s. It is now well accepted that neurogenesis occurs in discrete regions of the adult brain, in various species including human, and newly generated neuronal cells in the adult brain originate from stem cells [4]. Though neural stem cells remain an elusive cell in the adult brain, newly generated neuronal cells have been characterized and researchers have attempted to identify their function in the brain. Newly generated neuronal cells establish

*Correspondence: 11 Jalan Tan Tock Seng, Singapore 308433. Tel. (65) 6357 - 7533. Fax (65) 6256 - 9178. Email obgpjt@nus.edu.sg.

functional connections and would be involved in physio- and pathological processes, like learning and memory, Alzheimer's and Huntington diseases, cerebral strokes, depression and epilepsy [6]. However, the mechanisms underlying the integration of newly generated neuronal cells in the adult brain remain poorly understood, and the contribution of adult neurogenesis to these physio- and pathlogical processes remains unclear.

In the DG, newly generated neuronal cells in the subgranular zone (SGZ) migrate to the granule layer, where they differentiate into neuronal cells, extend axonal projections to the region CA3 of the Ammon's horn and establish functional connections. In the SVZ, newly generated neuronal cells migrate through the rostro-migratory stream, where they mature into functional inteneurons of the olfactory bulb. Previous studies have reported that neurogenesis occurs in specific microenvironments or niches in the adult brain, the angiogenic and astrocytic niches for neurogenesis [7, 8]. These niches provide an environment for the generation and maturation of newly generated neuronal cells in the adult brain. Molecular studies have highlighted the importance and trophic factors/cytokines, like interleukins-1β and 6, in niches for neurogenesis [9]. However, the nature of the neurotransmitters released by newly generated neuronal cells and their functional and physiological activities on postsynaptic cells remain to be elucidated.

In the nervous system, glutamate (L-glutamic acid, Glu) is the main excitatory neurotransmitter and γ-aminobutyric acid (GABA) the main inhibitory neurotransmitter [10]. In the hippocampus, the nerve cells of the principal layers of the DG and CA, the granule and pyramidal cells, are excitatory glutamatergic, whereas the interneurons are inhibitory GABAergic [11, 12]. The activities of Glu and GABA are mediated through their interaction with ionotropic receptors, particularly the activity of GABA is mediated through GABA-(A) receptors (GABA-(A)Rs) [13, 14]. GABA-(A)R is a ligand gated Cl- channels [14].

In the adult brain, newly generated neuronal cells in the DG receive GABAergic innervations soon after their migration is completed [15]. The GABAergic synaptic input on neural precursor cells of the SVZ and DG has a depolarizing activity on these cells, providing an excitatory input on newly generated neuronal cells in the adult brain [16, 17], similar to what is observed during development.

During development, GABA elicits a transient excitatory activity on immature progenitor cells in the developing brain, particularly the hippocampus [18-20]. The reversal of the distribution of chloride (Cl⁻) inside the cells underlies the depolarizing activity of GABA during development [21]. The depolarizing activity of GABA during development would contribute to an increase in nerve transmission activity, and synaptic integration of newly generated neuronal cells [22, 23].

The depolarizing activity of GABA on newly generated neuronal cells in the adult brain would result from increased chloride levels in immature neuronal cells, as during development. It would contribute to an increase in nerve transmission activity, and synaptic integration of newly generated neuronal cells [24].

In all, GABA exerts excitatory activities on newly generated neuronal cells during development and in the adult brain, and adult neurogenesis may follow a similar mechanism than during development. Whether adult neurogenesis follows a developmental process remains to be further evaluated. Indeed, during development, astrogenesis precedes neurogenesis, in contrast newly generated neuronal cells in the adult brain are generated in an environment of mature glial cells [8]. The understanding of the mechanism underlying adult neurogenesis will contribute to the understanding of the role of newly generated neuronal cells in the adult brain, and their contribution to the functioning and physiopathology of the nervous system, particularly the hippocampus.

REFERENCES

[1]   Gaarskjaer FB. (1986) The organization and development of the hippocampal mossy fiber system. *Brain Res*. 396, 335-57.

[2]   Gage FH. (2000) Mammalian neural stem cells. *Science.* 287, 1433-8.

[3]   Gross CG. (2000) Neurogenesis in the adult brain: death of a dogma. *Nat. Rev. Neurosci.* 1, 67-73.

[4]   Taupin P, Gage FH. (2002) Adult neurogenesis and neural stem cells of the central nervous system in mammals. *J. Neurosci. Res.* 69, 745-9.

[5]   Altman J. (1962) Are new neurons formed in the brains of adult mammals? *Science.*135, 1127-8.

[6]   Taupin P. Adult neurogenesis and neural stem cells in mammals. Publisher: Nova Science Publishers (January 2007).

[7]   Palmer, T.D., Willhoite, A.R. and Gage, F.H. (2000). Vascular niche for adult hippocampal neurogenesis. *J. Comp. Neurol.* 425, 479-94.

[8]   Song H, Stevens CF, Gage FH. (2002) Astroglia induce neurogenesis from adult neural stem cells *Nature* 417, 39-44.

[9]   Barkho BZ, Song H, Aimone JB, Smrt RD, Kuwabara T, Nakashima K, Gage FH, Zhao X. (2006) Identification of astrocyte-expressed factors that modulate neural stem/progenitor cell differentiation. *Stem Cells Dev.* 15, 407-21.

[10]   Curtis DR, Johnston GA. (1974) Amino acid transmitters in the mammalian central nervous system. *Ergeb. Physiol.* 69, 97-188.

[11]   Seress L, Ribak CE. (1983) GABAergic cells in the dentate gyrus appear to be local circuit and projection neurons. *Exp. Brain Res.* 50, 173-82.

[12]   Cotman CW, Flatman JA, Ganong AH, Perkins MN. (1986) Effects of excitatory amino acid antagonists on evoked and spontaneous excitatory potentials in guinea-pig hippocampus. *J. Physiol.* (London). 378, 403-15.

[13]   Monaghan D T, Bridges RJ, Cotman C W. (1989) The excitatory amino acid receptors: their classes, pharmacology, and distinct properties in the function of the central nervous system. *Ann. Rev. Pharmacol Toxicol.* 29, 365-402.

[14]   Sivilotti L, Nistri A. (1991) GABA receptor mechanisms in the central nervous system. *Progress in Neurobiology.* 36, 35-92.

[15]   Wang LP, Kempermann G, Kettenmann H. (2005) A subpopulation of precursor cells in the mouse dentate gyrus receives synaptic GABAergic input. *Mol. Cell. Neurosci.* 29, 181-9.

[16]   Wang DD, Krueger DD, Bordey A. (2003) GABA depolarizes neuronal progenitors of the postnatal subventricular zone via GABAA receptor activation. *J. Physiol.* 550, 785-800.

[17]   Ge S, Goh EL, Sailor KA, Kitabatake Y, Ming GL, Song H. (2005) GABA regulates synaptic integration of newly generated neurons in the adult brain. *Nature.* 439, 589-93.

[18]   LoTurco JJ, Owens DF, Heath MJ, Davis MB, Kriegstein AR. (1995) GABA and glutamate depolarize cortical progenitor cells and inhibit DNA synthesis. *Neuron.* 15, 1287-98.

[19]   Ben-Ari Y, Cherubini E, Corradetti R, Gaiarsa JL. (1989) Giant synaptic potentials in immature rat CA3 hippocampal neurones. *J. Physiol.* 416, 303-25.

[20]   Cherubini E, Rovira C, Gaiarsa JL, Corradetti R, Ben Ari Y. (1990) GABA mediated excitation in immature rat CA3 hippocampal neurons. *Int. J. Dev. Neurosci.* 8, 481-90.

[21]   Ben-Ari Y. (2002) Excitatory actions of gaba during development: the nature of the nurture. *Nat. Rev. Neurosci.* 3, 728-39.

[22]   Ben-Ari Y, Tseeb V, Raggozzino D, Khazipov R, Gaiarsa JL. (1994) Gamma-Aminobutyric acid (GABA): a fast excitatory transmitter which may regulate the development of hippocampal neurones in early postnatal life. *Prog. Brain Res.* 102, 261-73.

[23]   Ben-Ari Y. (2001) Developing networks play a similar melody. *Trends Neurosci.* 24, 353-60.

[24]   Tozuka Y, Fukuda S, Namba T, Seki T, Hisatsune T. (2005) GABAergic excitation promotes neuronal differentiation in adult hippocampal progenitor cells. *Neuron.* 47, 803-15.

In: Progress in Cell Growth Process Research
Editor: Takumi Hayashi, pp. 5-10

ISBN 978-1-60456-325-2
© 2008 Nova Science Publishers, Inc.

Short Communication A

DEPOLARIZING ACTIVITY OF GABA IN CA3 PYRAMIDAL NEURONS DURING DEVELOPMENT

Philippe Taupin [1, 2, 3*]
[1] National Neuroscience Institute, Singapore
[2] National University of Singapore
[3] Nanyang Technological University, Singapore

ABSTRACT

L-glutamic acid (glutamate, Glu) and γ-aminobutyric acid (GABA) are the main fast-acting amino acid neurotransmitters of the nervous system; Glu is the main excitatory neurotransmitter and GABA the main inhibitory neurotransmitter. In the hippocampus, the granule and pyramidal cells, the nerve cells of the principal layers of the dentate gyrus (DG) and Ammon's horn (CA) respectively, are glutamatergic excitatory and GABA is the neurotransmitter of inhibitory interneurons. The activities of the fast-acting neurotransmitters, Glu and GABA, are mediated through interaction with ionotropic receptors on postsynaptic cells. Particularly, the activity of the inhibitory neurotransmitter GABA is mediated by GABA-(A) receptors (GABA-(A)Rs). GABA-(A)Rs are ligand gated chloride ion (Cl⁻) channels. During development, GABA elicits an excitatory activity on pyramidal cells. The excitatory activity of the neurotransmitter GABA during development originates from a reversal in the distribution of Cl⁻ in nerve cells. GABA originating from interneurons transiently depolarizes CA pyramidal cells, an activity that would contribute to an increase in nerve transmission activity, synaptic integration and maturation of hippocampal pyramidal cells.

[*]Correspondence: 11 Jalan Tan Tock Seng, Singapore 308433. Tel. (65) 6357 - 7533. Fax (65) 6256 - 9178. Email obgpjt@nus.edu.sg.

INTRODUCTION

In the nervous system, fast-acting neurotransmitters mediate the transmission of nerve activity. Fast-acting neurotransmitters act through ionotropic receptors to mediate synaptic transmission. Ionotropic receptors are ligand gated ion channels, or receptors coupled to ion channels. The rapid opening of ion channels generates fast and large changes in the conductance of the membrane. Two kinds of fast-acting neurotransmitters exist in the nervous system, excitatory and inhibitory. Excitatory neurotransmitters depolarize the membrane potential of nerve cells and increase their excitability, leading to the propagation of nerve activity. Inhibitory neurotransmitters hyperpolarize the membrane potential and decrease the excitability of target cells [1].

In the mature vertebrate nervous system, Glu is the main excitatory neurotransmitters and GABA the main inhibitory neurotransmitter [2]. The activity of Glu is mediated through Glu ionotropic receptors, the N-methyl-D-aspartate (NMDA), α-amino-3-methyl-4-isoxazolepropionate (AMPA) and kainate receptors [3]. The activity of GABA is mediated through the GABA ionotropic receptors, the GABA-(A)Rs [4].

During development, GABA elicits an excitatory activity on pyramidal cells. The understanding of the mechanism underlying the excitatory activity of GABA is important for our understanding of the development and physiopathology of the developing brain, particularly the hippocampus.

GABA, AN INHIBITORY NEUROTRANSMITTER

The activity of GABA is mediated through the GABA ionotropic receptors, the GABA-(A)Rs. The GABA-(A)R is a ligand gated Cl⁻ channel. In nerve cells, Cl⁻ is actively transported by a potassium/chloride ion cotransporter (KCC) outside the cells [5]. The interaction of GABA with GABA-(A)Rs mediates the opening of Cl⁻ channels and the entrance of Cl⁻ inside the cells. The influx of Cl⁻ inside the cells hyperpolarizes the membrane potential of the postsynaptic membrane, leading to the inhibition of the transmission of nerve activity [6].

THE HIPPOCAMPUS

The hippocampus is an important memory center of the brain [7]. It is also involved in pathological processes, like Alzheimer's disease and epilepsy [8, 9]. The hippocampus is a highly distinctive and structured region of the cerebral cortex. It is divided into two regions, the DG and CA, each composed of a main cellular layer, the granule and pyramidal cell layers, respectively [10, 11]. Based on histological and genetic studies, the CA is divided into 3 regions, CA1, CA2 and CA3 [12, 13]. In the mature hippocampus, the granule and pyramidal cells, the nerve cells of the principal layers of the DG and CA respectively, are glutamatergic excitatory, and GABA is the neurotransmitter of inhibitory interneurons [14, 15].

The granule cells, the nerve cells of the principal layer of the DG, extend axonal projections, the mossy fibers (MFs), to the CA3 region and establish synaptic contacts with dendritic spines of the pyramidal cells [16]. In the CA regions, inhibitory interneurons, like basket cells, innervate the pyramidal cells with which they establish synaptic contact [17].

The pre- and postsynaptic terminals of the synapses MF-CA3 pyramidal cells are characterized by unique morphological features. The presynaptic terminals of the MF ending nerves are characterized by their large size, up to 10 μm diameter, high synaptic vesicles density and complex morphology, with dendritic spines invaginated in the boutons [16]. The postsynaptic terminals of the MF ending nerves are characterized by giant dendritic spines, named thorny excrescences [12, 16].

DEVELOPMENT OF THE HIPPOCAMPUS

During development of the nervous system, most nerve cells are born before birth [18]. In the hippocampus, the development of granule and pyramidal cells follows different patterns. In the CA, most pyramidal cells are born prenatally, like most others in the brain region [19]. The first precursor cells to be generated in the CA are as the precursor cells of the pyramidal cells of CA3. The maturation of newborn pyramidal cells extends until the postnatal period. The maturation process of the CA extends until 2-3 weeks after birth, with dendritic spines, including the thorny excrescences of CA3 pyramidal cells, formed around the second week postnatal [20].

In contrast to the CA and most other brain regions, the genesis of granule cells of the DG occurs mostly after birth [21]. Most of the granule cells, 70%, are born during the two first weeks of postnatal. The maturation of the MFs occurs mostly postnatally. Between day postnatal 10 and 14, the presynaptic terminals of the MF ending nerves become more complex, with increasing size and density of synaptic vesicles. At that time, concomitantly to the apparition of the dendritic spines on CA3 pyramidal cells, the MFs preterminals begin the process of invagination of the CA3 pyramidal cells' dendritic spines [21, 22].

DEPOLARIZING ACTIVITY OF GABAERGIC INTERNEURONS DURING DEVELOPMENT IN THE HIPPOCAMPUS

During the first week postnatal, contrary to the adult, GABA exerts a depolarizing activity on CA3 pyramidal cells [23, 24]. The excitatory activity of GABA during development becomes inhibitory as the neurons mature. From the second week postnatal, GABA exerts an inhibitory hyperpolarizing activity on CA3 pyramidal cells [25], at a time when pyramidal cells mature and acquire their adult features [22].

Pharmacological studies reveal that the excitatory activity of GABA on hippocampal pyramidal cells, during development, is mediated by GABA-(A)Rs [26]. In the rat hippocampus, the expression of an isoform of KCC, KCC2, begins around the first week after birth and reverses the cell's distribution of Cl⁻ inside the cells from high to low [27].

This shows that the excitatory activity of GABA on CA3 hippocampal pyramidal cells is mediated by GABA, through interaction with GABA-(A)Rs. As the expression of KCC2 correlates with the GABA activity switch from depolarizing to hyperpolarizing, it is proposed that a transient reversal in the distribution of Cl⁻ in immature nerve cells underlies the switch of GABA activity from hyperpolarizing to depolarizing, during development [28, 29]. GABA exerting a depolarizing activity onto CA3 pyramidal cells would originate from hilar and CA3 interneurons of the hippocampus.

CONCLUSION

In the nervous system, Glu and GABA are the main fast-acting amino acid neurotransmitters. In the mature nervous system, Glu is the main excitatory neurotransmitter and GABA the main inhibitory neurotransmitter. In the hippocampus, Glu is the neurotransmitters of the granule and pyramidal cells of the DG and CA, respectively, and GABA the inhibitory neurotransmitter of interneurons. During development, GABA elicits a transient excitatory activity on CA3 pyramidal cells. The depolarizing activity of GABA during development is mediated by GABA-(A)Rs. The reversal of the distribution of the Cl⁻ inside the cells underlies the depolarizing activity of GABA.

The function and physiological significance of the depolarizing activity of GABA during development and particularly in the hippocampus remain to be understood. The depolarizing activity of GABA may lead to an increase in nerve transmission activity [30]. In support of this contention, the depolarization of CA3 hippocampal neurons induced by GABA during the first week of development enables NMDA receptors to activate CA3 hippocampal neurons [31]. GABA may contribute to synaptic integration and survival of newly generated neuronal cells [32]. In support of this contention, GABA elicits trophic activities, particularly promoting neurite outgrowth [33, 34]. It is proposed that GABA excitatory activity would contribute to synaptic integration of newly generated neuronal cells in the CA, during development [29]. The physiopathological significance of the excitatory activity of GABA during development, and particularly the hippocampus, is yet to be determined.

REFERENCES

[1]   Nicoll RA. (1988) The coupling of neurotransmitter receptors to ion channels in the brain. *Science.* 241, 545-51.

[2]   Curtis DR, Johnston GA. (1974) Amino acid transmitters in the mammalian central nervous system. *Ergeb. Physiol.* 69, 97-188.

[3] Monaghan D T, Bridges RJ, Cotman C W. (1989) The excitatory amino acid receptors: their classes, pharmacology, and distinct properties in the function of the central nervous system. *Ann. Rev. Pharmacol Toxicol.* 29, 365-402.

[4] Mohler H. (2006) GABA(A) receptor diversity and pharmacology. *Cell Tissue Res.* 326, 505-16.

[5] Payne JA, Stevenson TJ, Donaldson LF. (1996) Molecular characterization of a putative K-Cl cotransporter in rat brain. A neuronal-specific isoform. *J. Biol. Chem.* 271, 16245-52.

[6] Sivilotti L, Nistri A. (1991) GABA receptor mechanisms in the central nervous system. *Progress in Neurobiology.* 36, 35-92.

[7] Sweatt JD. (2004) Hippocampal function in cognition. *Psychopharmacology* (Berl). 174, 99-110.

[8] Panegyres PK. (2004) The contribution of the study of neurodegenerative disorders to the understanding of human memory. *QJM.* 97, 555-67.

[9] Sloviter RS. (2005) The neurobiology of temporal lobe epilepsy: too much information, not enough knowledge. *C. R. Biol.* 328, 143-53.

[10] Ramon y Cajal S. Histologie du Système Nerveux de l'Homme et des Vertébrés, Vols. 1 and 2. A. Maloine. Paris (1911).

[11] Amaral DG. (1978) A Golgi study of cell types in the hilar region of the hippocampus in the rat. *J. Comp. Neurol.* 182, 851-914.

[12] Lorente de No R. (1934) Studies on the structure of the cerebral cortex. II. Continuation of the study of the ammonic system. *J. Psychol. Neurol.* (Lpz). 46, 113-77.

[13] Lein ES, Callaway EM, Albright TD, Gage FH. (2005) Redefining the boundaries of the hippocampal CA2 subfield in the mouse using gene expression and 3-dimensional reconstruction. *J. Comp. Neurol.* 485, 1-10.

[14] Seress L, Ribak CE. (1983) GABAergic cells in the dentate gyrus appear to be local circuit and projection neurons. *Exp. Brain Res.* 50, 173-82.

[15] Cotman CW, Flatman JA, Ganong AH, Perkins MN. (1986) Effects of excitatory amino acid antagonists on evoked and spontaneous excitatory potentials in guinea-pig hippocampus. *J. Physiol.* (London). 378, 403-15.

[16] Claiborne BJ, Amaral DG, Cowan WM. (1986) A light and electron microscopic analysis of the mossy fibers of the rat dentate gyrus. *J. Comp. Neurol.* 246, 435-58.

[17] Gamrani H, Onteniente B, Seguela P, Geffard M, Calas A. (1986) Gamma-aminobutyric acid-immunoreactivity in the rat hippocampus. A light and electron microscopic study with anti-GABA antibodies. *Brain Res.* 364, 30-8.

[18] Altman J. (1963) Autoradiographic investigation of cell proliferation in the brains of rats and cats. *Anat. Rec.* 145, 573-91.

[19] [19] Angevine JB. (1965) Time of neuron origin in the hippocampal region; an autoradiographic study in the mouse. *Exp. Neurol.* 13, 1-70.

[20] Bayer SA. (1980) Development of the hippocampal region in the rat. II. Morphogenesis during embryonic and early postnatal life. *J. Comp. Neurol.* 190, 115-34.

[21]   Gaarskjaer FB. (1986) The organization and development of the hippocampal mossy fiber system. *Brain Res* 396, 335-57.

[22]   Zimmer J. (1978) Development of the hippocampus and fascia dentata: morphological and histochemical aspects. *Prog. Brain Res.* 48, 171-90.

[23]   Ben-Ari Y, Cherubini E, Corradetti R, Gaiarsa JL. (1989) Giant synaptic potentials in immature rat CA3 hippocampal neurones. *J. Physiol.* 416, 303-25.

[24]   Cherubini E, Rovira C, Gaiarsa JL, Corradetti R, Ben Ari Y. (1990) GABA mediated excitation in immature rat CA3 hippocampal neurons. *Int. J. Dev. Neurosci.* 8, 481-90.

[25]   Gaiarsa JL, McLean H, Congar P, Leinekugel X, Khazipov R, Tseeb V, Ben-Ari Y. (1995) Postnatal maturation of gamma-aminobutyric acidA and B-mediated inhibition in the CA3 hippocampal region of the rat. *J. Neurobiol.* 26, 339-49.

[26]   Michelson HB, Wong RK. (1991) Excitatory synaptic responses mediated by GABAA receptors in the hippocampus. *Science.* 253, 1420-3.

[27]   Rivera C, Voipio J, Payne JA, Ruusuvuori E, Lahtinen H, Lamsa K, Pirvola U, Saarma M, Kaila K. (1999) The K+/Cl- co-transporter KCC2 renders GABA hyperpolarizing during neuronal maturation. *Nature.* 397, 251-5.

[28]   [28] Cherubini E, Gaiarsa JL, Ben-Ari Y. (1991) GABA: an excitatory transmitter in early postnatal life. *Trends Neurosci.* 14, 515-9.

[29]   Ben-Ari Y. (2002) Excitatory actions of gaba during development: the nature of the nurture. *Nat. Rev. Neurosci.* 3, 728-39.

[30]   Ben-Ari Y, Khazipov R, Leinekugel X, Caillard O, Gaiarsa JL. (1997) GABAA, NMDA and AMPA receptors: a developmentally regulated 'menage a trois'. *Trends Neurosci.* 20, 523-9.

[31]   Leinekugel X, Medina I, Khalilov I, Ben-Ari Y, Khazipov R. (1997) Ca2+ oscillations mediated by the synergistic excitatory actions of GABA(A) and NMDA receptors in the neonatal hippocampus. *Neuron.* 18, 243-55.

[32]   Ben-Ari Y, Tseeb V, Raggozzino D, Khazipov R, Gaiarsa JL. (1994) Gamma-Aminobutyric acid (GABA): a fast excitatory transmitter which may regulate the development of hippocampal neurones in early postnatal life. *Prog. Brain Res.* 102, 261-73.

[33]   Spoerri PE. (1988) Neurotrophic effects of GABA in cultures of embryonic chick brain and retina. *Synapse.* 2, 11-22.

[34]   Barbin G, Pollard H, Gaiarsa JL, Ben-Ari Y. (1993) Involvement of GABAA receptors in the outgrowth of cultured hippocampal neurons. *Neurosci. Lett.* 152, 150-4.

In: Progress in Cell Growth Process Research
Editor: Takumi Hayashi, pp. 11-20

ISBN 978-1-60456-325-2
© 2008 Nova Science Publishers, Inc.

Short Communication B

THE ROLE OF POLO-LIKE KINASES (PLKS) IN GYNECOLOGIC CANCERS

Noriyuki Takai[1], Kaei Nasu and Hisashi Narahara
Department of Obstetrics and Gynecology,
Oita University Faculty of Medicine, Oita, Japan

ABSTRACT

Deregulated centrosome duplication or maturation often results in increased centrosome size and/or centrosome number, both of which show a positive and significant correlation with aneuploidy and chromosomal instability, thus contributing to cancer formation. Given the role of Polo-like kinases (Plks) in the centrosome cycle, it is not unexpected that deregulated expression of Plks is detected in many types of cancer and is associated with oncogenesis. Plk1 has been closely linked to cellular proliferation, cancer development and cancer progression. There is no Plk1 expression in most differentiated cells in contrast to tissues with proliferative potential such as placenta and cancers. Many studies have shown that Plk1 expression is strongly correlated with aggressiveness and prognosis in gynecologic cancers. Plk1 gene and protein expression has been proposed as a new prognostic marker for gynecologic malignancies, and Plk1 is a potential target for cancer therapy. To date, several techniques and compounds to inhibit Plk1 have been identified and appear to be promising. In the future, methods for inhibition of Plk1 could be improved and applied in treatment of cancer patients. In contrast to Plk1, several studies have observed that Plk3 expression is negatively correlated with the development of certain cancers.

Keywords: Polo-like kinases, ovarian cancer, endometrial cancer.

---

[1] Correspondence to: Noriyuki Takai, M.D., Ph.D. Department of Obstetrics and Gynecology, Oita University Faculty of Medicine, 1-1 Idaigaoka, Hasama-machi, Oita 879-5593, Japan, Tel: 81-97-586-5922, Fax: 81-97-586-6687, E-mail: takai@med.oita-u.ac.jp.

INTRODUCTION

Polo-like kinases (Plks), which comprise a family of serine/threonine kinases, are highly conserved from yeasts to humans [1]. This family includes mammalian Plk1, Plk2 (serum-inducible kinase (Snk)), and Plk3 (fibroblast growth factor-inducible kinase (Fnk)/proliferation-related kinase (Prk)), Plk4 (Sak), Xenopus laevis Plx1, Drosophila melanogaster polo, Schizosaccharomyces pombe (fission yeast) Plo1, and Saccharomyces cerevisiae (budding yeast) Cdc5. These enzymes in addition to a conserved kinase domain at the N-terminus have highly conserved sequences of 30 amino acids, called polo-box(s) in the noncatalytic C terminal domain [2]. A polo-box mutant of Plk1 that does not affect its kinase activity but abolishes its subcellular relocalization is capable of abolishing its biological activity in vivo [3, 4]. These findings suggest that polo-box of Plk1 plays a critical role for Plk1 function, especially for its spatial distribution and physical interaction with substrates. Genetic and biochemical experiments in various organisms indicate that plks are important regulators of many cell-cycle-related events, including bipolar spindle formation [5, 6], chromosome segregation, centrosome maturation in late G2/early prophase [7], activation of Cdc2, regulation of anaphase-promoting complex, and execution of cytokinesis [2, 7, 8]. It is predominantly cytoplasmic during interphase but is associated with condensed chromosomes during mitosis [9] when its kinase activity is also at its peak [10]. It has been demonstrated that Plk1 mRNA expression is low at the G1/S transition, increases during S phase, and is maximally expressed during G2/M. The report of Kumagai and Dunphy [11] suggests that Plx1 is a critical trigger that initiates the onset of the G2/M transition through activating cdc25. During the metaphase–anaphase transition, Plx1 is required for the destruction of targets of the anaphase-promoting complex (APC) that drives mitotic exit [12]. Conversely, in myeloid leukemia cell lines undergoing terminal differentiation, Plk1 expression is drastically reduced [13].

Plk1 has been suggested to directly phosphorylate components of APC including Cdc27 and activate the latter [14]. Intranuclear Plk1 together with other signal proteins (p34 kinase, cyclin B, etc.) is responsible for mitotic progression. Increasing evidences support the concept that Plks regulate pivotal stages throughout mitosis including its initiation by activating Cdc2 through Cdc25 and direct phosphorylation of cyclin B1 targeting Cdc2/cyclin B1 to the nucleus [2, 15]. In addition, in a previous study [16], the level of Plk1 mRNA in cancer cells was associated with the extent of its interaction with heat-shock protein 90. Plk1-dependent phosphorylation of BRCA2 is enhanced during mitotic progression, or inhibited by DNA damage, suggesting that it serves to coordinate biological processes in which BRCA2 participates [17]. Still, recent data support a regulatory role of the mammalian Plk1 at the cell cycle G2 checkpoint [18, 19], although the finding that *Cdc25c -/-* mice did not display any obvious abnormalities in cellular response to DNA damage nor ability to activate Cdc2a [20] may argue against an essential function of Cdc25C in mammalian G2/M transition.

Plk1 has been closely linked to cellular proliferation. Therefore, it is not hard to imagine that Plk families could be associated with cancer development and progression. As a matter of fact, overexpression of murine Plk1 in NIH3T3 cells confers a transformed phenotype, which is manifested as foci capable of growth in soft agar and formation of tumors in nude mice [21]. It was further shown that cells isolated from the excised tumors continued to overexpress the Plk1 protein, and many of these cells were multinucleated [22]. As mentioned above, the expression and function of Plk1 have been analysed in cell lines from the viewpoint of physiological or pathological roles in vitro. In addition, Plk1 and Plk3 expressions have been widely examined in tumors from the cancer patients. Results from these studies indicate that overexpression of Plk1 is positively correlated with aggressiveness and prognosis in many cancers. In contrast, Plk3 is downregulated in carcinomas of the lung [23], head and neck [24], and the colon [25]. Moreover, inhibition of Plk1 with various techniques results in growth arrest or apoptosis for the cancer cells. Thus, Plk1 could be a novel prognostic marker and a good target for chemotherapeutic intervention.

OVARIAN CANCER

In tumor tissue from 17 patients with ovarian carcinoma, the percentage of Plk1-stained cells was $13.54 \pm 5.19\%$ in grade 1, $21.86 \pm 8.63\%$ in grade 2, and $35.03 \pm 5.20\%$ in grade 3, respectively. The number of Plk1-positive cells was significantly higher in ovarian cancers designated as grade 3 than in cancers designated as grade 1 ($P<0.001$). Furthermore, the percentage of Plk1-stained cells was $14.74 \pm 5.81\%$ in stage I, $23.00 \pm 9.61\%$ in stage II, $32.55 \pm 9.36\%$ in stage III, and 12.70% in stage IV. Percentage of Plk1-stained cells in each clinical stage. Plk1 expression was significantly higher in stage III and IV than in stage I and II ($p<0.01$) (Figure 1). [26]. Comparison of survival between low Plk1 expression ($<20\%$ of Plk1-stained cells, n=13) and high Plk1 expression ($\geq20\%$ of Plk1-stained cells, n=13), according to the Kaplan-Meier method. The prognosis of the patients with high levels of Plk1 expression was significantly worse than that of those with low Plk1 expression ($p<0.05$) (Figure 2).

In another report, the tissue specimens of normal ovaries (n=9), cystadenomas (n=17), borderline tumors (n=13), and ovarian carcinomas (n=77) were evaluated. The overexpression of Plk1 had an impact on patient prognosis with shortened survival time for patients with tumors positive for Plk1 (P=0.02), and Plk1 expression remained a prognostic factor in multivariate survival analysis (P=0.03) [27].

ENDOMETRIAL CANCER

In tumor tissue from 20 patients with endometrial carcinoma, the percentage of Plk1-stained cells was $13.48 \pm 4.86\%$ in grade 1, $17.51 \pm 6.71\%$ in grade 2, and $38.62 \pm 1.50\%$ in grade 3, respectively. The number of Plk1-positive cells was significantly higher in endometrial carcinomas designated as grade 3 than in carcinomas designated as grade 1 and 2 ($P<0.01$) (Figure 3) [28].

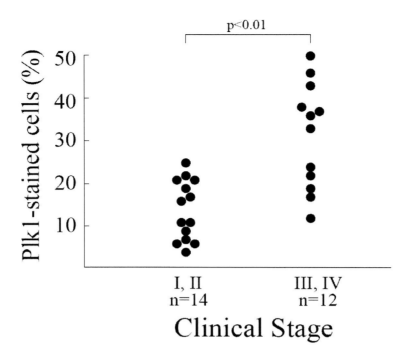

Figure 1. Percentage of Plk1-stained cells in each clinical stage. Plk1 expression was significantly higher in stage III and IV than in stage I and II (p<0.01).

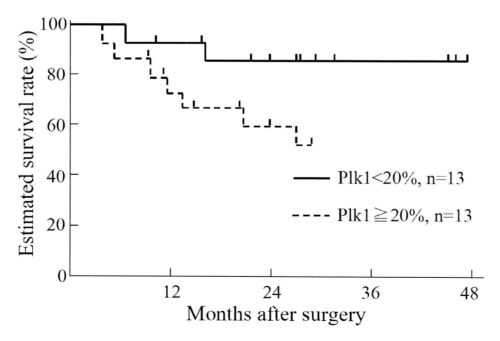

Figure 2. Comparison of survival between low Plk1 expression (<20% of Plk1-stained cells, n=13) and high Plk1 expression (≥20% of Plk1-stained cells, n=13), according to the Kaplan-Meier method. The prognosis of the patients with high levels of Plk1 expression was significantly worse than that of those with low Plk1 expression (p<0.05).

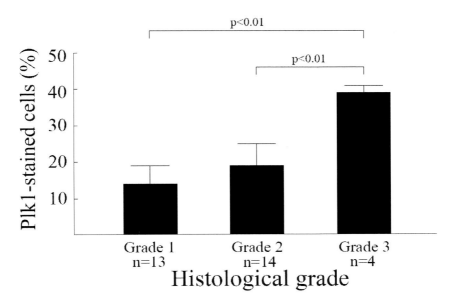

Figure 3. Percentage of Plk1-stained cells in each histological grade. Each bar represents the mean ± SD. Plk1 expression was significantly higher in grade 3 than in grade 1 and 2 (p<0.01).

Plk3 and Cancers

Mammalian Plk3 (alternatively named Prk [23] and Fnk [29] was originally shown to be an immediate early gene product. While initially linked to G1 phase, Plk3 protein can be detected throughout the cell cycle and, similar to Plk1, is actually found at its highest levels and activity from late S phase through M phase. Furthermore, in correlation with its activity, Plk3 is phosphorylated following growth stimulation and maximally during M phase [30]. Plk3, as well as Plk1, is capable of rescuing CDC5 temperature-sensitive (ts) mutants at restrictive temperature, indicating functional conservation of these kinases throughout evolution [31, 32]. In contrast to Plk1, several studies have observed that Plk3 expression is negatively correlated with the development of certain cancers, despite its original description as an immediate earlygene inducible by serum and cytokines [23]. Plk3 mRNA is either undetectable or markedly downregulated in lung carcinomas compared with the uninvolved 'normal tissues' of the same patients [23]. Several polymorphisms were identified in 40 lung tumor cell lines examined, although neither missense nor nonsense mutations were detected [33], suggesting that mutational inactivation of the coding sequence of the Plk3 gene is a rare event in lung cancer. The abundance of Plk3 mRNA is similarly reduced in HNSCC [24] and in carcinogeninduced rat colon tumors [25]. Consistent with these observations, ectopic expression of Plk3, but not that of a truncated, kinase-inactive mutant of this protein, reduces the rate of fibroblast cell proliferation in vitro [24]. Furthermore, enforced expression of constructs expressing kinase-active Plk3 induces the condensation of chromatin, rapid cell cycle arrest and apoptosis [34, 35].

Inhibition of Plk1

The use of different methods to abrogate the activity of Plk1 revealed its essential role for mitotic progression in mammalian cells. Microinjection of anti-Plk1 antibodies into both transformed HeLa cervical carcinoma cells and nontransformed (nonimmortalized) human Hs68 fibroblast cells disrupts these functions, resulting in a marked inhibition of cell cycle progression [7]. Antisense oligodeoxynucleotides (ODNs) to Plk1 have also been shown to be effective for inhibition of its expression in tumor cell lines, leading to loss of cell viability and even demonstrating an antitumor activity in A549 xenografts [36]. Results from transient expression of dominantnegative Plk1 differed from previous antibody microinjection experiments in that most of the mitotic HeLa cells were bipolar and cytokinesis seemed to be disrupted [37]. Expression of dominant-negative Plk1 via an adenoviral vector induces programmed cell death in most tumor cells but not in normal human mammary epithelial cells [34]. Polo-box, located in C-terminal region of Plk1, is thought to be important for subcelluar localization and interaction with substrate proteins. Yuan et al. have made fusion peptides of the polo-box with the homodomain of antennapedia to be internalized into cells. Membrane-permeable polo-box peptides inhibit cancer cell proliferation efficiently [38]. Overexpression of a kinase-inactive form of mammalian Plk1 in most tumor cell lines was shown to induce a centrosome maturation defect in combination with mitotic catastrophe and apoptosis [39]. Recently, a small interfering RNA (siRNA) technique has been developed to delete a specific mRNA. About half of the cells transiently treated with Plk1 siRNA arrest at G2/M with 4 N DNA content in FACS profiles and show the formation of a dumbbelllike DNA organization, suggesting that sister chromatids are not completely separated [40]. Plk1 depletion for extended period by vectorbased siRNA caused cell cycle arrest at mitosis and apoptosis in several cancer cells lines [40-42]. Moreover, the p53 pathway is shown to be involved in the apoptosis induced by Plk1 depletion [41].

Scytonemin, a yellow green pigment found only in the extracellular sheath of cyanobacteria, has been reported to be a low micromolar inhibitor of Plk1 that blocks proliferation of multiple cell types including rheumatoid synovial fibroblasts, normal human lung fibroblasts, human umbilical vein endothelial cells, and Jurkat cells [43]. The expression of Plk1 decreases following inhibition of PLCγ and PI3-kinase [44]. Expression of the Plk1 gene was significantly suppressed by β-hydroxyisovalerylshikonin (β-HIVS) in U937 and HL60 cells [45]. Treatment with Plk1-specific antisense ODNs sensitized K562 cells to β-HIVS-induced apoptosis, indicating that suppression of the expression and activity of Plk1 by β-HIVS is involved in apoptosis [45].

CONCLUSION

There is no Plk1 expression in most differentiated cells in contrast to tissues with proliferative potential such as placenta [46, 47], endometrium [48], and cancers. The expression of Plk1 is strongly correlated with aggressiveness and prognosis in many cancers. Therefore, Plk1 could be used as a novel diagnostic marker for several types of cancers, and inhibition of Plk1 function could be an important application for cancer therapy. To date, several techniques and compounds to inhibit Plk1 have been identified and appear to be promising. In the future, methods for inhibition of Plk1 could be improved and applied in treatment of cancer patients.

ACKNOWLEDGMENTS

The study was supported by a Grant-in-Aid (No. 16790961 to Noriyuki Takai) for Scientific Research from the Ministry of Education, Culture, Sports, Science, and Technology, Japan.

REFERENCES

[1]   Hamanaka, R; Maloid, S; Smith, MR; O'Connell, CD; Longo, DL; and Ferris, DK. (1994). Cloning and characterization of human and murine homologues of the Drosophila polo serine-threonine kinase. *Cell Growth Differ.*, 5, 249-257.

[2]   Glover, DM; Hagan, IM; and Tavares, AA. (1998). Polo-like kinases: a team that plays throughout mitosis. Genes Dev, 12, 3777-3787.

[3]   Lee, KS; Grenfell, TZ; Yarm, FR; and Erikson, RL. (1998). Mutation of the polo-box disrupts localization and mitotic functions of the mammalian polo kinase Plk. *Proc. Natl. Acad. Sci.* USA, 95, 9301-9306.

[4]   Lee, KS; Song, S; and Erikson, RL. (1999). The polo-box-dependent induction of ectopic septal structures by a mammalian polo kinase, plk, in Saccharomyces cerevisiae. *Proc. Natl. Acad. Sci.* USA, 96, 14360-14365.

[5]   Hamanaka, R; Smith, MR; O'Connor, PM; Maloid, S; Mihalic, K; Spivak, JL; Longo, DL; and Ferris, DK. (1995). Polo-like kinase is a cell cycle-regulated kinase activated during mitosis. *J. Biol. Chem.*, 270, 21086-21091.

[6]   Glover, DM; Ohkura, H; and Tavares, A. (1996). Polo kinase: the choreographer of the mitotic stage? *J. Cell Biol.*, 135, 1681-1684.

[7]   Lane, HA; and Nigg, EA. (1996). Antibody microinjection reveals an essential role for human polo-like kinase 1 (Plk1) in the functional maturation of mitotic centrosomes. *J. Cell. Biol.*, 135, 1701-1713.

[8]   Nigg, EA. (1998). Polo-like kinases: positive regulators of cell division from start to finish. *Curr. Opin. Cell. Biol.*, 10, 776-783.

[9]   Llamazares, S; Moreira, A; Tavares, A; Girdham, C; Spruce, BA; Gonzalez, C; Karess, RE; Glover, DM; and Sunkel, CE. (1991). polo encodes a protein kinase homolog required for mitosis in Drosophila. *Genes Dev.*, 5, 2153-2165.

[10]   Fenton, B; and Glover, DM. (1993). A conserved mitotic kinase active at late anaphase-telophase in syncytial Drosophila embryos. *Nature,* 363, 637-640.

[11]   Kumagai ,A; and Dunphy, WG. (1996). Purification and molecular cloning of Plx1, a Cdc25-regulatory kinase from Xenopus egg extracts. *Science*, 273, 1377-1380.

[12]　Descombes, P; and Nigg, EA. (1998). The polo-like kinase Plx1 is required for M phase exit and destruction of mitotic regulators in Xenopus egg extracts. *EMBO J.*, 17, 1328-1335.

[13]　Yuan, J; Horlin, A; Hock, B; Stutte, HJ; Rubsamen-Waigmann, H; and Strebhardt, K. (1997). Polo-like kinase, a novel marker for cellular proliferation. *Am. J. Pathol.*, 150, 1165-1172.

[14]　Kotani, S; Tugendreich, S; Fujii, M; Jorgensen, P; Watanabe, N; Hoog, C; Hieter, P; and Todokoro, K. (1998). PKA and MPF-activated polo-like kinase regulate anaphase-promoting complex activity and mitosis progression. *Mol. Cell.*, 1, 371-380.

[15]　Nigg, EA. (2001). Mitotic kinases as regulators of cell division and its checkpoints. Nat *Rev. Mol. Cell. Biol.*, 2, 21-32.

[16]　Shimizu, S; and Osada, H. (2000). Mutations in the Plk gene lead to instability of Plk protein in human tumour cell lines. *Nat. Cell Biol.*, 2, 852-854.

[17]　Lee, M; Daniels, MJ; and Venkitaraman, AR. (2004). Phosphorylation of BRCA2 by the Polo-like kinase Plk1 is regulated by DNA damage and mitotic progression. *Oncogene*, 23, 865-872.

[18]　Smits, VA; Klompmaker, R; Arnaud, L; Rijksen, G; Nigg, EA; and Medema, RH. (2000). Polo-like kinase-1 is a target of the DNA damage checkpoint. *Nat. Cell Biol.*, 2, 672-676.

[19]　vanVugt, MA; Smits, VA; Klompmaker, R; and Medema, RH. (2001). Inhibition of Polo-like kinase-1 by DNA damage occurs in an ATM- or ATR-dependent fashion. *J. Biol. Chem.*, 276, 41656-41660.

[20]　Chen, MS; Hurov, J; White, LS; Woodford-Thomas, T; and Piwnica-Worms, H. (2001). Absence of apparent phenotype in mice lacking Cdc25C protein phosphatase. *Mol. Cell Biol.*, 21, 3853-3861.

[21]　Smith, MR; Wilson, ML; Hamanaka, R; Chase, D; Kung, H; Longo, DL; and Ferris, DK. (1997). Malignant transformation of mammalian cells initiated by constitutive expression of the polo-like kinase. *Biochem. Biophys. Res. Commun.*, 234, 397-405.

[22]　Fisher, RAH; and Ferris, DK. (2002). *Curr. Med. Chem. Imun. Endoc. Metab. Agents*, 2, 1-10.

[23]　Li, B; Ouyang, B; Pan, H; Reissmann, PT; Slamon, DJ; Arceci, R; Lu, L; and Dai, W. (1996). Prk, a cytokine-inducible human protein serine/threonine kinase whose expression appears to be down-regulated in lung carcinomas. *J. Biol. Chem.*, 271, 19402-19408.

[24]　Dai, W; Li, Y; Ouyang, B; Pan, H; Reissmann, P; Li, J; Wiest, J; Stambrook, P; Gluckman, JL; Noffsinger, A; and Bejarano, P. (2000). PRK, a cell cycle gene localized to 8p21, is downregulated in head and neck cancer. *Genes Chromosomes Cancer*, 27, 332-336.

[25]　Dai, W; Liu, T; Wang, Q; Rao, CV; and Reddy, BS. (2002). Down-regulation of PLK3 gene expression by types and amount of dietary fat in rat colon tumors. *Int. J. Oncol.*, 20, 121-126.

[26]　Takai, N; Miyazaki, T; Fujisawa, K; Nasu, K; Hamanaka, R; and Miyakawa, I. (2001). Expression of polo-like kinase in ovarian cancer is associated with histological grade and clinical stage. *Cancer Lett*, 164, 41-49.

[27]   Weichert, W; Denkert, C; Schmidt, M; Gekeler, V; Wolf, G; Kobel, M; Dietel, M; and Hauptmann, S. (2004). Polo-like kinase isoform expression is a prognostic factor in ovarian carcinoma. *Br. J. Cancer*, 90, 815-821.

[28]   Takai, N; Miyazaki, T; Fujisawa, K; Nasu, K; Hamanaka, R; and Miyakawa, I. (2001). Polo-like kinase (PLK) expression in endometrial carcinoma. *Cancer Lett.*, 169, 41-49.

[29]   Donohue, PJ; Alberts, GF; Guo, Y; and Winkles, JA. (1995). Identification by targeted differential display of an immediate early gene encoding a putative serine/threonine kinase. *J. Biol. Chem.*, 270, 10351-10357.

[30]   Chase, D; Feng, Y; Hanshew, B; Winkles, JA; Longo, DL; and Ferris, DK. (1998). Expression and phosphorylation of fibroblast-growth-factor-inducible kinase (Fnk) during cell-cycle progression. *Biochem. J.*, 333, 655-660.

[31]   Lee, KS; and Erikson, RL. (1997). Plk is a functional homolog of Saccharomyces cerevisiae Cdc5, and elevated Plk activity induces multiple septation structures. *Mol. Cell Biol.*, 17, 3408-3417.

[32]   Ouyang, B; Pan, H; Lu, L; Li, J; Stambrook, P; Li, B; and Dai, W. (1997). Human Prk is a conserved protein serine/threonine kinase involved in regulating M phase functions. *J. Biol. Chem.*, 272, 28646-28651.

[33]   Wiest, J; Clark, AM; and Dai, W. (2001). Intron/exon organization and polymorphisms of the PLK3/PRK gene in human lung carcinoma cell lines. *Genes Chromosomes Cancer*, 32, 384-389.

[34]   Conn, CW; Hennigan, RF; Dai, W; Sanchez, Y; and Stambrook, PJ. (2000). Incomplete cytokinesis and induction of apoptosis by overexpression of the mammalian polo-like kinase, Plk3. *Cancer Res.*, 60, 6826-6831.

[35]   Wang, Q; Xie, S; Chen, J; Fukasawa, K; Naik, U; Traganos, F; Darzynkiewicz, Z; Jhanwar-Uniyal, M; and Dai, W. (2002). Cell cycle arrest and apoptosis induced by human Polo-like kinase 3 is mediated through perturbation of microtubule integrity. *Mol. Cell Biol.*, 22, 3450-3459.

[36]   Elez, R; Piiper. A; Giannini, CD; Brendel, M; and Zeuzem, S. (2000). Polo-like kinase1, a new target for antisense tumor therapy. *Biochem. Biophys. Res. Commun.*, 269, 352-356.

[37]   Mundt, KE; Golsteyn, R; Lane, HA; and Nigg, EA. (1997). On the regulation and function of human polo-like kinase 1 (PLK1): effects of overexpression on cell cycle progression. *Biochem. Biophys. Res. Commun.*, 239, 377-385.

[38]   Yuan, J; Kramer, A; Eckerdt, F; Kaufmann, M; and Strebhardt, K. (2002). Efficient internalization of the polo-box of polo-like kinase 1 fused to an Antennapedia peptide results in inhibition of cancer cell proliferation. *Cancer Res.*, 62, 4186-4190.

[39]   Cogswell, JP; Brown, CE; Bisi, JE; and Neill, SD. (2000). Dominant-negative polo-like kinase 1 induces mitotic catastrophe independent of cdc25C function. *Cell Growth Differ.*, 11, 615-623.

[40]   Liu, X; and Erikson, RL. (2002). Activation of Cdc2/cyclin B and inhibition of centrosome amplification in cells depleted of Plk1 by siRNA. *Proc. Natl. Acad. Sci. USA*, 99, 8672-8676.

[41]   Liu, X; and Erikson, RL. (2003). Polo-like kinase (Plk)1 depletion induces apoptosis in cancer cells. *Proc. Natl. Acad. Sci.* USA, 100, 5789-5794.

[42]   Spankuch-Schmitt, B; Bereiter-Hahn, J; Kaufmann, M; and Strebhardt, K. (2002). Effect of RNA silencing of polo-like kinase-1 (PLK1) on apoptosis and spindle formation in human cancer cells. *J. Natl. Cancer Inst.*, 94, 1863-1877.

[43]   Stevenson, CS. (1999). *Proceeding of 90th American Association for Cancer Research*, Washington DC.

[44]   Dietzmann, K; Kirches, E; von Bossanyi, P; Jachau, K; and Mawrin, C. (2001). Increased human polo-like kinase-1 expression in gliomas. *J. Neurooncol.*, 53, 1-11.

[45]   Masuda, Y; Nishida, A; Hori, K; Hirabayashi, T; Kajimoto, S; Nakajo, S; Kondo, T; Asaka, M; and Nakaya, K. (2003). Beta-hydroxyisovalerylshikonin induces apoptosis in human leukemia cells by inhibiting the activity of a polo-like kinase 1 (PLK1). *Oncogene,* 22, 1012-1023.

[46]   Takai, N; Yoshimatsu, J; Nishida, Y; Narahara, H; Miyakawa, I; and Hamanaka, R. (1999). Expression of polo-like kinase (PLK) in the mouse placenta and ovary. *Reprod. Fertil. Dev.*, 11, 31-35.

[47]   Yoshimatsu, J; Takai, N; Yoshimatsu, Y; Narahara, H; Miyakawa, I; and Hamanaka, R. (1999). Immunohistochemical localization of polo like kinase in early human placenta. *Res. Commun. Mol. Pathol. Pharmacol.*, 106, 3-12.

[48]   Takai, N; Miyazaki, T; Miyakawa, I; and Hamanaka, R. (2000). Polo-like kinase expression in normal human endometrium during the menstrual cycle. *Reprod. Fertil. Dev.*, 12, 59-67.

In: Progress in Cell Growth Process Research
Editor: Takumi Hayashi, pp. 21-64

ISBN 978-1-60456-325-2
© 2008 Nova Science Publishers, Inc.

Chapter 1

ENDOTHELIAL CELLS IN CARDIOVASCULAR RESEARCH – ASSESSMENT OF ORGAN- AND DISEASE-SPECIFIC ENDOTHELIAL CELLS IN VITRO FOR THERAPEUTIC INTERVENTION

Karla Lehle[1], Leoni A. Kunz-Schughart[2] and Christof Schmid[1]

[1] Dept. of Cardiothoracic Surgery, University of Regensburg Medical Center, Franz-Josef-Strauss-Allee 11, D-93053 Regensburg, Germany
[2] OncoRay - Center for Radiation Research in Oncology, Medical Faculty Carl Gustav Carus, TU Dresden, Fetscherstr. 74, PF86, D-01307 Dresden, Germany

ABSTRACT

The endothelium can no longer be regarded as an inert layer of cells lining the inside surface of the vascular system. It is now becoming clear that endothelial cells (EC) actively and reactively participate in multifaceted reactions and can mount anti- and pro-inflammatory and protective responses depending on environmental conditions. Endothelial cell dysfunction or activation also contributes to a variety of disease states. Considering the role of the endothelium in the initiation and propagation of vascular wall injury, there is a need for the discovery of validated biomarkers to serve as predictors for activation of inflammatory cascades in the development of vascular injury. Among the laboratory methods available for the detection of endothelial dysfunction, the use of species- and disease-specific endothelial cell culture models enables the presentation of heterogenous endothelial phenotypes and the assessment of environmental conditions on endothelial cell function. This review describes various in vitro EC culture systems with respect to developing therapeutic interventions in cardiovascular diseases. Understanding the mechanisms of EC dysfunction is a prerequisite for EC-targeted therapy to reduce the incidence of cardiovascular diseases.

OVERVIEW OF THE EC SOURCES FOR TESTING THERAPEUTIC INTERVENTIONS IN VITRO

1. Introduction: Endothelial Functions in Cardiovascular Disease

Cardiovascular disease (CVD) is the leading cause of death and disability in the developed world, and is projected to soon overtake infectious disease as the preeminent cause of death worldwide. Accounting for 49% of all deaths in Europe and 30% of all deaths before the age of 65 years, it contributes substantially to the escalating cost of health care [Murray and Lopez, 1997; De Backer et al., 2004; Goodacre et al., 2005]. The reasons for this generally reflect an increasing prevalence of several known CVD risk factors: obesity and insulin resistance, diabetes, smoking, hypertension, poor diet, and an increasing aging population [EUROASPIRE, 2001; De Backer et al., 2004]. The spectrum of CVD is broad and includes coronary artery disease (CAD), peripheral vascular disease (PVD), congestive heart failure, atrial fibrillation (AF), and stroke, in addition to the major risk factors of hypertension, hypercholesterolemia, smoking, and diabetes mellitus. The common factor between these conditions is the loss of appropriate endothelial physiology and function (damage/injury, leading to dysfunction) that is paramount to the maintenance of vascular hemostasis and blood pressure control [Blann, 2003]. The growing interest in the role of endothelium in physiological and pathological conditions has led to an increased demand for specific in vitro model systems for vascular tone, blood coagulation, angiogenesis, lymphocyte adhesion as well as signalling and transport routes across blood- and lymphatic-vessel walls. The goal of this article is to underscore the relevance and the complexity of the endothelium in vascular diseases and to introduce species- and disease-specific EC culture systems as important tools for the investigation of therapeutic interventions.

2. Heterogeneity of the Endothelium

2.1. Endothelial Phenotypes: Morphology and Function

Endothelial cells (EC) form the inner lining of blood vessels and traverse each and every tissue. They are highly active metabolically and play an important role in many physiological functions (e. g. control of vasomotor tone, blood cell trafficking, hemostatic balance, permeability, proliferation, survival, innate and adaptive immunity). Despite a number of common features, EC phenotypes are differentially regulated in space and time [Aird, 2003].

The structural heterogeneity of EC is based on histological findings and cell culture analysis demonstrating that EC from different sites across the vascular tree are different in size, shape, thickness, and orientation. As early as the seventies, some studies were describing major differences in the dimension and shape of EC from the aorta, arteries, veins or capillaries. EC from the rabbit inferior vena cave, for example, are broad and short (108x15 µm), whereas the aortic EC are long and narrow (96x11 µm) [Silkworth and Stehbens, 1975]. The fluid sheer stress and thus the nuclear and cellular orientation parallel to the axis of blood flow is another characteristic feature of EC from different tissues[Dewey et al., 1981]. Cells and their nuclei are aligned in the direction of blood flow in straight segments of arteries, but not at branch points [Passerini et al., 2004; Lupu C et al., 2005]. The nature of the EC junctions varies between different segments of the vascular tree: Tight junctions, which are usually found at the apical region of the intercellular cleft, form a barrier to transport between EC and help to maintain cell polarity between the luminal and abluminal side of the cells. Macrovascular arterial EC display a well developed system of these junctions, as might be predicted by the conduit function of these vessels and their exposure to high rates of pulsatile blood flow. The density of tight junctions in the microvasculature is very different: it is at a maximum in the micro-vessels of the blood-brain barrier and the arterioles; decreased in capillaries, and quite sparse in the venules. Furthermore, endothelium may be continuous or discontinuous, fenestrated or non-fenestrated, depending on the location in different vessels and organs as comprehensively reviewed by Aird [Aird, 2007b].

The expression pattern of the EC is also heterogenous. Table 1 summarizes the most relevant endothelial markers [Garlanda and Dejana, 1997]. Other EC-specific characteristics are the Weibel-Palade bodies [Weibel and Palade, 1964] and the EC "cobblestone morphology." Figure 1 demonstrates the cobblestone structure and representative EC markers. As shown in Figure 2, EC are also able to create tube-like structures, which were used as an in vitro model for angiogenesis. Also, vessel-specific cellular markers are documented for arteries and veins [Chi et al., 2003]. Genes that are preferentially expressed in arterial EC include ephrinB2 [Gale et al., 2001], Delta-like 4 (Ell4) [Krebs et al., 2000], activin-receptor-like kinase 1 (Alk1) [Seki et al., 2003], endothelial PAS domain protein 1 (EPAS-1) [Tian e t al., 1997], Hey1 and Hey2 [Nakagawa et al., 1999], neuropilin-1 (NRP1) [Mukouyama et al., 2005], and decidual protein induced by progesterone (Depp) [Shin and Anderson, 2005]. Venous EC-specific genes include EphB4 [Gerety et al., 1999], neuropilin 2 (NRP2) [Yuan et al., 2002], and COUP-TFII [You et al., 2005]. Furthermore, Deng et al. used microarray analysis to demonstrate specific gene expression profiles in arterial versus venous EC that contribute to differences in atherosclerotic disease susceptibility [Deng et al., 2006].

The principle functions of the endothelium – the control of hemostasis, vasomotor tone, cell and nutrient trafficking, barrier function, and angiogenesis – are performed by specific subsets of blood vessel types or vascular beds [Rosenberg and Aird, 1999; Gross and Aird, 2000; Aird, 2002]. Some of the EC functions are discussed below. Shear stress, for example, induces site-specific NO-dependent dilatation as shown in porcine epicardial arterioles compared with venules [Boegehold, 1998]. Differences in acetylcholine-induced NO activity and angiotensin conversion were seen in distinct segments of serially-arranged arterioles in the hamster cheek pouch approach as an example for vascular bed-specific control of vasomotor tone [Tang and Joyner, 1992; Tang et al. 1995]. The leukocyte trafficking involves a multistep adhesion cascade that includes initial attachment, rolling, arrest and transmigration. The molecular basis of this process is believed to involve CD99, PECAM-1/CD31 and the junctional adhesion molecule-1 (JAMA-1) [Springer, 1994; Aurrand-Lions et al., 2002; Nourshargh et al., 2006]. Moreover, EC activation results in stimulus- and organ-specific induction of the various adhesion molecules [Eppihimer et al., 1996; Henninger et al., 1997; Bauer et al., 2000].

Table 1. A choice of selected endothelial markers

EC-marker	Expression on other cell types	function	Reference
CD146, S-ENDO1, MUC18, MCAM	Activated T-cells	Cell-cell contact, adhesion molecule	Shih, 1999; Bardin et al., 2001
PECAM-1, CD31	Platelets, megakaryocytes, B and T lymphocytes, monocytes, neutrophils	Cell adhesion molecule, adhesion of leukocytes	DeLisser et al., 1993; Wong et al., 2000
Endoglin, CD105	Monocyte-macrophages, B lymphocytes, syncytiotrophoblasts,	regulating the sensitivity to TGF-β	Altomote et al., 1996; Wikström et al., 2002
Von Willebrand factor	Platelets, megakaryocytes	Regulation in hemostasis	Wagner & Bonfanti, 1991; Denis, 2002
Vascular endothleial-Cadherin (CD144)	Trophoblasts, PLN sinus macrophages	Cell-cell junctional protein, angiogenesis	Dejana et al., 2001 ; Fukuhra et al., 2006
Flt-1 (VEGFR-1)	Hematopoetic stem cells	Regulation of angiogenesis	Sawano et al., 2001; Shibuja, 2006
KDR/Flk-1 (VEGFR-2)	Hematopoetic stem cells	Regulation of angiogenesis	Kappel et al., 1999, Sawano et al., 2001
Thrombomodulin, CD141		potent natural anticoagulant	Yonezawa et al., 1987
UEA-1, Ulex europaeus I agglutinin binding	Erythrocytes	Binding of fucose residues on EC surface	Jackson et al., 1990; Anthony & Ramani, 1991; Oxhorn et al., 2002
Tie-1	Hematopoetic stem cells, embryonic EC	endothelial-cell-specific tyrosine kinase receptor, capillary sprouting	Boutet et al., 2001;
PAL-E, pathologische anatomie Leiden-endothelium	Only vascular endothelium	unknown	Niemelä et al., 2005
E-selectin, CD62E		Leukocyte trafficking	Kansas, 1996
acetylated-low density lipoprotein (dil-Ac-LDL)	Macrophages, SMCs pericytes, fibroblasts	metabolism of Ac-LDL	Voyta et al., 1984
Angiotensin-converting enzyme (ACE)	Epithelial cells, monoycyte-macrophages, T lymphocytes	Regulation of renin-angiotensin-system	Belloni & Tressler, 1990
ICAM-1, CD54	Dendritic cells, monocytes, lymmphocytes, peritoneal macrophages	Neutrophil-endothelial interaction	Tonnesen, 1989
p-Selectin, GMP140, CD62P	Activated platelets	Platelet activation	Blann et al., 2003

SMC = Smooth muscle cells

A common function of the endothelium is the maintenance of blood fluidity. However, the distribution of hemostatic factors depends on the vascular beds, e.g. endothelial protein C receptor (EPCR) is expressed predominantly in large arteries and veins, most arterioles, and some postcapillary venules, but not in capillary EC [Laszik et al., 1997].

In contrast, thrombomodulin is detected in high concentrations in both large vessels and capillary endothelium. More details on vascular bed-specific differences in the structure and function of EC were referenced and discussed in an interesting review series by Aird [Aird, 2002; Aird, 2007a; Aird, 2007b]. Another informative overview was published in 2006 by Pries and Kuebler [Pries and Kuebler, 2006]. These authors also emphasize the organ-specific functional heterogeneity which is discussed in the following section.

2.2. Organ-Specific Approaches to the Endothelium

Research over the past several decades has revealed that EC heterogeneity occurs between different organs, within the vascular loop to a given organ, and even between neighboring EC of a single blood vessel. Organ-specific approaches to the endothelium have gained deeper insight in the variability of EC phenotypes. Accordingly, cardiologists who focus primarily on the coronary arteries, neurologists who are interested in the cerebral circulation/blood-brain barrier, hepatologists investigating liver circulation and dermatologists monitoring skin micro-vasculature should each apply their own particular organ-specific EC to in vitro studies. Given the diversity of the vascular channels and the associated differences in hemodynamics, structure, and embryonic origins, it is not surprising that the EC lining vessels of different organs exhibit regional specializations in morphology and function. Systemic identification of the specific molecular features of specialized components of the vascular network will not only enhance our understanding of vascular development, lymphocyte homing, and various disease processes, but may also provide the potential for site-specific delivery of therapeutic agents. A variety of approaches have been applied to identify molecular markers for specific vessels or vascular beds, including the Stamper-Woodruff assay [Mitsuoka et al., 1997], monoclonal antibodies [Zannettino et al., 2007], phage display [Zhang et al., 2005], SAGE analysis [St Croix et al., 2000; De Waard et al., 1999], and microarray [Podgrabinska et al., 2002]. The latter method was used to demonstrate that EC from different blood vessels or anatomical sites are indeed distinct differentiated cell types with correspondingly characteristic gene expression programs. Chi et al. demonstrated a tissue-specific gene expression profile in different microvascular EC tissue [Chi et al., 2003]. Hendrickx et al. analyzed, among others, 10 genes which were highly expressed in heart ventricles, but nearly absent in aortic EC, and confirmed these genes in cultures of ventricular endocardial endothelium, underscoring the concept that an intrinsic genetic "endocardial" program may exist in these EC. They also demonstrated that some genes (e.g. GATA-GT2, oxidized low-density lipoprotein receptor 1, apolipoprotein E, creatine kinase brain type, parathyroin hormone receptor and UDP guanosyltransverase 1) are preserved in cardiac microvascular EC and endocardial EC [Hendrickx et al., 2004]. This may provide new insights into the functional adaptations of the EC subtype to its intracavity localization and to its role in the control of ventricular performance.

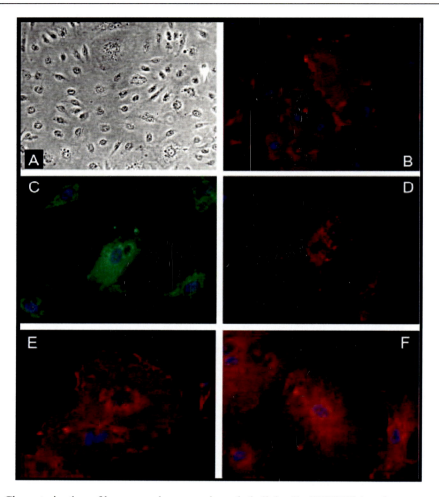

Figure 1. Characterization of human saphenous vein endothelial cells (HSVEC) by phase contrast and fluorescence microscopy. (A) "Cobblestone morphology". (B) Binding of monoclonal antibody CD31 (PECAM)-Texas red. (C) Interaction of Ulex europaeus lectin-1-FITC. (D) Presence of von Willebrand factor-Texas red. (E) Binding of monoclonal antibody CD146-Texas red. (F) Binding of monoclonal antibody CD62E (E-Selectin)-Texas red on TNF-stimulated EC.

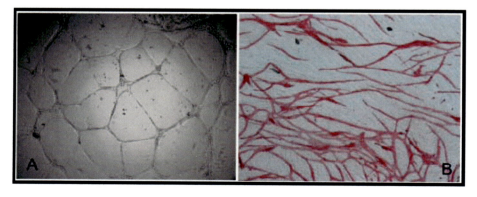

Figure 2. Formation of tube-like structures (A) within MatrigelR and (B) in a coculture model with human fibroblasts (kindly provided by Kunz-Schughart et al. (2006)).

In addition to the analysis of tissue-specific gene expression profiles, some scientific groups have demonstrated the organ-specific function of EC from different origins. To gain a better understanding as to how EC vary in their immunological properties, Hillyer et al. examined primary human dermal microvascular EC (DMVEC), lung microvascular EC (LMVEC), saphenous vein EC (HSVEC), human umbilical vein EC (HUVEC), and bone marrow EC (BMEC) [Hillyer et al., 2003]. They could show that the variation between endothelia in chemokine secretion was much greater than the variation in the expression of adhesion molecules, both on resting cells and following cytokine stimulation. The authors supported the theory that tissue-specific patterns of leukocyte migration are determined, at least in part, by the differentiated endothelium found in each tissue.

Considering the importance of understanding the mechanisms that regulate EC functions, due to its critical role in many important human pathologies, the possibility of isolating different EC phenotypes within the same individual may represent a unique and important tool for identifying organ-specific human markers of endothelium. However, since diverse human tissue specimens from the same subject are difficult to obtain, comprehensive studies of EC derived from different organs or tissues are subject to enormous variability as a consequence of the differences among donors (sex, age, pathologies, etc.). To avoid this problem, Invernici et al. isolated human fetal EC derived from different organs (brain, heart, lung, liver, kidney, aorta) of the same embryos [Invernici et al., 2005]. These cultures showed organ-specific differences with respect to morphological appearance, growth rate and expression of cellular adhesion molecules (CAM) before and after stimulation by inflammatory cytokines. For instance, TNF showed a specific effect on fetal heart EC by stimulating E-selectin expression. This might be particularly important for the heart since studies demonstrate a correlation between the expression of TNF and the severity of the rejection episode [Turner et al., 1995; Azzawi et al., 1999]. One limitation of such studies is certainly the ethical restriction and the authorization to use human embryonic tissue for research experiments.

These few examples should provide an indication of the capability of identifying organ-specific EC markers and help initiate the discovery of new approaches in therapeutic interventions.

3. Endothelial Function and Model Systems

3.1. Animal Models

Studies on vascular function and pathomechanisms in vascular diseases require the appropriate in vitro and in vivo models. For certain study designs, non-human model systems are obligatory. Although bound by ethical restrictions, animal experiments allow the progression of kinetic studies, e.g. cytotoxic and pharmacologic trials, or the investigation of new strategies in surgery. Other advantages of animal models are easy tissue recruitment, genetically identical mice or rats enable the realization of progression studies (e.g. time shape, dose effects), analysis of multiorgan effects, etc. However, the problem of species differences makes data interpretation and extrapolation to the clinical situation of humans problematic. In addition, the heterogeneity of a particular cell type requires careful attention to the choice of both animal type and cell source.

A wide variety of animal models including small animals such as mice, rats, and rabbits or larger ones such as pigs, goats, and calfs allows the investigation of specific vascular problems. Animal models have proven to be a very valuable resource for the study of atherosclerosis and cardiac allograft vasculopathy (CAV). The role of the endothelium, smooth muscle cells and the extracellular matrix in both diseases was described in a review of relevant rabbit as well as rat and mouse models by Rahmani et al. [Rahmani et al., 2006]. This review summarizes the current understanding of the risk factors and pathophysiological similarities and differences between CAV and atherosclerosis. Furthermore, the regenerative potential of cardiac progenitor cells were tested in respective animal models. Recent data from animal models suggest that a variety of cell types, including unfractionated bone marrow mononuclear cells and those obtained by ex vivo expansion of human peripheral blood or enriched progenitors, can function as endothelial progenitor cells (EPC) to promote tissue vasculogenesis, regeneration, and repair when introduced in vivo [Young et al., 2007]. Animal models were also necessary for pharmacokinetic and pharmacodynamic studies for cardiovascular interventions (e. g. immunosuppressive drugs, antihypertensiva, ß-blocker, etc.). Biemond et al., for example, used two well-established rabbit models for experimental thrombosis to demonstrate that the orally available selective direct factor-Xa inhibitor rivaroxaban is effective in the prevention and treatment of venous thrombosis [Biemond et al., 2007]. A transgenic mouse model for atherosclerosis, in which mechanical injury to the aortic endothelium was induced by several passages of a guidewire into the aorta, was used to demonstrate that albumin-encapsulated microbubbles adhere to the vascular endothelium via a complement-dependent mechanism, both early in the atherosclerotic process and in the development of plaque. In addition to their ability to bind selectively to plaque, these microbubbles also bind to therapeutic agents which could be used as a drug-specific delivery system. The advantage of this method lies in the verification of the localization of the bubbles by ultrasound [Anderson et al., 2007]. Another interesting approach is the investigation of neointima hyperplasia using drug-eluting stents in a pig model. Blindt et al. deployed integrin-binding cyclic Arg-Gly-Asp peptide loaded stents in porcine coronary arteries and could show that neointimal hyperplasia was significantly reduced after 12 weeks [Blindt et al., 2006]. In addition, the endothelial coverage was reached 4 weeks after implantation of the stents and consisted of attracted endothelial progenitor cells.

The use of animal models is obligatory in cardiovascular research such as atherosclerosis, allograft vasculopathy, hypertension, cardiac repair after myocardial infarction, etc. However, EC culture techniques are useful adjuncts to this research and allow the investigation of simple and complex mechanisms at the endothelial level.

3.2. EC Functions in Vitro

To exclude restricted functional and morphological properties of immortalized cell lines, the usage of primary cell cultures is mandatory. Many studies have been performed in 2-d assays to analyze different aspects of EC characteristics. The growth-modulating effects of several molecules like the VEGF family or fibroblast growth factor can be investigated in monolayer EC assays by direct or indirect counting [Mawatari et al., 1989; Pepper et al.,

1992]. In addition, cytotoxicity of drugs with a known potential for vascular damage could be detected in standardized screening tests in a 96-well format. The release of lactate dehydrogenase in the supernatant (cell lysis), cell staining with trypane blue or calcein-AM (viability), the incorporation of propidium iodide (PI) in the DNA and the induction of apoptosis (e.g. caspase activity, cell cycle analysis, DAPI-staining) or necrosis are only a small selection of available in vitro tests. The migratory potential of EC was analyzed in 2-d trans-well assays with EC being seeded in the upper well of a Transwell insert system or a modified Boyden chamber [Mawatari et al., 1991]. Chemotaxis could be evaluated by counting cells passing through an insert (e.g. Boyden chamber) or directly observing cell cultures (e.g. Dunn chamber), both in response to stationary concentration gradients. Furthermore, these chemotactic assays allow the analysis of the role of proteases in endothelial migration and the influence of inhibitors on EC invasion. A flow chamber apparatus might also allow the transendothelial migration of shear-promoted leukocytes combined with signals from basal chemokines [Cinamon and Alon, 2003].

The endothelial reaction to proinflammatory stimuli, such as tumor necrosis factor (TNF), interleukin-1ß (IL-1ß) and bacterial endothoxin (LPS, lipopolysaccharide), could be verified by measuring the expression of cell adhesion molecules (CAM) using the cellular ELISA-technique or flow cytometry, the release of cytokines/chemokines or soluble CAM in the supernatant of cell cultures, or the adhesion or transmigration of peripheral mononuclear blood cells (PBMC). The heterogeneity of the EC specified the extent of the inflammatory reactions: For example, HUVEC (human umbilical vein EC) showed a more marked reaction than HPMEC (human pulmonary microvascular EC). However, heat shock proteins (HSPs) under metal ion induction gave similar patterns [Wagner et al., 1999]. Other functional parameters are the expression of tissue factor, thrombomodulin, metalloproteinases (MMPs), the release of prostaglandin E2 (PGE2), nitric oxide (NO), growth factors (VEGF, vascular endothelial growth factor), etc.

The sheer stress on EC as a result of blood flow could be demonstrated in relevant in vitro assays. Comparative studies demonstrated that EC under dynamic flow conditions have a different morphology (orientation in flow direction) and functional status than EC under static monolayer culture [Malek et al., 1993; Nerem, 1993; Dieterich et al., 2000]. Interactions between biomaterials and cells, for example EC or blood cells, can be studied under shear stress using a parallel plate flow chamber with integrated video microscopy and computer-controlled image analysis systems [Otto et al., 1997; Otto et al., 2001], a rotating disc [Kao, 2000], or a plate and cone rheometer [Furukawa et al., 2000; Furukawa et al., 2003].

3.3. Animal EC Cultures

Due to the availability of bed-specific vessels and relevant isolation strategies, primarily EC from porcine pulmonary arteries or aorta and aortic EC from mice and rats were prepared and used as a model system to investigate principle mechanisms, e.g. the interaction of EC and leucocytes in the inflammatory cascade [DiCorleto and de la Motte, 1985]. The following references give a selection of the broad range of available animal endothelial models. Immortal mouse cell lines were derived from endotheliomas [Obeso et al., 1990] and the myocard [Plendl et al., 1995]. Primary mouse EC were isolated from brain, ovary and lung [Auerbach et al., 1985] or pathologic mouse endothelium [Moyer et al., 1992; Langley et al., 2003]. An immortalized rat bone marrow EC line [Miyata et al., 2005], primary rat heart EC [Diglio et al., 1988; Derhaag et al., 1996] and immortalized rat brain EC [Régina et al., 1999] were described. Bovine primary aortic EC [Lokeshwar et al., 1996], fetal bovine bone EC [Streeten et al., 1989] as well as immortalized bovine brain capillary EC [Durieu-Trautmann et al., 1991] have been isolated. Other authors describe immortalized porcine aortic [Maher et al., 1996] and liver EC [Sepp et al., 1997], as well as primate (rhesus monkey) primary corpus luteum EC [Christenson and Stouffer, 1996]. Costa et al. implanted porcine aortic EC under the kidney capsule of BALB/c and BALB/c SCID mice and could show that control cells were rejected within 2-4 weeks, whereas rejection of genetically modified PAEC (including a human chimeric molecule hCD152-hCD59 to block pCD86) was significantly delayed [Costa et al., 2004]. The authors postulated that CD86 contributes to the rejection of porcine xenografts. In addition, most organ-specific heterogenous endothelial functions were discovered not by the isolation and cultivation of EC from different vascular beds and organs, but from the same organism. Plendl et al. isolated vital EC from the thoracic aorta, brain, myocardium, ovary and testis from fetal pigs and showed that these cells express organ- and tissue specific heterogeneity [Plendl et al., 1996].

The results obtained from animal cells may be more easily compared with in vivo data from experiments of the same species. Animal cells were not taken into account since human EC presumably reflect the human in situ situation incompletely, but better than EC from any other organism.

3.4. Immortalized Human EC Lines

As suggested in section 3.2, different sources and types of EC are available as an in vitro model. The species-specific heterogeneity of animal EC cultures requires the use of human culture systems.

Due to the difficulties associated with acquisition of human tissue for primary culture and further passage, as well as the considerable biological variability between individual donors, it has long been a goal to develop immortalized cell lines, which have the advantage of reducing experimental costs, improving intra- and interlaboratory variation and permitting more rapid advancement in the research field by facilitating more experiments per unit of time. Bouis et al. presented a list of the most frequently used human cell lines [Bouis et al., 2001]. The best characterized macro- and micro-vascular EC lines are EA.hy926 (fusion of HUVEC with the human lung carcinoma cell line A549) [Edgell et al., 1983] and HMEC-1 (transfection of human dermal EC with large T antigens of SV40) [Ades et al., 1992]. The former has been used for adhesion assays with several human leukocyte cell lines [Thornhill et al., 1993], and human peripheral blood mononuclear cells (PBMC) in the presence of blocking monoclonal antibodies [Brown et al., 1993], unstimulated human neutrophiles in the presence of dexamethasone [Burke-Gaffney and Hellewell, 1996] and murine T cells [Kita et al., 1996]. The principal disadvantage of such permanent cell lines is that the most effective induction methodologies are generally associated with massive loss of phenotype and function. For example, immortalized human saphenous EC (HSVEC) have been created, which are clearly convenient for large-scale experiments [Scoumanne et al., 2002]. Unfortunately, these cells show significant morphological and functional differences from primary EC lines [Scoumanne et al., 2002]. In selecting an appropriate EC line, the goal is to identify the cell line having most of the desired primary characteristics with as few tumor cell traits as possible. Scientists looking for blood-endothelium interactions, for example, would prefer cell lines that express specific adhesion molecules or members of the coagulation cascade like tissue factor (TF) or tissue-type plasminogen activator (tPA), or those that show lymphocyte adhesion.

3.5. Sophisticated EC Models

Angiogenesis and vascular maturation require a complex series of biological reactions from different cell types to form new microvascular branches or sprouts from the pre-existing vasculature that finally develop into fully functional vessels. EC respond to receptor-mediated pro-angiogenic signals and undergo cytoskeletal reorganization and breakdown of their own basement membrane, followed by migration and proliferation to form new sprouts. Extracellular matrix lysis occurs during these invasive phases, while matrix neosynthesis and remodeling are important during the final stages of new blood vessel formation. After this period of remodeling, the vasculature matures into a stationary state by recruitment of perivascular and smooth muscle cells. Vascular maturation is associated with arrest of angiogenesis as manifested by contact inhibition of EC proliferation, e.g. when co-cultured with pericytes (PCs) or smooth muscle cells [Orlidge and D'Amore, 1987; Nehls et al., 1994]. In addition to their role in mediating angiostasis and survival, PCs and smooth muscle cells are important for regulating hemodynamics by providing the vessels with the capability to respond to vasoreactive signals [Kelley et al., 1987; Kelley et al., 1988].

Based on these complex processes, numerous advanced in vitro model systems were established over the past three decades to reflect and study the underlying mechanisms, and they have also become the basis for many approaches in vascular engineering. The aim of the present article is not to give a comprehensive overview of all complex in vitro culture models available, since there are a number of books and book chapters available that more than adequately summarize this issue [Mironov et al., 1998; Murray, 2001] However, we intend to make the reader more aware of such applications, since they clearly go beyond the classical monolayer system.

It is well accepted that the ECM is not just a scaffold, but ECM compounds signal towards the vasculature and remodel in response to signals from the vasculature [Davis and Senger, 2005; Rhodesand Simons, 2007], Accordingly, extracellular matrix (ECM) culture systems have been developed to simulate interactions between cells and their extracellular environment. In the simplest approach, EC are seeded onto collagen, fibrin, or matrigel gels and invasion of cells into the gel and the formation of tube-like structures by EC is documented by microscopy or immunohistochemical staining [Madri et al., 1988; Fukushima et al., 2005; Sorrell et al., 2007]. Gel type assays are commercially available from various sources and are most frequently applied to monitor the effects of pro- or anti-angiogenic factors and drug candidates.

In light of the observation that EC seeded onto such gels form cord-like structures but not real tubules, and with the knowledge of blood vessel formation to require stromal cells, gel-based assays have progressed into real three-dimensional systems with EC dispersed in the gels or onto beads, and have also been combined with various cell types for EC co-culturing

[Sieminski et al., 2005; Martineau and Doillon, 2007; Nillesen et al., 2007]. Indeed, cells applied in direct co-culture with endothelial cells to support either vascular sprouting and tube formation or vascular maturation for tissue engineering purposes and to optimize angiogenesis assaying, primarily include smooth muscle cells [Korff et al. 2001; Burch et al., 2005; Heydarkhan-Hagvall et al., 2003; Dietrich and Lelkes, 2006; Niwa et al., 2007; Wallace et al., 2007a; Wallace et al., 2007b; Wu et al., 2007,], pericytes [Dente et al., 2001; Edelman et al., 2007; Anfuso et al., 2007] or fibroblasts [Nehls et al., 1998; Bishop et al., 1999; Donovan et al., 2001; Saito et al., 2003; Wenger et al., 2005; Kunz-Schughart et al., 2006, Schmid et al., 2007]. Some of the referenced co-culture approaches are known to form multilayers or are particularly designed to produce spherical shaped non-adherent cultures, e.g. fibroblast-EC [Wenger et al., 2005; Kunz-Schughart, et al., 2006] or smooth muscle cell-EC spheroid co-cultures [Korff et al., 2001]. The spheroid model has entered various domains of biomedical research, but still receives particular interest (i) in the field of oncology with multicellular tumor cell spheroids studied as an in vitro model of avascular tumor sites (for review [Mueller-Klieser, 1997; Kunz-Schughart, 1999; Mueller-Klieser, 2000; Kunz-Schughart et al., 2004]) and (ii) in stem cell research with so-called embryoid bodies (= embryonal stem cell spheres) or neurospheres being able to maintain stem or progenitor cell properties in vitro [Valliers and Pedersen, 2005; Jensen and Parmar, 2006; Marshall et al., 2007; Kurosawa, 2007] . Embryoid bodies have also been applied in confrontation culture, e.g. with tumor spheroids as an angiogenesis model [Wartenberg et al., 2001; Wartenberg et al. 2006; Goodwin, 2007]. On the other hand, EC in co-culture, with or without smooth muscle cells, also form free-floating spheroids [Korff and Augustin, 1998; Korff et al., 2001] that may then be embedded in ECM gels, i.e. collagen, to monitor EC sprouting [Vernon and Sage, 1999].

It is beyond the scope of this article to discuss further advanced approaches for in vitro vascular engineering. However, it is noted that there has been an exponential increase in relevant literature in the past few years, in particular with the application of perfused culture devices. In lieu of such systems that are not feasible for disease-related (cardiovascular) research, we want to highlight a recently published study that attempted to simulate the morphology of a normal muscular artery in order to investigate initial events in atherosclerosis. Dorweiler and coworkers used a modified fibrin gel as a scaffold for multilayer growth of SMC covered by an EC layer. Lipoprotein insudation was investigated under simulated hypo-, normo- and hypercholesterolemic conditions through addition of LDL to the medium with subsequent time and dose-dependent insudation of LDL. When human monocytes were added to the culture medium, infiltration and foam cell formation of macrophages and SMCs as well as expression of IL-8 was demonstrated. The authors even suggested that this in vitro model is suitable for the study of pivotal events in atherosclerotic plaque development. [Dorweiler et al., 2006].

The usage of such complex in vitro culture models to study the pathomechanisms of cardiovascular diseases requires information about the responses of the individual cell types involved. Therefore, the focus of the next section is the presentation of human EC cultures including the well-known organ specificity as mentioned above. In addition, we introduce disease-specific EC to document the endothelial dysfunction of vascular diseases under in vitro conditions.

4. Primary Cultures of Human EC for Cardiovascular Research

Vascular endothelial pathology is central to a range of diseases, e.g. atherosclerosis, tumor angiogenesis, metastasis, diabetes mellitus, and chronic allograft rejection. Thus, endothelial dysfunction refers to the broad alterations in endothelial phenotype that contribute to the development and clinical expression of vascular diseases. It is therefore important to isolate primary EC in order to establish in vitro models to study the properties of vascular endothelium. The most widespread EC culture system used in this area is HUVEC. However, these cells are close to senescence and are cultured from hypoxic vessels [Garlanda and Dejana, 1997]. Therefore, HUVEC are introduced in this section only as an example, with the main focus being on organ-specific and disease-related EC cultures. However, the use of the latter requires the availability of the respective human vessel material corresponding to the underlying vascular disease. Suitable models of human "pathological endothelium" (isolated from patient lesions) may greatly expand our knowledge of the mechanisms responsible for initiation and progression of endothelial dysfunction. In this context, this section introduces disease-related EC models from available vessels in cardiovascular surgery. We discuss, among other models, the "diabetic human saphenous vein EC" which is isolated from vein grafts for cardiac bypass operations from diabetic patients. In contrast, human coronary artery and aortic EC represent organ-specificity of EC for cardiovascular research. Cardiac microvascular EC were introduced to demonstrate the endothelial response in small vessel EC. Finally, exemplary data of circulating EC (CEC) and endothelial progenitor cells (EPC) are discussed in the context of new therapeutic strategies for therapeutic interventions in endothelial repair and angiogenesis. The extent of published in vitro studies using these specific cells mainly depends on the availability of the respective vessel material.

4.1. Human Umbilical Vein Endothelial Cells (HUVEC)

The first successful isolation and characterization of EC from the umbilical vein in culture was reported in 1973 and 1974 by Jaffe et al. [Jaffe et al., 1973] and Gimbrone et al. [Gimbrone et al., 1974]. The ability to culture EC allowed investigators to manipulate – in a controlled manner – the extracellular environment and to study cell biology in far greater detail. Among the seminal findings of that time was the observation that incubation of cultured EC with inflammatory mediators or bacterial products induced proadhesive, antigen-presenting and procoagulant activities, a phenomenon that was termed "EC activation" [Pober and Gimbrone, 1982; Gamble et al., 1985; Bevilacqua et al., 1986; Pober et al., 1986; Schleimer and Rutledge, 1986; Bevilacqua et al. 1987; Bevilacqua et al., 1989]. Since then, EC derived from the human umbilical vein (HUVEC) have been the major source of primary EC, mainly because umbilical cords are readily available and ethically unproblematic. HUVEC have been used to study a range of important patho-physiological processes, including immune-endothelial interactions, endothelial dysfunction related to atheroma formation and tumor metastasis. The literature is filled with studies using the HUVEC model. HUVEC and immortalized EC lines are also used for routine cytotoxicity studies. The pharmaceutical industry has established in vitro screening assays for drug candidates using human EC as a model for vascular injury after intravenous application. L´Azou et al. used standardized vascular EC models (HUVEC, EA-hy926, HBMEC) to test the toxic effects of cyclosporine A and cadmium [L´Azou et al., 2005]. Schleger et al. tested 5 compounds (cyclosporine A, mitomycin C, menadione, amrinone and rolipram) based on their known effects on the vasculature [Scheger et al., 2004]. Despite a similar cytotoxicity for all these drugs, they documented a dose-dependent decrease in transendothelial resistance and an increase in FITC-dextran permeability. They postulated more functional assays on EC for more detailed characterization of individual compounds. Nevertheless, the applicability of these cells in cardiovascular research failed. HUVEC are derived from immune-privileged fetal tissue [French et al., 1996] and may not be representative of adult endothelium. HUVEC express a high level of CD95 (Fas) ligand, which contributes to fetal immune privilege. CD95L induces apoptosis in activated CD95+ lymphocytes, which may limit the availability of HUVEC to support inflammation [Guller and LaChapelle, 1999]. Hence, HUVEC are not suited for cardiovascular research.

4.2. Human Saphenous Vein Endothelial Cells (HSVEC)

4.2.1. Rationale f HSVEC Cultures

Adult EC may have been subjected to prolonged exposure to cytokines, hormones and other stimuli, potentially resulting in an altered phenotype. For this reason, there is a pressing need to develop a primary cell culture for adult large vessel endothelium. Human saphenous vein EC (HSVEC) are an obvious candidate due to the availability of saphenous veins. These are routinely removed in varicose vein surgery and during many vascular and coronary artery bypass operations. Culture of HSVEC has been previously performed by several groups, but their utility has been limited by the failure to maintain pure cultures for a reasonable period of time [Scoumanne et al., 2002]. Tan et al. characterized this alternative model and provided a detailed functional comparison with HUVEC [Tan et al., 2004]. Compared with HUVEC, HSVEC showed an increased sensitivity to ox-LDL and a reduced response to cytokines, as indicated by adhesion molecule expression as well as leukocyte adhesion and transmigration. With respect to their ability to present antigen, HSVEC have a higher level of HLA-DR, CD40 and ICOS-L following cytokine stimulation. In addition, HSVEC up-regulate the costimulatory ligand CD80 following CD40 ligation, and support allogeneic T cell proliferation, while HUVEC fail to express CD80. Due to differential expression of adhesion molecules, poorly differentiated tumor cell lines also showed more adhesion to HSVEC than to HUVEC [Tan et al., 2004]. They also documented a functional similarity of HSVEC and arterial EC. Venous/arterial identity was also supported by cell culture studies in which flow induces an arterial phenotype in venous EC [Tsukurov et al., 2000; Dai et al., 2004]. Furthermore, when veins are grafted into the arterial circulation, they acquire arterial-like properties, including a thickened wall and, in animal models, reduced permeability [Kwei et al., 2004]. In these and other in vivo studies, venous arterialization is adaptive and primarily mediated by differences in sheer stress and the microenvironment [Golledge et al., 1997; Mavromatis et al., 2000; Rabkin-Aikawa et al., 2004]. It was concluded that HSVEC are a robust model for studying most vascular pathophysiology.

Therefore, HSVEC cultures are mainly used in two different applications: (1) As a therapeutic tool for seeding human vascular cells onto vascular grafts in tissue engineering studies, and (2) as an in vitro model to study EC responses in conjunction with elucidation of the mechanisms of vascular diseases.

4.2.2. HSVEC for Tissue Engineering

EC seeding of biomaterial vascular grafts and scaffolds to improve device thrombogenicity is a popular strategy, which presumes that EC cultured on biomaterials will express a non-thrombogenic phenotype [McGuigan and Sefton, 2007]. For patients who lack autologous vascular tissue vital for successful surgery, the currently available prosthetic, biologic and allograft alternatives are less than satisfactory. Early tissue engineering strategies to solve this problem involved seeding nonabsorbable prosthetic grafts with vascular cells [Bordenave et al., 1999]. Although these conduits have shown promise, they have not achieved widespread clinical acceptance [Lamm et al., 1999]. In 12 patients undergoing coronary artery bypass grafting (CABG), the short segments of the patients' vein were harvested and the human autologous vein EC were cultured and subsequently seeded onto acellularized cryopreserved vein allografts. The 3-year primary graft patency rate was shown to be 87%. The main problems of these ex vitro seeding experiments are obvious: an additional surgery to remove vein segments, time consuming isolation and cultivation of patient-derived endothelial cells, endothelialization of vascular grafts under GMP (good medical practice) guidelines, and danger of infection.

Novel concepts of cardiovascular tissue engineering were reviewed by Vara et al. [Vara et al. ,2005]: For coronary and vascular bypass, 3 types of tissue-engineered grafts exist: biodegradable scaffold [Niklason et al., 1999], bioresistant scaffold such as polyurethane [Miwa et al. 1993], and decellularized matrix tube [Sacks and Gloeckner, 1999; Trantina-Yates et al., 2001]. The lumen of the grafts were lined with smooth muscle cells, myofibroblasts, chondrocytes or other extracellular basement membrane proteins and seeded with EC [Gulbins et al. 2005].

The static cell culture model with HSVEC allows a primary evaluation of the adhesive properties and functional retention of the EC on different biomaterials. For example, this technique enables the investigation of the endothelilaization potential of titanium-coated synthetic polymers [Lehle et al., 2003; Lehle et al., 2004] and of decellularized glutaraldehyde-fixed animal pericardium for human heart valve replacement. This in vitro technique eliminates non-biocompatible materials from tissue engineering studies, and therefore restricted the number of animal experiments. Moreover, as mentioned above, seeding of grafts with patient-derived vascular cells may improve the anti-thrombogenicity of the biomaterials.

4.2.3. HSVEC for Disease-Related Research

Primary success in clarifying pathways in the "EC activation" by using HUVEC are now adapted to the known organ-specific heterogeneity of EC as documented in vascular diseases. This section focuses on the usage of patient- and especially disease-specific HSVEC (isolated from patients with coronary heart disease) for cardiovascular research.

To avoid immunological reactions, patient-derived EC were favored for seeding of vascular grafts [Lamm et al., 1999]. Only a few scientific groups used patient-derived EC as an in vitro model to correlate the endothelial function and the individual characteristics of the cell donors. In this context, and due to the known heterogeneity of human EC from different vascular beds, our group compared the "endothelial activation" of different human macrovascular EC under identical cell culture conditions [Lehle et al., 2007b]. In this study, we compared, to our knowledge for the first time, the patient characteristics of our cell donors with EC functions and responses. Neither demographic data nor the basal disease (coronary heart disease) correlated with the activation status of the patient-derived EC cultures.

As mentioned above, one more tool for studying the mechanisms of cardiovascular diseases is the use of disease-specific EC culture models. This approach tends to be very interested in the investigation of drug effects on specific EC functions. Thus Roccaro et al. showed that bortezomib, a potent and selective inhibitor of the proteasome, targets angiogenesis in multiple myeloma by a direct effect on multiple myeloma patient-derived EC (MMEC) functions associated with angiogenesis both in vitro in proliferation, chemotaxis, adhesion on fibronectin, capillary formation on Matrigel assay, and in vivo in the chorioallantoic membrane assay [Roccaro et al., 2006]. Drug-related down-regulation of genes mandatory for autocrine and paracrine growth of EC, including VEGF, IL-6, IGF-1, Ang1, and Ang2, was observed. In addition, these translated proteins decreased in MMEC conditioned media. These data therefore show that bortezomib acts both directly and indirectly against MMEC, defining another mechanism which may contribute to its anti-multiple myeloma activity.

Another disease-specific model is the "diabetic EC" [Lehle et al., 2007a]. The diabetic endothelial dysfunction was, among other things, characterized by a chronic inflammatory state in the vessel wall, thus accelerating the development of macrovascular complications [Park et al., 1998; Schmidt et al., 2000; Schmidt and Stern, 2000a; Schmidt and Stern, 2000b]. Despite extensive animal studies, the extent of chronic vascular inflammation in diabetic patients remains largely unknown for lack of a reliable and noninvasive method to assess vascular inflammation. Feng et al. offers a minimally invasive method consisting of a catheter and a guide wire-based endothelial biopsy to obtain a few EC from patients [Feng et al., 2005]. These cells were characterized with respect to molecular phenotypes under the influence of both genetic and environmental factors. Strong associations were observed between induction of receptors for advanced glycation end products (RAGEs) mRNA and diabetes and between induction of RAGE and MCP-1 (monocyte chemoattractant protein-1) transcripts. Another scientific approach to expand our knowledge of the mechanisms responsible for initiation and progression of diabetic endothelial dysfunction is the isolation and cultivation of human EC from diabetic patients. Bolego et al. reported that EC from insulin-dependent diabetic patients feature a down-regulated expression of cyclooxygenase-2 (COX-2) and endothelial nitric oxide synthase (eNOS) enzyme proteins, whose products strategically cooperate in the protection of the vessel wall [Bolego et al., 2006]. These findings may have clinical relevance given the critical role of the endothelium in the development of cardiovascular disease whereby diabetes represents a significant factor.

The inflammatory response of the endothelium could be verified in the EC culture model [Pober and Cotran, 1990] by measuring the release of cytokines/chemokines and the expression of cellular adhesion molecules, both important factors in the inflammatory cascade. In the case of diabetic patients, the clinical manifestation of the endothelial dysfunction was based on increased concentrations of soluble adhesion molecules and cytokines in the plasma and atherosclerotic malformations in the arterial wall. With a disease-specific in vitro model – the "diabetic EC" – our group postulated that EC isolated from saphenous veins from diabetic patients remember their dysfunction in vitro [Lehle et al., 2007a]. To verify our hypothesis we analyzed the growth characteristics and the inflammatory status of non-diabetic and diabetic HSVEC. In a comparative experimental trial, we reported that the diabetic HSVEC showed delayed growth kinetics with reduced cell densities of about 40%. We speculate that a successful regeneration of denuded areas in the endothelial layer of an atherosclerotic stressed diabetic vessel may be time-retarded and incomplete. Our hypothesis was supported by a reduced proliferation potential of endothelial progenitor cells isolated from diabetic patients [Sorrentino et al., 2007; Capla et al., 2007]. In addition, during exponential growth of the diabetic EC, the surface expression of adhesion molecules was increased 10-fold. Under non-stimulating conditions the release of soluble E-selectin, VCAM-1 (vascular cellular adhesion molecule-1), IL-6 and MCP-1 was also significantly increased, whereas the concentration of IL-8 and soluble ICAM-1 (intracellular adhesion molecule-1) in the supernatant of diabetic and non-diabetic EC were comparable. Thus, our data suggest a link between the pathologically proinflammatory basic state of diabetic EC and the endothelial dysfunction in diabetic disease. The reasons for the altered phenotype of the diabetic EC may be the prolonged exposure to hyperglycaemia, AGES (advanced glycation end products), and other stimuli [Basta et al., 2004]. From several in vitro studies we know that high concentrations of glucose and AGES induce the expression of adhesion molecules in "healthy" HUVEC [Takami et al., 1998; Altannavch et al., 2004; Quagliaro et al., 2005]. Glucose treatment of the diseased diabetic EC resulted in an isolated increase in the VCAM-1 expression by 10-20%, and an enhancement in the release of MCP-1 by 40-70%. In contrast to the "healthy" EC, the expression of ICAM-1 and E-selectin and the release of IL-6 and IL-8 of diabetic EC was not affected [Haubner et al., 2007]. In addition to glucose, other factors in the serum of diabetic serum influenced the response of diabetic EC. Diabetic serum (without glucose and oral antidiabetic drugs) showed unchanged surface expression of adhesion molecules and elevated levels of soluble ICAM-1 in HSVEC of all donors. In addition, the proinflammatory basic state of diabetic EC characterized by increased levels of cytokines was compensated [Münzel et al., 2007]. We concluded that even under normoglycemic conditions the serum itself contains critical factors leading to abnormal regulation of inflammation in diabetics. Consequently, future studies should identify these specific factors in diabetic serum to develop therapeutic interventions. These findings could potentially be used to scientific advantage in the monitoring of potential therapeutic agents specifically targeted to the reduction of vascular inflammation. In contrast to former pharmacologic studies using HUVEC or immortalized EC, our disease-specific EC model will provide more diabetic-specific results and seems to be more appropriate for drug screening tests.

4.3. Human Arterial Endothelial Cells

4.3.1. Rationale of Arterial EC Cultures

Atherosclerosis is primarily a disease of large conduit arteries and rarely affects the veins. Differences in hemodynamic environments between veins and arteries may play an important role in the development of atherosclerosis, but cannot fully explain the differences in predisposition to atherosclerosis between different vascular beds. The proximal left anterior descending coronary artery in the coronary circulation, the proximal portions of the renal arteries, the carotid bifurcation in the extracranial circulation, and the aorta exhibit a particular predilection for atherosclerosis. Therefore, there is an increasing trend to use arterial EC derived from the coronary artery [Zhang et al., 2001; Deng et al., 2006] and aorta [Honda et al., 1999; Shih et al., 1999] to study the pathogenesis of atherosclerosis in vitro. Unfortunately, the limited supply of these tissues - especially from humans - makes their application difficult and impractical in many centers. Nevertheless, both distinct and characteristic gene expression profiles [Chi et al., 2003] and the functional heterogeneity of arterial EC [Aird, 2002; Aird, 2007b] were supported, which necessitates the discussion of the arterial EC culture.

4.3.2. Isolation of Arterial EC for Pure Cell Cultures

Besides the limited availability of respective vessel material, the isolation of pure cultures of human arterial EC is another problem in the use of such cultures for cardiovascular research. Literature shows isolation of cardiovascular EC by perfusion of hearts or large heart-derived vessels with digesting enzymes [Grafe et al., 1994]. In such preparations primary EC cultures were often overgrown by fibroblasts, smooth muscle cells or pericytes. This phenomenon was aggravated by using tissue material from explanted hearts. Sclerotic and calcified vessel materials from diseased elderly donors with coronary artery disease, and/or diabetes mellitus yielded only purities of 5% to 50% EC in the primary cultures [Lehle et al., 2007a]. Therefore, separation protocols including magnetic bead isolation strategies [Grafe et al., 1994; Conrad-Lapostolle et al., 1996] and flow cytometric sorting procedures (FACS) [Craig et al., 1998; Nistri et al., 2002; Oxhorn et al., 2002; Huang et al., 2003] using antibodies against EC surface markers (CD31, CD105, CD146) were published. Commonly used magnetic bead isolation techniques are from Dynal (Hamburg, Germany; Dynabeads), Miltenyi (Bergisch Gladbach, Germany; MACS micro-beads), and others. As a representative example, Table 2 presents our data from experiments separating EC from a mixture of EC and fibroblasts using different labeling strategies for MACS separation. According to the manufacturer's instructions, EC were labeled with anti-CD31-FITC antibody and anti-FITC-MACS-microbeads (1) or with anti-CD105-microbeads (2), or fibroblasts were labeled with anti-fibroblast-MACS-microbeads (3). In either case, the percentage of CD31-positive cells (= EC) was increased, but failed to reach 100%. In addition, the recovery (meaning the amount of cells after separation relative to the introduced EC before separation) of EC ranged between 60% and 96%. After recultivation, only a small amount of fibroblasts (≥5%) was sufficient to overgrow the separated EC fraction preventing long-term cultivation. In contrast, FACSorting using anti-human CD31-labeling resulted in purities of ≥99% and a cell loss of less than 20% [Lehle et al., 2007b]. This method benefits from the single cell sorting technique. Both magnetic cell separation and FACSorting were shown to alter membrane physiology of sensitive cells, which was discussed as a sort-induced stress syndrome due to exposure to hydrodynamic forces or magnetic fields [Seidl et al., 1999]. However, for EC neither magnetic cell separation nor FACSorting affected morphology, growth or function of these cells [Grafe et al., 1994; Craig et al., 1998; Lehle et al., 2007b]. These isolation strategies may allow the application of arterial EC for functional analysis in vitro.

4.3.3. Characteristic Features of Arterial EC

Preferentially, bovine, porcine, or rat aortic EC and coronary artery EC were used for in vitro vascular research. However, for human studies commercially available primary arterial EC cultures were purchased from Clonetics (San Diego, CA, USA), Promocell (Heidelberg, Germany) or Provitro (Berlin, Germany). These preparations originate from brain death organ donors. The complex isolation of arterial EC from patient vessels (e.g. from explanted hearts) primarily prevented its usage in cardiovascular research.

In this context, a recent gene expression profiling study by Deng et al. compared the genes of EC from human saphenous veins and coronary arteries in response to various atherogenic stimuli [Deng et al., 2006]. They identified 285 genes that were more highly expressied in HSVEC, and 111 genes that were more highly expressed in HCAEC. The vein EC-selective transcripts were enriched for genes involved in inhibiting reactive oxygen species (ROS), attenuating the inflammatory response, and promoting proliferation. The artery-selective genes included inhibitors of cell proliferation and lipid metabolism. In response to ox-LDL, many more genes were upregulated and downregulated in venous compared with arterial cells, whereas TNF and IL-1 induced similar gene expression responses in both cell types. In venous EC, ox-LDL-activated genes involved protective pathways, whereas arterial EC demonstrated upregulation of cell adhesion molecules and genes involved in proliferation and apoptosis. The differential effect of ox-LDL on HCAEC versus HSVEC proliferation was validated in functional assays.

Vascular bed-specific responses of EC to TNF and IL-1 were also documented by Briones et al. [Briones et al., 2001]. Upon in vitro stimulation with TNF and IL-1, the production of RANTES (regulated-upon-activated-normal-T-cells expressed and secreted protein) by HCAEC was significantly increased relative to that by HUVEC. The opposite effect, however, was noted for levels of MCP-1 (monocyte chemoattractant protein-1) and IP-10 (gamma interferon-inducible protein-10). These data provide evidence for their potential to contribute to site-specific and possibly selective recruitment of leukocytes in coronary artery vessels. A multifunctional cytokine expression profile by HCAEC and its regulation by monokines and glucocorticoids was also introduced by Krishnaswamy et al. [Krishnaswamy et al., 1998].

Furthermore, EC from coronary arteries signalized a higher synthesis rate of IL-6 compared to venous macrovascular EC and EC from arteria thoracica interna [Lehle et al., 2007a]. This intrinsic property of HCAEC might be a source for increased concentrations of IL-6 in the plasma of patients with coronary heart disease. However, in the current state a distinct correlation of the in vitro and the in vivo data is very difficult and dangerous. The evolutionary selective development of unique chemokine profiles of different vascular beds during inflammatory stress can ultimately be measured in terms of survival benefits to the host.

4.3.4. Arterial EC for Application in Cardiovascular Research

The coronary artery is the most important vascular bed with respect to the problem of cardiovascular risk. Therefore, HCAEC were used increasingly as an in vitro model to demonstrate early events in the pathogenesis of atherosclerosis on the level of the endothelium. Inflammatory activation of EC is a critical step in the development of atherosclerosis [Shi et al., 2000], and the agents responsible are being sought. Arterial EC cultures were used (1) to identify plasma compounds and its effects on EC structure and function, and (2) to evaluate therapeutic interventions on the cellular level.

The identification of plasma components that are responsible for exchange of EC structure and function is important in light of their potential application as pathogenic atherosclerosis markers, predictors or therapeutic targets. A large number of different compounds have been investigated in the past. However, the present review focuses on only a few examples in recently published studies. The effect of enterobacterial endotoxin on EC activation and its role as contributor to atherosclerosis is well characterized (as reviewed by [Stoll et al., 2004]). However, much less is known about the effects on the vasculature of non-enterobacterial endotoxins, which are likely to contribute a much larger fraction to the circulating endotoxin pool [Berg, 1996; Geerts et al., 2002]. Thus, Erridge et al. could show that endotoxins of P. gingivalis, P. aeruginosa and B. fragilis are capable of stimulating activation of coronary artery EC, whereas the proinflammatory response of HUVEC was not affected [Erridge et al., 2007]. These in vitro experiments reflect the responsiveness of HCAEC and the underestimated impact of non-enterobacterial endotoxins on EC which may contribute to the development of atherosclerosis. Other important components in human plasma which seem to be responsible for lesion formation/development in atherosclerosis are lipids and/or protein oxidation products (as reviewed by Refs. [Jessup et al., 2004; Nakajima et al., 2006]). This idea was stimulated by the pro-atherogenic properties of these molecules: Recent studies showed that carbamylated low-density lipoproteins (LDL) and non modified LDLs induced a variety of damaging stimuli to HCAEC and vascular smooth muscle cells, all of which attributed to atherosclerosis [Apostolov et al., 2007a; Apostolov et al., 2007b]. Moreover, not only the concentration but also the composition of LDL appears to be important in alteration of adhesive properties and proinflammatory responses of EC (e.g. monocyte adhesion and induction of intracellular adhesion molecule-1 and vascular cellular adhesion molecule-1 in HCAEC) [Marschang et al., 2006]. Another interesting field is diabetes research and the development of the metabolic syndrome. The impact of high glucose concentration and advanced glycation end products (AGES) on the activation status of EC was discussed in numerous studies [Federici and Lauro, 2005; Yun et al., 2006]. Furthermore, Staiger et al. [Staiger et al., 2004] documented the effect of high levels of the plasma free fatty acid (FFA) palmitate on the inflammatory induction of IL-6, which is an important player in the pathogenesis of the metabolic syndrome [McGarry, 2002].

The arterial EC cultures were also used to evaluate the therapeutic relevance of different cardiovascular drugs. One focus is the reduction of inflammatory reactions (e.g. adherence of leukocytes, expression of adhesion molecules, and release of proinflammatory cytokines/chemokines). In this context, incubation of arterial EC with phytotherapeutica, such as garlic and garlic extracts, decreased the IL-1-induced expression of ICAM-1 and VCAM-1 and the adhesion of monocytes, thus potentially contributing to the beneficial effects traditionally attributed to garlic [Rassoul et al., 2006]. In addition, the culture model was used to analyze the effect of immunosuppressive drugs on coronary artery EC activation which could be responsible for endothelial activation during the process of chronic heart disease. Due to the class of immunosuppressive drugs – calcineurin or mTOR inhibitor – the inflammatory response of both HSVEC and HCAEC were comparable: Neither calcineurin inhibitors (cyclosporine A, tacorlimus) nor mTOR inhibitors (Sirolimus, Everolimus) affected the basal expression of cellular adhesion molecules (E-selectin, VCAM-1, ICAM-1) and the release of IL-8 and MCP-1. However, incubation with mTOR inhibitors inhibited the TNF-induced production of IL-6. This was a time- and dose-dependent effect [Lehle et al., 2005; Schreml et al., 2007]. In addition, due to the known increased synthesis rate of IL-6 by HCAEC [Lehle et al., 2007b], incubation with mTOR inhibitors resulted in an inhibition of its basal release of IL-6 [Schreml et al., 2007]. Our data clearly show a vessel-specific reaction to mTOR inhibitors and additionally an anti-inflammatory effect of mTOR inhibitors on the endothelial level. We hypothesize that the documented anit-inflammatory impact of mTOR inhibitors supports the process of reduced transplant vasculopathy as a positive side-effect of this new class of immunosuppressive drugs.

Glucocorticoids, which have various anti-inflammatory effects, are widely used clinically for the treatment of inflammatory and autoimmune disorders. In HCAEC exposed to TNF, intravenous immunglobulin (IVIG) and dexamethasone inhibited IL-6 production to a similar degree, whereas the expression of E-selectin was inhibited more strongly by IVIG [Ichiyama et al., 2004; Makata et al., 2006]. Furthermore, high-dose IVIG inhibits the activation of monocytes/macrohages and HCAEC to a greater degree than T cells, whereas dexamethasone inhibits the activation of all three cell types. This cell type-specific therapy may allow the treatment of acute Kawasaki disease (KD) in which monocytes, macrophages, but not T lymphocytes are activated [Makata et al., 2006].

Lipid-lowering agents such as statins also possess broad immunomodulatory and anti-inflammatory properties. Recent studies investigating how these drugs modify EC function demonstrate that the therapeutic effect of statins can be attributed, in part, to their action on the endothelium. Greenwood and Mason reviewed the effects of statins on vascular endothelial inflammatory response [Greenwood and Mason, 2007]. They also referred, for example, to a study from Li et al. providing direct evidence that ox-LDL via LOX-1 (lectin-like receptors fro ox-LDL) activation induces ACE (angiotensin converting enzyme) gene expression in HCAEC, and MAPK (mitogen-activated protein kinase) activation plays a signal transduction role in this process [Li et al., 2003].

4.4. Human Microvascular Cardiac EC

4.4.1. Rationale of Cardiac Microvascular EC and its Isolation

The mechanisms leading to preferential localization of atherosclerotic lesions are less well understood. To further define these mechanisms, especially in the context of microvascular damage, HCAEC and cardiac microvascular EC (HHMEC) were isolated and cultured under identical conditions [Nishida et al., 1993; Gräfe et al., 1994; McDouall et al., 1996]. The isolation strategy for human microvascular cardiac EC is based on the perfusion of donor hearts resulting in a mixture of micro- and macrovascular EC [Gräfe et al., 1994; McDouall et al., 1996]. Another possibility for obtaining the microvascular cells is the proteolytical digestion of endomyocardial biopsies. However, the small amount of biopsy material prevents usable yields of pure EC cultures. Only 40% to 50% of the preparations resulted in the mixed cultures needed further purification. Successful FACSorting, as described above, depended on the proportion of contaminated cells. In addition, each purification/separation step increased the passage number and increased the risk of dedifferentiation of the cells. Recently, human microvascular cardiac EC have been made commercially available (Promocell, Heidelberg, Germany), which offers the possibility of withdrawing the cardiac microvessels.

4.4.2. Functional Characteristics of Human Microvascular Cardiac EC

Cardiac arterial EC (HCAEC, HHMEC) constitutively express both VCAM-1 and E-selecitn, bind more PMBC under non-stimulating and TNF-stimulating conditions, and were more sensitive to TNF than aortic EC [Farrar et al., 2000; McDouall et al., 2001]. The authors hypothesize that EC in different regions of the coronary tree express different patterns of basal and cytokine-stimulated adhesion molecule expression. Incubation of EC with oxidized LDL induced a significant increase in plasminogen-activator inhibitor (PAI-1) activity in HCAEC. This stimulatory effect of ox-LDL was less developed in HHMEC. Stimulation with angiotensin II induced expression of E-selectin more effectively in macrovascular than in microvascular EC. In addition, angiotensin II-induced E-selectin expression led to increased E-selectin-dependent adhesion of HL60 cells to HCAEC under flow conditions, while only minor effects were observed with HHMEC. In contrast, L-selectin-dependent adhesion, which has been shown to play an important role in inflammatory reactions, was preferentially observed in cardiac microvascular EC and could only be stimulated with TNF, not by angiotensin II. Therefore, these cellular differences may, in part, explain specific properties of cardiac EC: Such as atherosclerotic lesions are localized in macrovascular vessel segments, whereas inflammatory responses are predominantly found in the microvasculature [Gräfe et al., 1998].

Human cardiac microvascular EC can be used in cardiovascular research. In a co-culture system using HHMEC and HIV-infected leukocytes, Sundstrom et al. determined that norepinephrine (NE), a stress-associated autonomic nervous system neurotransmitter, can promote increased leukocyte interactions with the cardiac microvascular endothelium and suggested a mechanism by which NE may influence the progression of AIDS-related heart disease [Sundstrom et al., 2003]. In view of the role of EC as initiators of allograft rejection, McDouall et al. was interested in the regulation of MHC class II regulation by HHMEC [McDouall et al., 1997]. They could show that (1) class II expression was maintained longer in HHMEC compared with HUVEC; (2) NK cells and supernatants from HHMEC/NK cultures induced MHC class II antigens on HHMEC with an enhanced sensitivity compared with HUVEC. This observation has implications for therapeutic interventions.

4.5. Human Endothelial Progenitor Cells (EPC)

The important role of the vascular endothelium in cardiovascular health/disease is becoming increasingly recognized. Quantification of circulating endothelial cells (CEC) in peripheral blood is developing as a novel and reproducible method of assessing endothelial damage/injury (as reviewed by Refs. [Boos et al., 2006; Erdbruegger et al., 2006]). It was postulated that CEC have detached from the intimal monolayer in response to endothelial injury and emerged in the circulation. In cardiovascular diseases CEC have been found to be elevated in acute myocardial infarction [Heloire et al., 2003], after coronary angioplasty for stable angina [Heloire et al., 2003], in acute coronary syndrome [Boos et al., 2006], in acute and chronic coronary heart disease [Zal et al., 2004], in acute ischemic stroke [Numaguchi et al., 2006], in pulmonary hypertension [Sata, 2006], diabetes mellitus [Thum et al., 2007], etc. Boos et al. present an overview of the pathophysiology of CEC in the setting of cardiovascular disease [Boos et al., 2006].

In contrast, endothelial progenitor cells (EPC) are non-leukocytes derived from the bone marrow that are believed to have proliferative potential and may be important in vascular regeneration. It has been suggested that these cells might not only be responsible for the continuous recovery of the endothelium after injury/damage, but also might take part in angiogenesis, giving the hope of new treatment opportunities. There have been no studies to date that have actually attempted to quantify both CEC and EPC simultaneously in the same patient population. The definition of each cell type is the initial problem which aggravates the isolation of these small cell populations: i.e. CD146 for CEC and any combination of CD34, CD133, VEGFR-2, and so on, for EPC [George et al., 1992; Rafii et al., 1994; Asahara et al., 1997; Boyer et al., 2000; Hristov et al., 2003; Bompais et al., 2004]. Additional phenotyping and the endothelioid nature of CEC and EPC are generally presumed by staining for vWF, lectins (UEA-1), endothelial nitric oxide synthase (eNOS), and acetylated low-density lipoprotein cholesterol [Blann et al., 2005; Walenta et al., 2005]. In addition, a microvascular marker, CD36, and the expression of E-selectin and ICAM-1 were discussed as markers for CEC. The use of CD45 to exclude a leukocyte origin for these cells is common [Mancuso et al., 2001; Del Papa et al., 2004; Lee et al., 2005]. EPC possess the commonality of being capable of augmenting revascularization and endothelial regeneration. This effect was identified under different names: endothelial outgrowth cells [Lin et al., 2000], circulating angiogenetic cells [Rehman et al., 2003] or endothelial-like cells [Pujol et al., 2000].

The clinical role of EPC and perspectives for treatment of cardiovascular disorder was reviewed in detail by Shantsila et al. [Shantsila et al., 2007]. An increasing body of evidence suggests that cardiovascular risk factors affect the number and properties of EPC. An inverse correlation is found between the number and functional activity of EPC and cardiovascular risk factors among apparently healthy people and in patients with coronary artery disease [Vasa et al., 2001; Hill et al., 2003]. One highlight of EPC as a therapeutic intervention is EPC transplantation. It is increasingly recognized that EPCs are recruited to sites of injury and participate in the repair of damaged tissues and neovascularization in ischemic myocardium [Wang and LI, 2007], hind limb [Kolvenbach et al., 2007], and brain [Liu et al., 2007]. The therapeutic efficacy of EPC was demonstrated in many animal models for ischemic disorder and vascular injury [Caballero et al., 2007]. However, the precise role of EPCs in ischemic heart and cerebral disease and their therapeutic potential still remain to be explored [Ding et al., 2007]. Another therapeutic approach of EPC is the usage of EPC from the individual patients for in vitro and spontaneous endothelialization of graft materials [Dzau et al., 2005; Miller-Kasprzak and Jagodzinski 2007].

Healthy EPC may be able to replace the dysfunctional endothelium through endogenous repair mechanisms. Therefore, strategies to augment cell function, survival, and homing could be crucial in improving success rates for cell therapy. Experimental studies have provided novel options for improving survival and function by transduction of stem or progenitor cells with prosurvival genes [Seeger et al., 2007].

5. Overview of the EC Sources for Testing Therapeutic Interventions in Vitro

Within the same species, EC differ in terms of phenotype, growth, antigenic composition, basal release of endothelial-derived factors, and sensitivity to agonists. Moreover, vascular diseases selectively target and alter the function of certain regions of the endothelium. An understanding of the differences of EC functions in various regions of the vasculature and in disease states, and the recognition of the anatomic variations could not only lead to more insight into cardiovascular physiology, but also open new therapeutic approaches that could selectively take advantage of unique targets. The development and evaluation of organ-specific and also of disease-specific EC culture systems may allow the realization of such objectives. Finally, Table 3 summarizes the main sources of human EC and their usage for therapeutic interventions or research studies in cardiovascular diseases.

REFERENCES

Ades, EW; Candal, FJ; Swerlick, RA; George, VG; Summers, S; Bosse, DC; Lawley, TJ. HMEC-1: establishment of an immortalized human microvascular endothelial cell line. *J. Invest. Dermatol.*, 1992, 99(6), 683-90.

Aird, WC. Endothelial cell dynamics and complexity theory. *Crit. Care Med,* 2002, 30(5 Suppl), S180-5.

Aird WC. Endothelial cell heterogeneity. *Crit. Care Med.,* 2003, 31(4 Suppl), S221-30.

Aird, WC. Phenotypic heterogeneity of the endothelium: I. Structure, function, and mechanisms. *Circ. Res,* 2007a, 100(2), 158-73.

Aird, WC. Phenotypic heterogeneity of the endothelium: II. Representative vascular beds. *Circ. Res.,* 2007b, 100(2), 174-90.

Altannavch, TS; Roubalová, K; Kucera, P; Andel, M. Effect of high glucose concentrations on expression of ELAM-1, VCAM-1 and ICAM-1 in HUVEC with and without cytokine activation. *Physiol. Res.,* 2004, 53(1), 77-82.

Altomonte, M; Montagner, R; Fonsatti, E; Colizzi, F; Cattarossi, I; Brasoveanu, LI; Nicotra, MR; Cattelan, A; Natali, PG; Maio, M. Expression and structural features of endoglin (CD105), a transforming growth factor beta1 and beta3 binding protein, in human melanoma. *Br. J. Cancer,* 1996, 74(10), 1586-91.

Anderson, DR; Tsutsui, JM; Xie, F; Radio, SJ; Porter, TR. The role of complement in the adherence of microbubbles to dysfunctional arterial endothelium and atherosclerotic plaque. *Cardiovasc. Res.*, 2007, 73(3), 597-606.

Anfuso, CD; Lupo, G; Romeo, L; Giurdanella, G; Motta, C; Pascale, A; Tirolo, C; Marchetti, B; Alberghina, M. Endothelial cell-pericyte cocultures induce PLA2 protein expression through activation of PKCalpha and the MAPK/ERK cascade. *J. Lipid. Res.*, 2007, 48(4), 782-93.

Anthony, PP; Ramani, P. Endothelial markers in malignant vascular tumours of the liver: superiority of QB-END/10 over von Willebrand factor and Ulex europaeus agglutinin 1. *J. Clin. Pathol.*, 1991, 44(1), 29-32.

Apostolov, EO; Shah, SV; Ok, E; Basnakian, AG. Carbamylated low-density lipoprotein induces monocyte adhesion to endothelial cells through intercellular adhesion molecule-1 and vascular cell adhesion molecule-1. *Arterioscler. Thromb. Vasc. Biol.*, 2007a, 27(4), 826-32.

Apostolov, EO; Basnakian, AG; Yin, X; Ok, E; Shah, SV. Modified LDLs induce proliferation-mediated death of human vascular endothelial cells through MAPK pathway. *Am. J. Physiol Heart Circ. Physiol.*, 2007b, 292(4), H1836-46.

Asahara, T; Murohara, T; Sullivan, A; Silver, M; van der Zee, R; Li, T; Witzenbichler, B; Schatteman, G; Isner, JM. Isolation of putative progenitor endothelial cells for angiogenesis. *Science,* 1997, 275(5302), 964-7.

Auerbach, R; Alby, L; Morrissey, LW; Tu, M; Joseph, J. Expression of organ-specific antigens on capillary endothelial cells. *Microvasc. Res.*, 1985, 29(3), 401-11.

Aurrand-Lions, M; Johnson-Leger, C; Imhof, BA. The last molecular fortress in leukocyte trans-endothelial migration. *Nat. Immunol.*, 2002, 3(2), 116-8.

Azzawi, M; Hasleton, PS; Hutchinson, IV. TNF-alpha in acute cardiac transplant rejection. *Cytokines Cell Mol. Ther.*, 1999, 5(1), 41-9.

Basta, G; Schmidt, AM; De, Caterina R. Advanced glycation end products and vascular inflammation: implications for accelerated atherosclerosis in diabetes. *Cardiovasc. Res,* 2004 1, 63(4), 582-92.

Bardin, N; Anfosso, F; Massé, JM; Cramer, E; Sabatier, F; Le Bivic A; Sampol, J; Dignat-George, F. Identification of CD146 as a component of the endothelial junction involved in the control of cell-cell cohesion. *Blood,* 2001, 98(13), 3677-84.

Bauer, P; Lush, CW; Kvietys, PR; Russell, JM; Granger, DN. Role of endotoxin in the expression of endothelial selectins after cecal ligation and perforation. *Am. J. Physiol. Regulatory Integrative Comp. Physiol.*, 2000, 278, 1140-7.

Belloni, PN; Tressler, RJ. Microvascular endothelial cell heterogeneity: interactions with leukocytes and tumor cells. *Cancer Metastasis Rev.*, 1990, 8(4), 353-89.

Berg, RD. The indigenous gastrointestinal microflora. *Trends Microbiol.*, 1996, 4(11), 430-5.

Bevilacqua, MP; Pober, JS; Majeau, GR; Fiers, W; Cotran, RS; Gimbrone, MA Jr. Recombinant tumor necrosis factor induces procoagulant activity in cultured human vascular endothelium: characterization and comparison with the actions of interleukin 1. *Proc. Natl. Acad. Sci. USA,* 1986, 83(12), 4533-7.

Bevilacqua, MP; Pober, JS; Mendrick, DL; Cotran, RS; Gimbrone, MA Jr. Identification of an inducible endothelial-leukocyte adhesion molecule. *Proc. Natl. Acad. Sci. USA,* 1987, 84(24), 9238-42.

Bevilacqua, MP; Stengelin, S; Gimbrone, MA Jr; Seed, B. Endothelial leukocyte adhesion molecule 1: an inducible receptor for neutrophils related to complement regulatory proteins and lectins. *Science,* 1989, 243(4895), 1160-5.

Biemond, BJ; Perzborn, E; Friederich, PW; Levi, M; Buetehorn, U; Büller, HR. Prevention and treatment of experimental thrombosis in rabbits with rivaroxaban (BAY 597939)--an oral, direct factor Xa inhibitor. *Thromb. Haemost.,* 2007, 97(3), 471-7.

Bishop, ET; Bell, GT; Bloor, S; Broom, IJ; Hendry, NF; Wheatley, ND. An in vitro model of angiogenesis: basic features. *Angiogenesis,* 1999, 3, 335-44.

Blann, AD. Assessment of endothelial dysfunction: focus on atherothrombotic disease. *Pathophysiol. Haemost. Thromb,* 2003, 33(5-6), 256-61.

Blann, AD; Nadar, SK; Lip, GY. The adhesion molecule P-selectin and cardiovascular disease. *Eur. Heart J.,* 2003, 24(24), 2166-79.

Blann, AD; Woywodt, A; Bertolini, F; Bull, TM; Buyon, JP; Clancy, RM; Haubitz, M; Hebbel, R; Lip, GYH; Mancuso, P; Sampol, J; Solovey, A; Dignat, F. Circulating endothelial cells Biomarker of vascular disease. *Thromb Haemost.,* 2005, 93(2), 228-235.

Blindt, R; Vogt, F; Astafieva, I; Fach, C; Hristov, M; Krott, N; Seitz, B; Kapurniotu, A; Kwok, C; Dewor, M; Bosserhoff, AK; Bernhagen, J; Hanrath, P; Hoffmann, R; Weber, C. A novel drug-eluting stent coated with an integrin-binding cyclic Arg-Gly-Asp peptide inhibits neointimal hyperplasia by recruiting endothelial progenitor cells. *J. Am. Coll. Cardiol.,* 2006, 47(9), 1786-95.

Boegehold, MA. Heterogeneity of endothelial function within the circulation. *Curr. Opin. Nephrol. Hypertens.,* 1998, 7(1), 71-8.

Bolego, C; Buccellati, C; Radaelli, T; Cetin, I; Puglisi, L; Folco, G; Sala, A. eNOS; COX-2, and prostacyclin production are impaired in endothelial cells from diabetics. *Biochem. Biophys. Res. Commun.,* 2006, 339(1), 188-90.

Bompais, H; Chagraoui, J; Canron, X; Crisan, M; Liu, XH; Anjo, A; Tolla-Le, PC; Leboeuf, M; Charbord, P; Bikfalvi, A; Uzan, G. Human endothelial cells derived from circulating progenitors display specific functional properties compared with mature vessel wall endothelial cells. *Blood,* 2004, 103(7), 2577-84.

Boos, CJ; Lip, GY; Blann, AD. Circulating endothelial cells in cardiovascular disease. *J. Am. Coll .Cardiol.,* 2006, 48(8), 1538-47.

Bordenave, L; Rémy-Zolghadri, M; Fernandez, P; Bareille, R; Midy, D. Clinical performance of vascular grafts lined with endothelial cells. *Endothelium,* 1999, 6(4), 267-75.

Bouis, D; Hospers, GA; Meijer, C; Molema, G; Mulder, NH. Endothelium in vitro: a review of human vascular endothelial cell lines for blood vessel-related research. *Angiogenesis,* 2001, 4(2), 91-102.

Boutet, SC; Quertermous, T; Fadel, BM. Identification of an octamer element required for in vivo expression of the TIE1 gene in endothelial cells. *Biochem. J,* 2001, 360(Pt1), 23-9.

Boyer, M; Townsend, LE; Vogel, LM; Falk, J; Reitz-Vick, D; Trevor, KT; Villalba, M; Bendick, PJ; Glover, JL. Isolation of endothelial cells and their progenitor cells from human peripheral blood. *J. Vasc. Surg,* 2000, 31(1 Pt 1), 181-9.

Briones, MA; Phillips, DJ; Renshaw, MA; Hooper, WC. Expression of chemokine by human coronary-artery and umbilical-vein endothelial cells and its regulation by inflammatory cytokines. *Coron. Artery Dis.*, 2001, 12(3), 179-86.

Brown, KA; Vora, A; Biggerstaff, J; Edgell, CJ; Oikle, S; Mazure, G; Taub, N; Meager, A; Hill, T; Watson, C; et al. Application of an immortalized human endothelial cell line to the leucocyte:endothelial adherence assay. *J. Immunol. Methods*, 1993, 163(1), 13-22.

Burch, MG; Pepe, GJ; Dobrian, AD; Lattanzio, FA Jr; Albrecht, ED. Development of a coculture system and use of confocal laser fluorescent microscopy to study human microvascular endothelial cell and mural cell interaction. *Microvasc. Res.*, 2005, 70(1-2), 43-52.

Burke-Gaffney, A; Hellewell, PG. Regulation of ICAM-1 by dexamethasone in a human vascular endothelial cell line EAhy926. *Am. J. Physiol.*, 1996, 270(2 Pt 1), C552-61.

Caballero, S; Sengupta, N; Afzal, A; Chang, KH; Li, Calzi S; Guberski, DL; Kern, TS; Grant, MB. Ischemic vascular damage can be repaired by healthy, but not diabetic, endothelial progenitor cells. *Diabetes*, 2007, 56(4), 960-7.

Capla, JM; Grogan, RH; Callaghan, MJ; Galiano, RD; Tepper, OM; Ceradini, DJ; Gurtner, GC. Diabetes impairs endothelial progenitor cell-mediated blood vessel formation in response to hypoxia. *Plast Reconstr. Surg.*, 2007, 119(1), 59-70.

Chi, JT; Chang, HY; Haraldsen, G; Jahnsen, FL; Troyanskaya, OG; Chang, DS; Wang, Z; Rockson, SG; van de Rijn, M; Botstein, D; Brown, PO. Endothelial cell diversity revealed by global expression profiling. *Proc. Natl .Acad. Sci. USA*, 2003, 100(19), 10623-8.

Christenson, LK; Stouffer, RL. Isolation and culture of microvascular endothelial cells from the primate corpus luteum. *Biol. Reprod.* 1996, 55(6), 1397-404.

Cinamon, G; Alon, R. A real time in vitro assay for studying leukocyte transendothelial migration under physiological flow conditions *J. Immunol. Meth.*, 2003, 273(1-2), 53-62.

Cola, C; Almeida, M; Li, D; Romeo, F; Mehta, JL. Regulatory role of endothelium in the expression of genes affecting arterial calcification. *Biochem. Biophys. Res. Commun.*, 2004, 320(2), 424-7.

Conrad-Lapostolle, V; Bordenave, L; Baquey, C. Optimization of use of UEA-1 magnetic beads for endothelial cell isolation. *Cell Biol. Toxicol.*, 1996, 12, 189-197.

Costa, C; Pizzolato, MC; Shen, Y; Wang, Y; Fodor, WL. CD86 blockade in genetically modified porcine cells delays xenograft rejection by inhibiting T-cell and NK-cell activation. *Cell Transplant.*, 2004, 13(1), 75-87.

Craig, LE; Spelman, JP; Strandberg, JD; Zink, MC. Endothelial cells from diverse tissues exhibit differences in growth and morphology. *Microvasc. Res.*, 1998, 55, 65-76.

Csiszar, A; Labinskyy, N; Smith, KE; Rivera, A; Bakker, EN; Jo, H; Gardner, J; Orosz, Z; Ungvari, Z. Downregulation of bone morphogenetic protein 4 expression in coronary arterial endothelial cells: role of shear stress and the cAMP/protein kinase A pathway. *Arterioscler. Thromb. Vasc. Biol.*, 2007, 27(4), 776-82.

Dai, G; Kaazempur-Mofrad, MR; Natarajan, S; Zhang, Y; Vaughn, S; Blackman, BR; Kamm, RD; García-Cardeña, G; Gimbrone, MA Jr. Distinct endothelial phenotypes evoked by arterial waveforms derived from atherosclerosis-susceptible and -resistant regions of human vasculature. *Proc. Natl. Acad. Sci. USA*, 2004, 101(41), 14871-6.

Davis, GE; Senger, DR. Endothelial extracellular matrix: biosynthesis, remodeling, and functions during vascular morphogenesis and neovessel stabilization. *Circ. Res.,* 2005, 97(11), 1093-107.

De Backer, G; Ambrosioni, E; Borch-Johnsen, K; Brotons, C; Cifkova, R; Dallongeville, J; Ebrahim, S; Faergeman, O; Graham, I; Mancia, G; et al. European guidelines on cardiovascular disease prevention in clinical practice<SBT>Third Joint Task Force of European and other Societies on Cardiovascular Disease Prevention in Clinical Practice (constituted by representatives of eight societies and by invited experts). *Atherosclerosis,* 2004, 173(2), 379-89.

Dejana, E; Spagnuolo, R; Bazzoni, G. Interendothelial junctions and their role in the control of angiogenesis, vascular permeability and leukocyte transmigration. *Thromb Haemost.,* 2001, 86(1), 308-15.

DeLisser, HM; Newman, PJ; Albelda, SM. Platelet endothelial cell adhesion molecule (CD31). *Curr. Top Microbiol. Immunol.,* 1993, 184, 37-45.

Del Papa, N; Colombo, G; Fracchiolla, N; Moronetti, LM; Ingegnoli, F; Maglione, W; Comina, DP; Vitali, C; Fantini, F; Cortelezzi, A. Circulating endothelial cells as a marker of ongoing vascular disease in systemic sclerosis. *Arthritis. Rheum.,* 2004, 50(4), 1296-304.

Denis, CV. Molecular and cellular biology of von Willebrand factor. *Int. J. Hematol.,* 2002, 75(1), 3-8.

Deng, DX; Tsalenko, A; Vailaya, A; Ben-Dor, A; Kundu, R; Estay, I; Tabibiazar, R; Kincaid, R; Yakhini, Z; Bruhn, L; Quertermous, T. Differences in vascular bed disease susceptibility reflect differences in gene expression response to atherogenic stimuli. *Circ. Res.,* 2006, 98(2), 200-8.

Dente, CJ; Steffes, CP; Speyer, C; Tyburski, JG. Pericytes augment the capillary barrier in in vitro cocultures. *J. Surg. Res.,* 2001, 97(1), 85-91.

Derhaag, JG; Duijvestijn, AM; Emeis, JJ; Engels, W; van Breda Vriesman, PJ. Production and characterization of spontaneous rat heart endothelial cell lines. *Lab. Invest.,* 1996, 74(2), 437-51.

de Waard, V; van den Berg, BM; Veken, J; Schultz-Heienbrok, R; Pannekoek, H; van Zonneveld, AJ. Serial analysis of gene expression to assess the endothelial cell response to an atherogenic stimulus. *Gene,* 1999, 226(1), 1-8.

Dewey, CF Jr; Bussolari, SR; Gimbrone, MA; Davies, PF. The dynamic response of vascular endothelial cells to fluid shear stress. *J. Biomech. Eng.,* 1981, 103, 177–85.

DiCorleto, PE; de la Motte, CA. Characterization of the adhesion of the human monocytic cell line U937 to cultured endothelial cells. *J. Clin. Invest.,* 1985, 75(4), 1153-61.

Dieterich, P; Odenthal-Schnittler, M; Mrowietz, C; Krämer, M; Sasse, L; Oberleithner, H; Schnittler, HJ. Quantitative morphodynamics of endothelial cells within confluent cultures in response to fluid shear stress. *Biophys. J.,* 2000, 79(3), 1285-97.

Dietrich, F; Lelkes, PI. Fine-tuning of a three-dimensional microcarrier-based angiogenesis assay for the analysis of endothelial-mesenchymal cell co-cultures in fibrin and collagen gels. *Angiogenesis,* 2006, 9(3), 111-25.

Diglio, CA; Grammas, P; Giacomelli, F; Wiener, J. Rat heart-derived endothelial and smooth muscle cell cultures: isolation, cloning and characterization. *Tissue Cell*, 1988, 20(4), 477-92.

Donovan, D; Brown, NJ; Bishop, ET; Lewis, CE. Comparison of three in vitro human 'angiogenesis' assays with capillaries formed in vivo. *Angiogenesis*, 2001, 4, 113-121.

Dorweiler, B; Torzewski, M; Dahm, M; Ochsenhirt, V; Lehr, HA; Lackner, KJ; Vahl, CF. A novel in vitro model for the study of plaque development in atherosclerosis. *Thromb. Haemost.*, 2006, 95(1), 182-9.

Durieu-Trautmann, O; Foignant-Chaverot, N; Perdomo, J; Gounon, P; Strosberg, AD; Couraud, PO. Immortalization of brain capillary endothelial cells with maintenance of structural characteristics of the blood-brain barrier endothelium. *In Vitro Cell Dev. Biol.*, 1991, 27A(10), 771-8.

Dzau, VJ; Gnecchi, M; Pachori, AS; Morello, F; Melo, LG. Therapeutic potential of endothelial progenitor cells in cardiovascular diseases. *Hypertension*, 2005, 46(1), 7-18.

Edelman, DA; Jiang, Y; Tyburski, JG; Wilson, RF; Steffes, CP. Lipopolysaccharide activation of pericyte's Toll-like receptor-4 regulates co-culture permeability. *Am. J. Surg.*, 2007, 193(6), 730-5.

Edgell, CJ; McDonald, CC; Graham, JB. Permanent cell line expressing human factor VIII-related antigen established by hybridization. *Proc. Natl .Acad. Sci. USA*, 1983, 80(12), 3734-7.

Eppihimer, MJ; Wolitzky, B; Anderson, DC; Labow, MA; Granger, DN. Heterogeneity of expression of E- and P-selectins in vivo. *Circ. Res.*, 1996, 79(3), 560-9.

Erdbruegger, U; Haubitz, M; Woywodt, A. Circulating endothelial cells: a novel marker of endothelial damage. *Clin. Chim. Acta*, 2006, 373(1-2), 17-26.

Erol, A; Cinar, MG; Can, C; Olukman, M; Ulker, S; Koşay, S. Effect of homocysteine on nitric oxide production in coronary microvascular endothelial cells. *Endothelium*, 2007 14(3), 157-61.

Erridge, C; Spickett, CM; Webb, DJ. Non-enterobacterial endotoxins stimulate human coronary artery but not venous endothelial cell activation via Toll-like receptor 2. *Cardiovasc. Res*, 2007, 73(1), 181-9.

EUROASPIRE II Euro Heart Survey Programme. Lifestyle and risk factor management and use of drug therapies in coronary patients from 15 countries. *Eur. Heart J.*, 2001, 22, 554-72.

Farrar, MW; McDouall, R; Khan, S; Yacoub, MH; Allen, SP. Serum activation unmasks unique sensitivities to adhesion molecule expression in human coronary artery and heart microvascular endothelial cells. *Microvasc. Res.*, 2000, 59(3), 338-44.

Federici, M; Lauro, R. Review article: diabetes and atherosclerosis--running on a common road. *Aliment. Pharmacol. Ther.*, 2005, 22 Suppl 2, 11-5.

Feng, L; Matsumoto, C; Schwartz, A; Schmidt, AM; Stern, DM; Pile-Spellman, J. Chronic vascular inflammation in patients with type 2 diabetes: endothelial biopsy and RT-PCR analysis. *Diabetes Care*, 2005, 28(2), 379-84.

French, LE; Hahne, M; Viard, I; Radlgruber, G; Zanone, R; Becker, K; Müller, C; Tschopp, J. Fas and Fas ligand in embryos and adult mice: ligand expression in several immune-privileged tissues and coexpression in adult tissues characterized by apoptotic cell turnover. *J. Cell Biol.*, 1996, 133(2), 335-43.

Fukuhra, S; Sakurai, A; Yamagishi, A; Sako, K; Mochizuki, N. Vascular endothelial cadherin-mediated cell-cell adhesion regulated by a small GTPase, Rap1. *J. Biochem. Mol. Biol.*, 2006, 39(2), 132-9.

Fukushima, K; Miyamoto, S; Tsukimori, K; Kobayashi, H; Seki, H; Takeda, S; Kensuke, E; Ohtani, K; Shibuya, M; Nakano, H. Tumor necrosis factor and vascular endothelial growth factor induce endothelial integrin repertories, regulating endovascular differentiation and apoptosis in a human extravillous trophoblast cell line. *Biol. Reprod.*, 2005, 73(1), 172-9.

Furukawa, KS; Ushida, T; Sugano, H; Tamaki, T; Ohshima, N; Tateishi, T. Effect of shear stress on platelet adhesion to expanded polytetrafluoroethylene, a silicone sheet, and an endothelial cell monolayer. *ASAIO J.*, 2000, 46(6), 696-701.

Furukawa, KS; Ushida, T; Noguchi, T; Tamaki, T; Tateishi, T. Development of cone and plate-type rheometer for quantitative analysis of endothelial cell detachment by shear stress. *Int. J. Artif. Organs.*, 2003, 26(5), 436-41.

Gale, NW; Baluk, P; Pan, L; Kwan, M; Holash, J; DeChiara, TM; McDonald, DM; Yancopoulos, GD. Ephrin-B2 selectively marks arterial vessels and neovascularization sites in the adult, with expression in both endothelial and smooth-muscle cells. *Dev. Biol.*, 2001, 230(2), 151-60.

Gamble, JR; Harlan, JM; Klebanoff, SJ; Vadas, MA. Stimulation of the adherence of neutrophils to umbilical vein endothelium by human recombinant tumor necrosis factor. *Proc. Natl. Acad. Sci. USA.* 1985, 82(24), 8667-71.

Garlanda, C; Dejana, E. Heterogeneity of endothelial cells. Specific markers. *Arterioscler. Thromb. Vasc. Biol.*, 1997, 17(7), 1193-202.

Geerts, SO; Nys, M; De, MP; Charpentier, J; Albert, A; Legrand, V; Rompen, EH. Systemic release of endotoxins induced by gentle mastication: association with periodontitis severity. *J. Periodontol.*, 2002, 73(1), 73-8.

George, F; Brisson, C; Poncelet, P; Laurent, JC; Massot, O; Arnoux, D; Ambrosi, P; Klein-Soyer, C; Cazenave, JP; Sampol, J. Rapid isolation of human endothelial cells from whole blood using S-Endo1 monoclonal antibody coupled to immuno-magnetic beads: demonstration of endothelial injury after angioplasty. *Thromb, Haemost,* 1992, 67(1), 147-53.

Gerety, SS; Wang, HU; Chen, ZF; Anderson, DJ. Symmetrical mutant phenotypes of the receptor EphB4 and its specific transmembrane ligand ephrin-B2 in cardiovascular development. *Mol. Cell,* 1999, 4(3), 403-14.

Gimbrone, MA Jr; Cotran, RS; Folkman, J. Human vascular endothelial cells in culture. Growth and DNA synthesis. *J. Cell Biol.*, 1974, 60(3), 673-84.

Golledge, J; Turner, RJ; Harley, SL; Springall, DR; Powell, JT. Circumferential deformation and shear stress induce differential responses in saphenous vein endothelium exposed to arterial flow. *J. Clin. Invest.*, 1997, 99(11), 2719-26.

Goodacre, S; Cross, E; Arnold, J; Angelini, K; Capewell, S; Nicholl, J. The health care burden of acute chest pain. *Heart,* 2005, 91, 229-30.

Goodwin, AM. In vitro assays of angiogenesis for assessment of angiogenic and anti-angiogenic agents. *Microvasc. Res.,* 2007, in press.

Gräfe, M; Auch-Schwelk, W; Graf, K; Terbeek, D; Hertel, H; Unkelbach, M; Hildebrandt, A; Fleck, E. Isolation and characterization of macrovascular and microvascular endothelial cells from human hearts. *Am. J. Physiol.,* 1994, 267(6 Pt 2), H2138-48.

Gräfe, M; Auch-Schwelk, W; Hertel, H; Terbeek, D; Steinheider, G; Loebe, M; Fleck, E. Human cardiac microvascular and macrovascular endothelial cells respond differently to oxidatively modified LDL. *Atherosclerosis,* 1998, 137(1), 87-95.

Greenwood, J; Mason, JC. Statins and the vascular endothelial inflammatory response. *Trends Immunol.,* 2007, 28(2), 88-98.

Gross, PL; Aird, WC. The endothelium and thrombosis. *Semin. Thromb Hemost.,* 2000, 26(5), 463-78.

Gulbins, H; Pritisanac, A; Uhlig, A; Goldemund, A; Meiser, BM; Reichart, B;, Daebritz, S. Seeding of human endothelial cells on valve containing aortic mini-roots: development of a seeding device and procedure. *Ann. Thorac. Surg.,* 2005, 79(6), 2119-26.

Guller, S; LaChapelle, L. The role of placental Fas ligand in maintaining immune privilege at maternal-fetal interfaces. *Semin. Reprod. Endocrinol.,* 1999, 17(1), 39-44.

Haubner, F; Lehle, K; Münzel, D; Schmid, C; Birnbaum, DE; Preuner, JG. Hyperglycemia increases the levels of vascular cellular adhesion molecule-1 and monocyte-chemoattractant-protein-1 in the diabetic endothelial cell. *Biochem. Biophys. Res. Commun.,* 2007, 360(3), 560-5.

Heloire F, Weill B, Weber S, Batteux F. Aggregates of endothelial microparticles and platelets circulate in peripheral blood. Variations during stable coronary disease and acute myocardial infarction. *Thromb. Res.* 2003; 110(4): 173-80.

Hendrickx, J; Doggen, K; Weinberg, EO; Van Tongelen, P; Fransen, P; De Keulenaer, GW. Molecular diversity of cardiac endothelial cells in vitro and in vivo. *Physiol. Genomics,* 2004, 19(2), 198-206.

Henninger, DD; Panes, J; Eppihimer, M; Russell, J; Gerritsen, M; Anderson, DC; Granger, DN. Cytokine-induced VCAM-1 and ICAM-1 expression in different organs of the mouse *J. Immunol.,* 1997, 158, 1825-32.

Heydarkhan-Hagvall, S; Helenius, G; Johansson, BR; Li, JY; Mattsson, E; Risberg, B. Co-culture of endothelial cells and smooth muscle cells affects gene expression of angiogenic factors. *J. Cell Biochem.,* 2003, 89(6), 1250-9.

Hill, JM; Zalos, G; Halcox, JP; Schenke, WH; Waclawiw, MA; Quyyumi, AA; Finkel, T. Circulating endothelial progenitor cells, vascular function, and cardiovascular risk. *N. Engl. J. Med.* 2003, 348(7), 593-600.

Hillyer, P; Mordelet, E; Flynn, G; Male, D. Chemokines, chemokine receptors and adhesion molecules on different human endothelia: discriminating the tissue-specific functions that affect leucocyte migration. *Clin. Exp. Immunol.,* 2003, 134(3), 431-41.

Honda, HM; Leitinger, N; Frankel, M; Goldhaber, JI; Natarajan, R; Nadler, JL; Weiss, JN; Berliner, JA. Induction of monocyte binding to endothelial cells by MM-LDL: role of lipoxygenase metabolites. *Arterioscler. Thromb. Vasc. Biol.,* 1999, 19(3), 680-6.

Hristov, M; Erl, W; Weber, PC. Endothelial progenitor cells: mobilization, differentiation, and homing. *Arterioscler. Thromb. Vasc. Biol.*, 2003, 23(7), 1185-9.

Huang, H; McIntosh, J; Hoyt, DG. An efficient, nonenzymatic method for isolation and culture of murine aortic endothelial cells and their response to inflammatory stimuli. *In Vitro Cell. Dev. Biol. Anim.,* 2003, 39(1-2), 43-50.

Ichiyama, T; Ueno, Y; Isumi, H; Niimi, A; Matsubara, T; Furukawa, S. An immunoglobulin agent (IVIG) inhibits NF-kappaB activation in cultured endothelial cells of coronary arteries in vitro. *Inflamm. Res.*, 2004, 53(6), 253-6.

Invernici, G; Ponti, D; Corsini, E; Cristini, S; Frigerio, S; Colombo, A; Parati, E; Alessandri, G. Human microvascular endothelial cells from different fetal organs demonstrate organ-specific CAM expression. *Exp. Cell Res.,* 2005, 308(2), 273-82.

Jackson, CJ; Garbett, PK; Nissen, B; Schrieber, L. Binding of human endothelium to Ulex europaeus I-coated Dynabeads: application to the isolation of microvascular endothelium. *J. Cell Sci.*; 1990; 96(Pt2); 257-62.

Jaffe, EA; Hoyer, LW; Nachman, RL. Synthesis of antihemophilic factor antigen by cultured human endothelial cells. *J. Clin. Invest.,* 1973, 52(11), 2757-64.

Jensen, JB; Parmar, M. Strengths and limitations of the neurosphere culture system. *Mol. Neurobiol.,* 2006, 34(3), 153-61.

Jessup, W; Kritharides, L; Stocker, R. Lipid oxidation in atherogenesis: an overview. *Biochem. Soc. Trans.,* 2004, 32(Pt 1), 134-8.

Justice, JM; Tanner, MA; Myers, PR. Endothelial cell regulation of nitric oxide production during hypoxia in coronary microvessels and epicardial arteries. *J. Cell Physiol.,* 2000, 182(3), 359-65.

Kansas, GS. Selectins and their ligands: current concepts and controversies. *Blood,* 1996; 88, 3259-87.

Kao, WJ. Evaluation of leukocyte adhesion on polyurethanes: the effects of shear stress and blood proteins. *Biomaterials,* 2000, 21(22), 2295-303.

Kappel, A; Rönicke, V; Damert, A; Flamme, I; Risau, W; Breier, G. Identification of vascular endothelial growth factor (VEGF) receptor-2 (Flk-1) promoter/enhancer sequences sufficient for angioblast and endothelial cell-specific transcription in transgenic mice. *Blood,* 1999, 93(12), 4284-92.

Kelley, C; D'Amore, P; Hechtman, HB; Shepro, D. Microvascular pericyte contractility in vitro: comparison with other cells of the vascular wall. *J. Cell Biol.*, 1987, 104(3), 483-90.

Kelley, C; D'Amore, P; Hechtman, HB; Shepro, D. Vasoactive hormones and cAMP affect pericyte contraction and stress fibres in vitro. *J. Muscle Res. Cell Motil.,* 1988, 9(2), 184-94.

Kita, M; Eguchi, K; Kawabe, Y; Tsukada, T; Migita, K; Kawakami, A; Matsuoka, N; Nagataki, S. Staphylococcal enterotoxin B-specific adhesion of murine splenic T cells to a human endothelial cell line. *Immunology,* 1996, 88(3), 441-6.

Kolvenbach, R; Kreissig, C; Ludwig, E; Cagiannos, C. Stem cell use in critical limb ischemia. *J. Cardiovasc. Surg. (Torino),* 2007, 48(1), 39-44.

Korff, T; Augustin, HG. Integration of endothelial cells in multicellular spheroids prevents apoptosis and induces differentiation. *J. Cell Biol.,* 1998, 143(5), 1341-52.

Korff, T; Kimmina, S; Martiny-Baron, G; Augustin, HG. Blood vessel maturation in a 3-dimensional spheroidal coculture model: direct contact with smooth muscle cells regulates endothelial cell quiescence and abrogates VEGF responsiveness. *FASEB J.,* 2001, 15(2), 447-57

Krebs, LT; Xue, Y; Norton, CR; Shutter, JR; Maguire, M; Sundberg, JP; Gallahan, D; Closson, V; Kitajewski, J; Callahan, R; Smith, GH; Stark, KL; Gridley, T. Notch signaling is essential for vascular morphogenesis in mice. *Genes Dev.,* 2000, 14(11), 1343-52.

Krishnaswamy, G; Smith, JK; Mukkamala, R; Hall, K; Joyner, W; Yerra, L; Chi, DS. Multifunctional cytokine expression by human coronary endothelium and regulation by monokines and glucocorticoids. *Microvasc. Res.,* 1998, 55(3), 189-200.

Kunz-Schughart, LA. Multicellular tumor spheroids: intermediates between monolayer culture and in vivo tumor. *Cell Biol. Int.,* 1999, 23(3), 157-61.

Kunz-Schughart, LA; Freyer, JP; Hofstaedter, F; Ebner, R. The use of 3-D cultures for high-throughput screening: the multicellular spheroid model. *J. Biomol. Screen,* 2004, 9(4), 273-85.

Kunz-Schughart, LA; Schroeder, JA; Wondrak, M; van Rey, F; Lehle, K; Hofstaedter, F; Wheatley, DN. Potential of fibroblasts to regulate the formation of three-dimensional vessel-like structures from endothelial cells in vitro. *Am. J. Physiol. Cell Physiol.,* 2006, 290(5), C1385-98.

Kurosawa, H. Methods for inducing embryoid body formation: in vitro differentiation system of embryonic stem cells. *J. Biosci. Bioeng.,* 2007, 103(5), 389-98.

Kwei, S; Stavrakis, G; Takahas, M; Taylor, G; Folkman, MJ; Gimbrone, MA Jr; García-Cardeña, G. Early adaptive responses of the vascular wall during venous arterialization in mice. *Am. J. Pathol.,* 2004, 164(1), 81-9.

Lamm, P; Juchem, G; Weyrich, P; Nees, S; Reichart, B. New alternative coronary bypass graft: first clinical experience with an autologous endothelialized cryopreserved allograft. *J. Thorac. Cardiovasc. Surg,* 1999, 117(6), 1217-9.

Langley, RR; Ramirez, KM; Tsan, RZ; Van Arsdall, M; Nilsson, MB; Fidler, IJ. Tissue-specific microvascular endothelial cell lines from H-2K(b)-tsA58 mice for studies of angiogenesis and metastasis. *Cancer Res.,* 2003, 63(11), 2971-6.

Laszik, Z; Mitro, A; Taylor, FB Jr; Ferrell, G; Esmon, CT. Human protein C receptor is present primarily on endothelium of large blood vessels: implications for the control of the protein C pathway. *Circulation,* 1997, 96(10), 3633-40.

L'Azou, B; Fernandez, P; Bareille, R; Beneteau, M; Bourget, C; Cambar, J; Bordenave, L. In vitro endothelial cell susceptibility to xenobiotics: comparison of three cell types. *Cell Biol. Toxicol.,* 2005, 21(2), 127-37.

Lee, KW; Lip, GY; Tayebjee, M; Foster, W; Blann, AD. Circulating endothelial cells, von Willebrand factor, interleukin-6, and prognosis in patients with acute coronary syndromes. *Blood,* 2005, 105(2), 526-32.

Lehle, K; Buttstaedt, J; Birnbaum, DE. Expression of adhesion molecules and cytokines in vitro by endothelial cells seeded on various polymer surfaces coated with titaniumcarboxonitride. *J. Biomed. Mater. Res. A,* 2003, 65(3), 393-401.

Lehle, K; Lohn, S; Reinerth, GG; Schubert, T; Preuner, JG; Birnbaum, DE. Cytological evaluation of the tissue-implant reaction associated with subcutaneous implantation of polymers coated with titaniumcarboxonitride in vivo. *Biomaterials,* 2004, 25(24), 5457-66.

Lehle, K; Birnbaum, DE; Preuner, JG. Predominant inhibition of interleukin-6 synthesis in patient-specific endothelial cells by mTOR inhibitors below a concentration range where cell proliferation is affected and mitotic arrest takes place. *Transplant Proc.,* 2005, 37(1), 159-61.

Lehle, K; Haubner, F; Münzel, D; Birnbaum, DE; Preuner, JG. Development of a disease-specific model to evaluate endothelial dysfunction in patients with diabetes mellitus. *Biochem. Biophys. Res. Commun.,* 2007a, 357(1), 308-13.

Lehle, K; Kunz-Schughart, LA; Kuhn, P; Schreml, S; Birnbaum, DE; Preuner, JG. Validity of a patient-derived system of tissue-specific human endothelial cells: interleukin-6 as a surrogate marker in the coronary system. *Am. J. Physiol. Heart Circ. Physiol,* 2007b, 293(3), H1721-8.

Li, D; Singh, RM; Liu, L; Chen, H; Singh, BM; Kazzaz, N; Mehta, JL. Oxidized-LDL through LOX-1 increases the expression of angiotensin converting enzyme in human coronary artery endothelial cells. *Cardiovasc. Res.,* 2003, 57(1), 238-43.

Lin, Y; Weisdorf, DJ; Solovey, A; Hebbel, RP. Origins of circulating endothelial cells and endothelial outgrowth from blood. *J. Clin. Invest.,* 2000, 105(1), 71-7.

Liu, L; Liu, H; Jao, J; Liu, H; Bergeron, A; Dong, JF; Zhang, J. Changes in circulating human endothelial progenitor cells after brain injury. *J. Neurotrauma.,* 2007, 24(6), 936-43.

Li, ZZ; Bai, SG; Huang, J; Qian, HY. Trans-coronary transplantation may be an optimal route in cellular cardiomyoplasty with stem cells. *Med. Hypotheses*, 2007, in press.

Lokeshwar, VB; Iida, N; Bourguignon, LY. The cell adhesion molecule, GP116, is a new CD44 variant (ex14/v10) involved in hyaluronic acid binding and endothelial cell proliferation. *J. Biol. Chem.,* 1996, 271(39), 23853-64.

Lupu, C; Westmuckett, AD; Peer, G; Ivanciu, L; Zhu, H; Taylor, FB Jr; Lupu, F. Tissue factor-dependent coagulation is preferentially up-regulated within arterial branching areas in a baboon model of Escherichia coli sepsis. *Am. J. Pathol.,* 2005, 167(4), 1161-72.

Madri, JA; Pratt, BM; Tucker, AM. Phenotypic modulation of endothelial cells by transforming growth factor-beta depends upon the composition and organization of the extracellular matrix. *J. Cell Biol.,* 1988, 106(4), 1375-84.

Maher, SE; Karmann, K; Min, W; Hughes, CC; Pober, JS; Bothwell, AL. Porcine endothelial CD86 is a major costimulator of xenogeneic human T cells: cloning, sequencing, and functional expression in human endothelial cells. *J. Immunol.,* 1996, 157(9), 3838-44.

Makata, H; Ichiyama, T; Uchi, R; Takekawa, T; Matsubara, T; Furukawa, S. Anti-inflammatory effect of intravenous immunoglobulin in comparison with dexamethasone in vitro: implication for treatment of Kawasaki disease. *Naunyn Schmiedebergs Arch. Pharmacol.,* 2006, 373(5), 325-32.

Malek, AM; Gibbons, GH; Dzau, VJ; Izumo, S. Fluid shear stress differentially modulates expression of genes encoding basic fibroblast growth factor and platelet-derived growth factor B chain in vascular endothelium. *J. Clin. Invest.,* 1993, 92(4), 2013-21.

Mancuso, P; Burlini, A; Pruneri, G; Goldhirsch, A; Martinelli, G; Bertolini, F. Resting and activated endothelial cells are increased in the peripheral blood of cancer patients. *Blood,* 2001, 97(11), 3658-61.

Marschang, P; Götsch, C; Kirchmair, R; Kaser, S; Kähler, CM; Patsch, JR. Postprandial but not postabsorptive low-density lipoproteins increase the expression of intercellular adhesion molecule-1 in human aortic endothelial cells. *Atherosclerosis,* 2006, 186(1), 101-6.

Marshall, GP 2nd; Reynolds, BA; Laywell, ED. Using the neurosphere assay to quantify neural stem cells in vivo. *Curr. Pharm .Biotechnol.,* 2007, 8(3), 141-5.

Martineau, L; Doillon, CJ. Angiogenic response of endothelial cells seeded dispersed versus on beads in fibrin gels. *Angiogenesis.* 2007, in press.

Mavromatis, K; Fukai, T; Tate, M; Chesler, N; Ku, DN; Galis, ZS. Early effects of arterial hemodynamic conditions on human saphenous veins perfused ex vivo. *Arterioscler. Thromb Vasc. Biol.,* 2000, 20(8), 1889-95.

Mawatari, M; Kohno, K; Mizoguchi, H; Matsuda, T; Asoh, K; Van Damme, J; Welgus, HG; Kuwano, M. Effects of tumor necrosis factor and epidermal growth factor on cell morphology, cell surface receptors, and the production of tissue inhibitor of metalloproteinases and IL-6 in human microvascular endothelial cells. *J. Immunol.,* 1989, 143(5), 1619-27.

Mawatari, M; Okamura, K; Matsuda, T; Hamanaka, R; Mizoguchi, H; Higashio, K; Kohno, K; Kuwano, M. Tumor necrosis factor and epidermal growth factor modulate migration of human microvascular endothelial cells and production of tissue-type plasminogen activator and its inhibitor. *Exp. Cell Res.,* 1991, 192(2), 574-80.

McGarry, JD. Banting lecture 2001: dysregulation of fatty acid metabolism in the etiology of type 2 diabetes. *Diabetes,* 2002, 51(1), 7-18.

McGuigan, AP; Sefton, MV. The influence of biomaterials on endothelial cell thrombogenicity. *Biomaterials,* 2007, 28(16), 2547-71.

McDouall, RM; Batten, P; McCormack, A; Yacoub, MH; Rose, ML. MHC class II expression on human heart microvascular endothelial cells, exquisite sensitivity to interferon-gamma and natural killer cells. T*ransplantation*, 1997, 64(8), 1175-80.

McDouall, RM; Farrar, MW; Khan, S; Yacoub, MH; Allen, SP. Unique sensitivities to cytokine regulated expression of adhesion molecules in human heart-derived endothelial cells. *Endothelium,* 2001, 8(1), 25-40.

McDouall, RM; Yacoub, M; Rose, ML. Isolation, culture, and characterisation of MHC class II-positive microvascular endothelial cells from the human heart. *Microvasc. Res.,* 1996, 51(2), 137-52.

Miller-Kasprzak, E; Jagodziński, PP. Endothelial progenitor cells as a new agent contributing to vascular repair. *Arch. Immunol. Ther .Exp. (Warsz),* 2007, 55(4), 247-59.

Mironov, V; Little, C; Sage, H (Eds). Vascular Morphogenesis: in vivo, in vitro, in mente. Birkhäuser, Boston, 1998.

Mitsuoka, C; Kawakami-Kimura, N; Kasugai-Sawada, M; Hiraiwa, N; Toda, K; Ishida, H; Kiso, M; Hasegawa, A; Kannagi, R. Sulfated sialyl Lewis X, the putative L-selectin ligand, detected on endothelial cells of high endothelial venules by a distinct set of anti-sialyl Lewis X antibodies. *Biochem. Biophys. Res. Commun.*, 1997, 230(3), 546-51.

Miwa, H; Matsuda, T; Tani, N; Kondo, K; Iida, F. An in vitro endothelialized compliant vascular graft minimizes anastomotic hyperplasia. *ASAIO J.*, 1993, 39(3), M501-5.

Miyata, T; Iizasa, H; Sai, Y; Fujii, J; Terasaki, T; Nakashima, E. Platelet-derived growth factor-BB (PDGF-BB) induces differentiation of bone marrow endothelial progenitor cell-derived cell line TR-BME2 into mural cells, and changes the phenotype. *J. Cell Physiol.*, 2005, 204(3), 948-55.

Moyer, CF; Huggins, E; Sarantopoulos, S; Lewis, JC; Sajuthi, D; Biron, CA; Reinisch CL. Cloned endothelium derived from autoimmune vascular disease retain structural and functional characteristics of normal endothelial cells. *Exp. Cell Res.* 1992;199(1):63-73.

Mueller-Klieser, W. Three-dimensional cell cultures: from molecular mechanisms to clinical applications. *Am. J. Physiol.*, 1997, 273(4 Pt 1), C1109-23.

Mueller-Klieser, W. Tumor biology and experimental therapeutics. *Crit. Rev. Oncol. Hematol.*, 2000; 36(2-3), 123-39.

Münzel, D; Lehle, K; Haubner, F; Schmid, C; Birnbaum, DE; Preuner, JG. Impact of diabetic serum on endothelial cells: An in-vitro-analysis of endothelial dysfunction in diabetes mellitus type 2. *Biochem. Biophys. Res. Commun,* 2007, 362(2), 238-44.

Mukouyama, YS; Gerber, HP; Ferrara, N; Gu, C; Anderson, DJ. Peripheral nerve-derived VEGF promotes arterial differentiation via neuropilin 1-mediated positive feedback. Development, 2005, 132(5), 941-52.

Murray, CJ; Lopez, AD. Global mortality, disability, and the contribution of risk factors: Global Burden of Disease Study. *Lancet,* 1997, 349(9063), 1436-42.

Murray, JC. (Ed). Angiogenesis Protocols. Methods in Molecular Medicine. Humana Press, Totowa, New Jersey, 2001.

Nakagawa, O; Nakagawa, M; Richardson, JA; Olson, EN; Srivastava, D. HRT1, HRT2, and HRT3: a new subclass of bHLH transcription factors marking specific cardiac, somitic, and pharyngeal arch segments. *Dev. Biol.*, 1999, 216(1), 72-84.

Nakajima, K; Nakano, T; Tanaka, A. The oxidative modification hypothesis of atherosclerosis: the comparison of atherogenic effects on oxidized LDL and remnant lipoproteins in plasma. *Clin. Chim. Acta,* 2006, 367(1-2), 36-47.

Nehls, V; Herrmann, R; Hühnken, M; Palmetshofer, A. Contact-dependent inhibition of angiogenesis by cardiac fibroblasts in three-dimensional fibrin gels in vitro: implications for microvascular network remodeling and coronary collateral formation. *Cell Tissue Res*, 1998, 293(3), 479-88.

Nehls, V; Schuchardt, E; Drenckhahn, D. The effect of fibroblasts, vascular smooth muscle cells, and pericytes on sprout formation of endothelial cells in a fibrin gel angiogenesis system. *Microvasc. Res*, 1994, 48(3), 349-63.

Nerem, RM. Hemodynamics and the vascular endothelium. *J. Biomech. Eng.*, 1993, 115(4B), 510-4.

Niemelä, H; Elima, K; Henttinen, T; Irjala, H; Salmi, M; Jalkanen, S. Molecular identification of PAL-E, a widely used endothelial-cell marker. *Blood*, 2005, 106(10), 3405-9.

Niklason, LE; Gao, J; Abbott, WM; Hirschi, KK; Houser, S; Marini, R; Langer, R. Functional arteries grown in vitro. *Science,* 1999, 284(5413), 489-93.

Nillesen, ST; Geutjes, PJ; Wismans, R; Schalkwijk, J; Daamen, WF; van Kuppevelt, TH. Increased angiogenesis and blood vessel maturation in acellular collagen-heparin scaffolds containing both FGF2 and VEGF. *Biomaterials,* 2007, 28(6), 1123-31.

Nishida, M; Carley, WW; Gerritsen, ME; Ellingsen, O; Kelly, RA; Smith, TW. Isolation and characterization of human and rat cardiac microvascular endothelial cells. *Am. J. Physiol.,* 1993, 264(2 Pt 2), H639-52.

Nistri, S; Mazzetti, L; Failli, P; Bani, D. High-Yield Method for Isolation and Culture of Endothelial Cells from Rat Coronary Blood Vessels Suitable for Analysis of Intracellular Calcium and Nitric Oxide Biosynthetic Pathways. *Biol .Proced. Online,* 2002, 4, 32-37.

Niwa, K; Sakai, J; Watanabe, T; Ohyama, T; Karino, T. Improved arterial wall model by coculturing vascular endothelial and smooth muscle cells. *In Vitro Cell Dev. Biol. Anim.,* 2007, 43(1), 17-20.

Nourshargh, S; Krombach, F; Dejana, E. The role of JAM-A and PECAM-1 in modulating leukocyte infiltration in inflamed and ischemic tissues. *J. Leukoc. Biol.,* 2006, 80(4), 714-8.

Numaguchi Y, Sone T, Okumura K, Ishii M, Morita Y, Kubota R, Yokouchi K, Imai H, Harada M, Osanai H, Kondo T, Murohara T. The impact of the capability of circulating progenitor cell to differentiate on myocardial salvage in patients with primary acute myocardial infarction. *Circulation.* 2006; 114(1 Suppl): I114-9.

Obeso, J; Weber, J; Auerbach, R. A hemangioendothelioma-derived cell line: its use as a model for the study of endothelial cell biology. Lab Invest, 1990, 63(2), 259-69.

Orlidge, A; D'Amore, PA. Inhibition of capillary endothelial cell growth by pericytes and smooth muscle cells. *J. Cell Biol.,* 1987, 105(3), 1455-62.

Otto, M; Bittinger, F; Kriegsmann, J; Kirkpatrick, CJ. Differential adhesion of polymorphous neutrophilic granulocytes to macro- and microvascular endothelial cells under flow conditions. *Pathobiology,* 2001, 69(3), 159-71.

Otto, M; Klein, CL; Köhler, H; Wagner, M; Röhrig, O; Kirkpatrick, CJ Dynamic blood cell contact with biomaterials: validation of a flow chamber system according to international standards. *J. Mater Sci. Mater Med.,* 1997, 8(3), 119-29.

Oxhorn, BC; Hirzel, DJ; Buxton, IL. Isolation and characterization of large numbers of endothelial cells for studies of cell signaling. *Microvasc. Res.,* 2002, 64(2), 302-15.

Passerini, AG; Polacek, DC; Shi, C; Francesco, NM; Manduchi, E; Grant, GR; Pritchard, WF; Powell, S; Chang, GY; Stoeckert, CJ Jr; Davies, PF. Coexisting proinflammatory and antioxidative endothelial transcription profiles in a disturbed flow region of the adult porcine aorta. *Proc. Natl. Acad. Sci. USA,* 2004, 101(8), 2482-7.

Park, HS; Chun, JN; Jung, HY; Choi, C; Bae, YS. Role of NADPH oxidase 4 in lipopolysaccharide-induced proinflammatory responses by human aortic endothelial cells. *Cardiovasc. Res.,* 2006, 72(3), 447-55.

Park, L; Raman, KG; Lee, KJ; Lu, Y; Ferran, LJ Jr; Chow, WS; Stern, D; Schmidt, AM. Suppression of accelerated diabetic atherosclerosis by the soluble receptor for advanced glycation endproducts. *Nat. Med.* 1998, 4(9), 1025-31.

Pepper, MS; Ferrara, N; Orci, L; Montesano, R. Potent synergism between vascular endothelial growth factor and basic fibroblast growth factor in the induction of angiogenesis in vitro. *Biochem. Biophys. Res .Commun.*, 1992, 189(2), 824-31.

Plendl, J; Neumüller, C; Vollmar, A; Auerbach, R; Sinowatz, F. Isolation and characterization of endothelial cells from different organs of fetal pigs. *Anat. Embryol. (Berl)*, 1996, 194(5), 445-56.

Plendl, J; Sinowatz, F; Auerbach, R. A transformed murine myocardial vascular endothelial cell clone: characterization of cells in vitro and of tumours derived from clone in situ. *Virchows Arch.*, 1995, 426(6), 619-28.

Pober, JS; Bevilacqua, MP; Mendrick, DL; Lapierre, LA; Fiers, W; Gimbrone, MA Jr. Two distinct monokines, interleukin 1 and tumor necrosis factor, each independently induce biosynthesis and transient expression of the same antigen on the surface of cultured human vascular endothelial cells. *J.Immunol*, 1986, 136(5), 1680-7.

Pober, JS; Cotran, RS. The role of endothelial cells in inflammation. *Transplantation,* 1990, 50(4), 537-44.

Pober, JS; Gimbrone, MA Jr. Expression of Ia-like antigens by human vascular endothelial cells is inducible in vitro: demonstration by monoclonal antibody binding and immunoprecipitation. *Proc. Natl. Acad. Sci. USA*, 1982, 79(21), 6641-5.

Podgrabinska, S; Braun, P; Velasco, P; Kloos, B; Pepper, MS; Skobe, M. Molecular characterization of lymphatic endothelial cells. *Proc. Natl. Acad. Sci. USA*, 2002, 99(25), 16069-74.

Prasad, CK; Jayakumar, K; Krishnan, LK. Phenotype gradation of human saphenous vein endothelial cells from cardiovascular disease subjects. *Endothelium*, 2006, 13(5), 341-52.

Pries, AR; Kuebler, WM. Normal endothelium. *Handb. Exp. Pharmacol.,* 2006, (176 Pt 1), 1-40.

Pujol, BF; Lucibello, FC; Gehling, UM; Lindemann, K; Weidner, N; Zuzarte, ML; Adamkiewicz,J; Elsässer, HP; Müller, R; Havemann, K. Endothelial-like cells derived from human CD14 positive monocytes. *Differentiation,* 2000, 65(5), 287–300.

Quagliaro, L; Piconi, L; Assaloni, R; Da Ros, R; Maier, A; Zuodar, G; Ceriello, A. Intermittent high glucose enhances ICAM-1, VCAM-1 and E-selectin expression in human umbilical vein endothelial cells in culture: the distinct role of protein kinase C and mitochondrial superoxide production. *Atherosclerosis,* 2005, 183(2), 259-67.

Rabkin-Aikawa, E; Aikawa, M; Farber, M; Kratz, JR; Garcia-Cardena, G; Kouchoukos, NT; Mitchell, MB; Jonas, RA; Schoen, FJ. Clinical pulmonary autograft valves, pathologic evidence of adaptive remodeling in the aortic site. *J. Thorac. Cardiovasc. Surg.,* 2004, 128(4), 552-61.

Rafii, S; Shapiro, F; Rimarachin, J; Nachman, RL; Ferris, B; Weksler, B; Moore, MA; Asch, AS. Isolation and characterization of human bone marrow microvascular endothelial cells: hematopoietic progenitor cell adhesion. *Blood,* 1994, 84(1), 10-9.

Rahmani, M; Cruz, RP; Granville, DJ; McManus, BM. Allograft vasculopathy versus atherosclerosis. *Circ. Res.,* 2006, 99(8), 801-15.

Rassoul, F; Salvetter, J; Reissig, D; Schneider, W; Thiery, J; Richter, V. The influence of garlic (Allium sativum) extract on interleukin 1alpha-induced expression of endothelial intercellular adhesion molecule-1 and vascular cell adhesion molecule-1. Phytomedicine, 2006, 13(4), 230-5.

Régina, A; Romero, IA; Greenwood, J; Adamson, P; Bourre, JM; Couraud, PO; Roux, F. Dexamethasone regulation of P-glycoprotein activity in an immortalized rat brain endothelial cell line, GPNT. J. Neurochem., 1999, 73(5), 1954-63.

Rehman, J; Li, J; Orschell, CM; March, KL. Peripheral blood "endothelial progenitor cells" are derived from monocyte/macrophages and secrete angiogenic growth factors. Circulation, 2003, 107(8), 1164-9.

Rhodes, JM; Simons, M. The extracellular matrix and blood vessel formation: not just a scaffold. Journal of Cellular and Molecular Medicine, 2007, 11(2), 176–205.

Roccaro, AM; Hideshima, T; Raje, N; Kumar, S; Ishitsuka, K; Yasui, H; Shiraishi, N; Ribatti, D; Nico, B; Vacca, A; Dammacco, F; Richardson, PG; Anderson, KC. Bortezomib mediates antiangiogenesis in multiple myeloma via direct and indirect effects on endothelial cells. Cancer Res., 2006, 66(1), 184-91

Rosenberg, RD; Aird, WC. Vascular-bed--specific hemostasis and hypercoagulable states. N. Engl. J. Med., 1999, 340(20), 1555-64.

Sacks, MS; Gloeckner, DC. Quantification of the fiber architecture and biaxial mechanical behavior of porcine intestinal submucosa. J. Biomed. Mater Res., 1999, 46(1), 1-10.

Saito, M; Hamasaki, M; Shibuya, M. Induction of tube formation by angiopoietin-1 in endothelial cell/fibroblast co-culture is dependent on endogenous VEGF. Cancer Sci., 2003, 94(9), 782-90.

Sata M. Role of circulating vascular progenitors in angiogenesis, vascular healing, and pulmonary hypertension: lessons from animal models. Arterioscler. Thromb. Vasc. Biol. 2006; 26(5): 1008-14.

Sawano, A; Iwai, S; Sakurai, Y; Ito, M; Shitara, K; Nakahata, T; Shibuya, M. Flt-1, vascular endothelial growth factor receptor 1, is a novel cell surface marker for the lineage of monocyte-macrophages in humans. Blood, 2001, 97(3), 785-91.

Schleger, C; Platz, SJ; Deschl, U. Development of an in vitro model for vascular injury with human endothelial cells. ALTEX, 2004, 21 Suppl 3, 12-9.

Schleimer, RP; Rutledge, BK. Cultured human vascular endothelial cells acquire adhesiveness for neutrophils after stimulation with interleukin 1, endotoxin, and tumor-promoting phorbol diesters. J. Immunol., 1986, 136(2), 649-54.

Schmid, SA; Gaumann, A; Wondrak, M; Eckermann, C; Schulte, S; Mueller-Klieser, W; Wheatley, DN; Kunz-Schughart, LA. Lactate adversely affects the in vitro formation of endothelial cell tubular structures through the action of TGF-beta1. Exp. Cell Res., 2007, 313(12), 2531-49.

Schmidt, AM; Hofmann, M; Taguchi, A; Yan, SD; Stern, DM. RAGE: a multiligand receptor contributing to the cellular response in diabetic vasculopathy and inflammation. Semin. Thromb Hemost. 2000, 26(5), 485-93.

Schmidt, AM; Stern, D. Atherosclerosis and diabetes: the RAGE connection. Curr. Atheroscler. Rep, 2000a, 2(5), 430-6.

Schmidt, AM; Stern, DM. RAGE: a new target for the prevention and treatment of the vascular and inflammatory complications of diabetes. *Trends Endocrinol. Metab.*, 2000b, 11(9), 368-75.

Schreml, S; Lehle, K; Birnbaum, DE; Preuner, JG. mTOR-inhibitors simultaneously inhibit proliferation and basal IL-6 synthesis of human coronary artery endothelial cells. *Int. Immunopharmacol*, 2007, 7(6), 781-90.

Scoumanne, A; Kalamati, T; Moss, J; Powell, JT; Gosling, M; Carey, N. Generation and characterisation of human saphenous vein endothelial cell lines. *Atherosclerosis*, 2002, 160(1), 59-67.

Seeger, FH; Zeiher, AM; Dimmeler, S. Cell-enhancement strategies for the treatment of ischemic heart disease. Nat. *Clin. Pract. Cardiovasc. Me*d., 2007, 4 Suppl 1, S110-3.

Seidl, J; Knuechel, R; Kunz-Schughart, LA. Evaluation of membrane physiology following fluorescence activated or magnetic cell separation. *Cytometry,* 1999, 36(2), 102-11.

Seki, T; Yun, J; Oh, SP. Arterial endothelium-specific activin receptor-like kinase 1 expression suggests its role in arterialization and vascular remodeling. *Circ. Res.*, 2003, 93(7), 682-9.

Sepp, A; Skacel, P; Lindstedt, R; Lechler, RI. Expression of alpha-1,3-galactose and other type 2 oligosaccharide structures in a porcine endothelial cell line transfected with human alpha-1,2-fucosyltransferase cDNA. *J. Biol. Chem.,* 1997, 272(37), 23104-10.

Shantsila, E; Watson, T; Lip, GY. Endothelial progenitor cells in cardiovascular disorders. *J. Am. Coll. Cardiol.,* 2007, 49(7), 741-52.

Shen, YH; Zhang, L; Utama, B; Wang, J; Gan, Y; Wang, X; Wang, J; Chen, L; Vercellotti, GM; Coselli, JS; Mehta, JL; Wang, XL. Human cytomegalovirus inhibits Akt-mediated eNOS activation through upregulating PTEN (phosphatase and tensin homolog deleted on chromosome 10). *Cardiovasc. Res.*, 2006, 69(2), 502-11.

Shibuya, M. Differential roles of vascular endothelial growth factor receptor-1 and receptor-2 in angiogenesis. *J. Biochem. Mol. Biol.*, 2006, 39(5), 469-78.

Shih, IM. The role of CD146 (Mel-CAM) in biology and pathology. *J. Pathol.*, 1999, 189(1), 4-11.

Shih, PT; Elices, MJ; Fang, ZT; Ugarova, TP; Strahl, D; Territo, MC; Frank, JS; Kovach, NL; Cabanas, C; Berliner, JA; Vora, DK. Minimally modified low-density lipoprotein induces monocyte adhesion to endothelial connecting segment-1 by activating beta1 integrin. *J. Clin .Invest.,* 1999, 103(5), 613-25.

Shin, D; Anderson, DJ. Isolation of arterial-specific genes by subtractive hybridization reveals molecular heterogeneity among arterial endothelial cells. Dev Dyn, 2005, 233(4), 1589-604.

Shi, W; Wang, NJ; Shih, DM; Sun, VZ; Wang, X; Lusis, AJ. Determinants of atherosclerosis susceptibility in the C3H and C57BL/6 mouse model: evidence for involvement of endothelial cells but not blood cells or cholesterol metabolism. *Circ. Res.,* 2000, 86(10), 1078-84.

Silkworth, JB; Stehbens, WE. The shape of endothelial cells in en face preparations of rabbit blood vessels. *Angiology*, 1975, 26, 474–87.

Sieminski, AL; Hebbel, RP; Gooch, KJ. Improved microvascular network in vitro by human blood outgrowth endothelial cells relative to vessel-derived endothelial cells. *Tissue Eng.,* 2005, 11(9-10), 1332-45.

Sorrell, JM; Baber, MA; Caplan, AI. A self-assembled fibroblast-endothelial cell co-culture system that supports in vitro vasculogenesis by both human umbilical vein endothelial cells and human dermal microvascular endothelial cells. *Cells Tissues Organs,* 2007, 186(3), 157-68.

Sorrentino, SA; Bahlmann, FH; Besler, C; Müller, M; Schulz, S; Kirchhoff, N; Doerries, C; Horváth, T; Limbourg, A; Limbourg, F; Fliser, D; Haller, H; Drexler, H; Landmesser, U. Oxidant stress impairs in vivo reendothelialization capacity of endothelial progenitor cells from patients with type 2 diabetes mellitus: restoration by the peroxisome proliferator-activated receptor-gamma agonist rosiglitazone. *Circulation,* 2007, 116(2), 163-73.

Springer, TA. Traffic signals for lymphocyte recirculation and leukocyte emigration: the multistep paradigm. *Cell,* 1994, 76(2), 301-14.

Staiger, H; Staiger, K; Stefan, N; Wahl, HG; Machicao, F; Kellerer, M; Häring, HU. Palmitate-Induced Interleukin-6 Expression in Human Coronary Artery Endothelial Cells. *Diabetes,* 2004, 53, 3209-3216.

St. Croix, B; Rago, C; Velculescu, V; Traverso, G; Romans, KE; Montgomery, E; Lal, A; Riggins, GJ; Lengauer, C; Vogelstein, B; Kinzler, KW. Genes Expressed in Human Tumor Endothelium. *Science,* 2000, 298, 1197-1202.

Stoll, LL; Denning, GM; Weintraub, NL. Potential role of endotoxin as a proinflammatory mediator of atherosclerosis. Arterioscler Thromb Vasc Biol, 2004, 24(12), 2227-36.

Streeten, EA; Ornberg, R; Curcio, F; Sakaguchi, K; Marx, S; Aurbach, GD; Brandi, ML. Cloned endothelial cells from fetal bovine bone. *Proc. Natl. Acad. Sci. USA,* 1989, 86(3), 916-20.

Sundstrom, JB; Martinson, DE; Mosunjac, M; Bostik, P; McMullan, LK; Donahoe, RM; Gravanis, MB; Ansari, AA. Norepinephrine enhances adhesion of HIV-1-infected leukocytes to cardiac microvascular endothelial cells. *Exp. Biol. Med. (Maywood),* 2003, 228(6), 730-40.

Takami, S; Yamashita, S; Kihara, S; Kameda-Takemura, K; Matsuzawa, Y. High concentration of glucose induces the expression of intercellular adhesion molecule-1 in human umbilical vein endothelial cells. *Atherosclerosis,* 1998, 138(1), 35-41.

Tang, T; Connelly, BA; Joyner, WL. Heterogeneity of endothelial cell function for angiotensin conversion in serial-arranged arterioles. *J. Vasc. Res.,* 1995, 32(2), 129-37.

Tang, T; Joyner, WL. Differential role of endothelial function on vasodilator responses in series-arranged arterioles. *Microvasc. Res.,* 1992, 44(1), 61-72.

Tan, PH; Chan, C; Xue, SA; Dong, R; Ananthesayanan, B; Manunta, M; Kerouedan, C; Cheshire, NJ; Wolfe, JH; Haskard, DO; Taylor, KM; George, AJ. Phenotypic and functional differences between human saphenous vein (HSVEC) and umbilical vein (HUVEC) endothelial cells. *Atherosclerosis,* 2004,173(2), 171-83.

Tatsumi, T; Ashihara, E; Yasui, T; Matsunaga, S; Kido, A; Sasada, Y; Nishikawa, S; Hadase, M; Koide, M; Nakamura, R; Irie, H; Ito, K; Matsui, A; Matsui, H; Katamura, M; Kusuoka, S; Matoba, S; Okayama, S; Horii, M; Uemura, S; Shimazaki, C; Tsuji, H;

Saito, Y; Matsubara, H. Intracoronary transplantation of non-expanded peripheral blood-derived mononuclear cells promotes improvement of cardiac function in patients with acute myocardial infarction. *Circ. J.*, 2007, 71(8), 1199-207.

Thornhill, MH; Li, J; Haskard, DO. Leucocyte endothelial cell adhesion: a study comparing human umbilical vein endothelial cells and the endothelial cell line EA-hy-926. *Scand J. Immunol.*, 1993, 38(3), 279-86.

Thum T, Fraccarollo D, Schultheiss M, Froese S, Galuppo P, Widder JD, Tsikas D, Ertl G, Bauersachs J. Endothelial nitric oxide synthase uncoupling impairs endothelial progenitor cell mobilization and function in diabetes. *Diabetes*. 2007; 56(3): 666-74.

Tian, H; McKnight, SL; Russell, DW. Endothelial PAS domain protein 1 (EPAS1), a transcription factor selectively expressed in endothelial cells. *Genes Dev.*, 1997, 11(1), 72-82.

Tonnesen, MG. Neutrophil-endothelial cell interactions: mechanisms of neutrophil adherence to vascular endothelium. *J. Invest .Dermatol.*, 1989, 93(2 Suppl), 53S-58S.

Trantina-Yates, AE; Human, P; Bracher, M; Zilla, P. Mitigation of bioprosthetic heart valve degeneration through biocompatibility: in vitro versus spontaneous endothelialization. *Biomaterials,* 2001, 22(13), 1837-46.

Tsukurov, OI; Kwolek, CJ; L'Italien, GJ; Benbrahim, A; Milinazzo, BB; Conroy, NE; Gertler, JP; Orkin, RW; Abbott, WM. The response of adult human saphenous vein endothelial cells to combined pressurized pulsatile flow and cyclic strain, in vitro. *Ann. Vasc. Surg,* 2000, 14(3), 260-7.

Turner, DM; Grant, SC; Lamb, WR; Brenchley, PE; Dyer, PA; Sinnott, PJ; Hutchinson, IV. A genetic marker of high TNF-alpha production in heart transplant recipients. *Transplantation,* 1995, 60(10), 1113-7.

Tyagi, N; Sedoris, KC; Steed, M; Ovechkin, AV; Moshal, KS; Tyagi, SC. Mechanisms of homocysteine-induced oxidative stress. *Am. J. Physiol. Heart Circ. Physiol.*, 2005, 289(6), H2649-56.

Vallier, L; Pedersen, RA. Human embryonic stem cells: an in vitro model to study mechanisms controlling pluripotency in early mammalian development. *Stem. Cell Rev.,* 2005, 1(2), 119-30.

van Vliet, P; Sluijter, JP; Doevendans, PA; Goumans, MJ. Isolation and expansion of resident cardiac progenitor cells. *Expert Rev. Cardiovasc. Ther.*; 2007; 5(1); 33-43.

Vara, DS; Salacinski, HJ; Kannan, RY; Bordenave, L; Hamilton, G; Seifalian, AM. Cardiovascular tissue engineering: state of the art. *Pathol. Biol. (Paris)*, 2005, 53(10), 599-612.

Vasa, M; Fichtlscherer, S; Aicher, A; Adler, K; Urbich, C; Martin, H; Zeiher, AM; Dimmeler, S. Number and migratory activity of circulating endothelial progenitor cells inversely correlate with risk factors for coronary artery disease. *Circ. Res,* 2001, 89(1), E1-7.

Vernon, RB; Sage, EH. A novel; quantitative model for study of endothelial cell migration and sprout formation within three-dimensional collagen matrices. *Microvasc. Res,*. 1999, 57(2), 118-33.

Voyta, JC; Via, DP; Butterfield, CE; Zetter, BR. Identification and isolation of endothelial cells based on their increased uptake of acetylated-low density lipoprotein. *J. Cell. Biol.*, 1984, 99(6), 2034-40.

Wagner; DD; Bonfanti, R. von Willebrand factor and the endothelium. *Mayo Clin. Proc.*, 1991, 66(6), 621-7.

Wagner, M; Hermanns, I; Bittinger, F; Kirkpatrick, CJ. Induction of stress proteins in human endothelial cells by heavy metal ions and heat shock. *Am. J. Physiol.*, 1999, 277(5 Pt 1), L1026-33.

Walenta, K; Friedrich, EB; Sehnert, F; Werner, N; Nickenig, G. In vitro differentiation characteristics of cultured human mononuclear cells-implications for endothelial progenitor cell biology. *Biochem. Biophys. Res. Commun.*, 2005, 333(2), 476-82.

Wallace, CS; Champion, JC; Truskey, GA. Adhesion and function of human endothelial cells co-cultured on smooth muscle cells. *Ann. Biomed. Eng.*, 2007a, 35(3), 375-86.

Wallace, CS; Strike, SA; Truskey, GA. Smooth muscle cell rigidity and extracellular matrix organization influence endothelial cell spreading and adhesion formation in coculture. *Am. J. Physiol. Heart Circ. Physiol.*, 2007b, 293(3), H1978-86.

Wang, H; Long, C; Duan, Z; Shi, C; Jia, G; Zhang, Y. A new ATP-sensitive potassium channel opener protects endothelial function in cultured aortic endothelial cells. *Cardiovasc. Res.*, 2007, 73(3), 497-503.

Wang, XJ; Li, QP. The roles of mesenchymal stem cells (MSCs) therapy in ischemic heart diseases. *Biochem. Biophys. Res. Commun.*, 2007, 359(2), 189-93.

Wartenberg, M; Dönmez, F; Budde, P; Sauer, H. Embryonic stem cells: a novel tool for the study of antiangiogenesis and tumor-induced angiogenesis. *Handb. Exp. Pharmacol.*, 2006, 174, 53-71.

Wartenberg, M; Dönmez, F; Ling, FC; Acker, H; Hescheler, J; Sauer, H. Tumor-induced angiogenesis studied in confrontation cultures of multicellular tumor spheroids and embryoid bodies grown from pluripotent embryonic stem cells. *FASEB J.*, 2001, 15(6), 995-1005.

Weibel, ER; Palade, GE. New cytoplasmatic components in arterial endothelia. *J. Cell Biol.*, 1964, 23, 101-12.

Wenger, A; Kowalewski, N; Stahl, A; Mehlhorn, AT; Schmal, H; Stark, GB; Finkenzeller, G. Development and characterization of a spheroidal coculture model of endothelial cells and fibroblasts for improving angiogenesis in tissue engineering. *Cells Tissues Organs*, 2005, 181(2), 80-8.

Wikström, P; Lissbrant, IF; Stattin, P; Egevad, L; Bergh, A. Endoglin (CD105) is expressed on immature blood vessels and is a marker for survival in prostate cancer. *Prostate*, 2002, 51(4), 268-75.

Wong, CW; Wiedle, G; Ballestrem, C; Wehrle-Haller, B; Etteldorf, S; Bruckner, M; Engelhardt, B; Gisler, RH; Imhof, BA. PECAM-1/CD31 trans-homophilic binding at the intercellular junctions is independent of its cytoplasmic domain; evidence for heterophilic interaction with integrin alphavbeta3 in Cis. *Mol. Biol .Cell*, 2000, 11(9), 3109-21.

Wu, HC; Wang, TW; Kang, PL; Tsuang, YH; Sun, JS; Lin, FH. Coculture of endothelial and smooth muscle cells on a collagen membrane in the development of a small-diameter vascular graft. *Biomaterials,* 2007, 28(7), 1385-92.

Yonezawa, S; Maruyama, I; Sakae, K; Igata, A; Majerus, PW; Sato, E. Thrombomodulin as a marker for vascular tumors. Comparative study with factor VIII and Ulex europaeus I lectin. *Am. J. Clin. Pathol.,* 1987, 88(4), 405-11.

You, LR; Lin, FJ; Lee, CT; DeMayo, FJ; Tsai, MJ; Tsai, SY. Suppression of Notch signalling by the COUP-TFII transcription factor regulates vein identity. *Nature,* 2005, 435(7038), 98-104.

Young, PP; Vaughan, DE; Hatzopoulos, AK. Biologic properties of endothelial progenitor cells and their potential for cell therapy. *Prog. Cardiovasc. Dis.,* 2007, 49(6), 421-9.

Yuan, L; Moyon, D; Pardanaud, L; Bréant, C; Karkkainen, MJ; Alitalo, K; Eichmann, A. Abnormal lymphatic vessel development in neuropilin 2 mutant mice. *Development,* 2002, 129(20), 4797-806.

Yun, MR; Im, DS; Lee, JS; Son, SM; Sung, SM; Bae, SS; Kim, CD. NAD(P)H oxidase-stimulating activity of serum from type 2 diabetic patients with retinopathy mediates enhanced endothelial expression of E-selectin. *Life Sci,* 2006, 78(22), 2608-14.

Zal B, Kaski JC, Arno G, Akiyu JP, Xu Q, Cole D, Whelan M, Russell N, Madrigal JA, Dodi IA, Baboonian C. Heat-shock protein 60-reactive CD4+CD28null T cells in patients with acute coronary syndromes. *Circulation.* 2004; 109(10): 1230-5.

Zannettino, AC; Paton, S; Arthur, A; Khor, F; Itescu, S; Gimble, JM; Gronthos, S. Multipotential human adipose-derived stromal stem cells exhibit a perivascular phenotype in vitro and in vivo. *J. Cell Physiol.,* 2007, in press.

Zhang, L; Hoffman, JA; Ruoslahti, E. Molecular profiling of heart endothelial cells. *Circulation,* 2005, 112, 1601-11.

Zhang, S; Day, I; Ye, S. Nicotine induced changes in gene expression by human coronary artery endothelial cells. *Atherosclerosis,* 2001, 154(2), 277-83.

In: Progress in Cell Growth Process Research
Editor: Takumi Hayashi, pp. 65-88

ISBN 978-1-60456-325-2
© 2008 Nova Science Publishers, Inc.

Chapter 2

REACTIVE OXYGEN SPECIES
DETERMINE CELL FATE

Ina Berniakovich[1], Mirella Trinei[2], Elena Beltrami[1],
Pier Giuseppe Pelicci[1] and Marco Giorgio[1]

[1] Department of Experimental Oncology, European Institute of Oncology, Milan-Italy,
[2] Congenia Srl, Milan-Italy

ABSTRACT

Intracellular redox balance, i.e. the ratio between oxidizing and reducing species within the cell, plays a significant role in the regulation of cellular processes. Redox balance results from the activities of enzymatic systems that produce or neutralize oxidizing species. Aerobic metabolism significantly affects intracellular redox balance through the formation of reactive oxygen species, ROS. ROS, including superoxide anion, singlet oxygen, hydrogen peroxide and hydroxyl radical, are potent oxidizing agents that largely alter redox balance and target a variety of cellular components. Mitochondrial respiration as well as cytosolic and membrane oxidases contribute largely to the regulation of intracellular redox balance.

In the past, intracellular accumulation of ROS was thought to lead exclusively to an unspecific damage to cellular components. Nowadays, the physiological relevance of redox balance regulation by ROS has been reevaluated. In fact, emerging data suggest that ROS function as signaling molecules that regulate cellular processes such as angiogenesis, fat development, stem cell renewal and apoptosis. Furthermore, ROS were shown to regulate stem cell pools maintenance and proliferation and to adjust their differentiation program.

Here we review the current knowledge about ROS control of cellular growth and differentiation, discuss the critical and context specific role of ROS in regulating cell processes and finally hypothesize that integration of the different tissue specific regulatory circuits with the alteration of redox balance induced by ROS accumulation determines cell fate.

OXIDATION REACTIONS, REDOX BALANCE AND ROS

O_2 can react with a number of molecules, even at the concentration found in the atmosphere (21%). The first evidence that some chemical species, upon reaction with O_2, form oxides led to naming the observed reactions of oxygen transfer "oxidation". Further studies established that oxidation is actually a loss of electrons and an increase in the "oxidation number" (a parameter that indicates the charge a chemical element in a complex or molecule would have if all its ligands were removed along with their electrons contributing to the chemical bonds). Oxidation can occur only in the presence of an element able to decrease its oxidation number in a reaction called "reduction". The ability of molecules to be oxidized or reduced is indicated by their oxidation/reduction (or redox) potential, a thermodynamic parameter expressed in Volt (V) that measures the avidity for electrons, as compared with hydrogen; the more positive the redox potential of a species, the greater its tendency to acquire electrons and thus to be reduced.

Redox reactions are also key in the metabolic intracellular pathways. In particular, some reduced compounds such as NADH and succinate can donate electrons to specific mitochondrial enzymes that form the respiratory chain, a group of proteins that undergo sequential redox reactions terminating in O_2 reduction to H_2O. This process is fundamental in cell physiology since it is accompanied by production of ATP, the main form of energy used by the cell.

In certain conditions (see further), reduction of O_2 to H_2O is not complete and some highly reactive intermediates called reactive oxygen species (ROS) can be formed. ROS is a collective term that includes highly unstable and reactive oxygen derivatives such as superoxide anion ($O_2 \cdot^-$), hydroxyl radical ($OH^\bullet$) and hydrogen peroxide (H_2O_2). ROS can be formed inside the cells where they can react with a variety of molecules. Among biologically relevant ROS H_2O_2 has the lowest redox potential (i.e. the lowest tendency to acquire electrons), the highest stability and the highest intracellular concentration (Figure 1). These properties allow in particular H_2O_2 to accumulate and diffuse in and out a cell thus becoming an oxidizing signal.

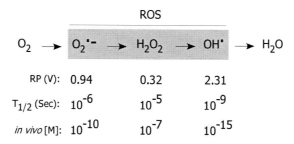

Figure 1. Oxygen reduction steps from molecular oxygen to water.

Redox potential (RP) is a measure of the affinity of a chemical element within a molecule for electrons, as compared with hydrogen (which is set at 0V). Half life ($T_{1/2}$; sec: seconds) indicates molecular stability and reactivity. The latter can also be evaluated from intracellular concentration (M: molar).

THE SOURCES OF CELLULAR ROS

It is established that about 85-90% of O_2 taken up by animals is utilized by mitochondria as the terminal electron acceptor of the electron transfer chain and 10-15% is used by a variety of oxidases and oxygenase enzymes as well as by direct chemical (non-enzymic) oxidation reactions (Figure 2) [55,114]. It has been estimated that a fraction of around 0.1% to 2% of the total oxygen consumed by a living cell is converted into ROS [17]. Cellular ROS are generated by specific enzymatic systems (Figure 2) or accidentally released as a consequence of incomplete oxygen reduction. All cell types can produce ROS in different cell compartments such as plasma membrane (phagocytic oxidases and NADPH oxidases), mitochondria ($O_2 \cdot -$ dismutases, mitochondrial respiratory chain, p66[Shc]/Cytochrome c enzymatic system and amine oxidase), peroxisome (peroxisomal oxidases), endoplasmic reticulum (sulfhydryl oxidase) and cytosol (aminoacid oxidases, cyclooxygenase, lipid oxygenase, xanthine oxidase and $O_2 \cdot -$ dismutases; figure 2).

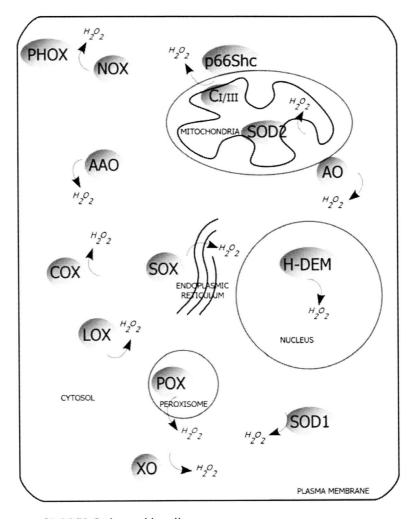

Figure 2. Sources of ROS/H2O2 in aerobic cells.

Specific sources of ROS are enzymes involved in cellular metabolism such as: D-amino acid oxidase that uses O_2 to oxidize unwanted D-amino acids; xanthine oxidase that oxidizes xanthine and hypoxanthine to produce uric acid; proline and lysine hydroxylase that add –OH group to collagen; tyrosine hydroxylase that uses O_2 to add –OH during the synthesis of adrenalin and noradrenalin; cytochromes P450, involved in the oxidation of a wide range of physiological substrates (bile acids, estrogens, testosterone) as well as molecules of exogenous origin (phenobarbital, amphetamine, methadone, paracetamol etc.) [56].

Despite the number of specific enzymatic sources of ROS, they have been traditionally regarded as by-products of aerobic metabolism and mitochondrial respiration is considered to be the major intracellular source of their accidental generation. Mitochondrial ROS production results from the leakage of electrons from the mitochondrial electron transport chain and their subsequent reaction with O_2 to form $O_2 \cdot^-$ [5]. It is estimated that up to 2% of the oxygen consumed by mitochondria is partially reduced to form $O_2 \cdot^-$, which is subsequently converted to H_2O_2 [55. 56].

Several enzymatic systems (indicated in gray) generate H2O2 within different cellular compartments, including plasma membrane: phagocytic oxidases (PHOX) and NADPH oxidases (NOX); mitochondria: $O2 \cdot^-$ dismutases (SOD2), mitochondrial respiratory complexes I/III (COXI/III), the $p66^{Shc}$/Cytochrome c enzymatic system and amine oxidase (AO); peroxisomes: peroxisomal oxidases (POX); endoplasmic reticulum: sulfhydryl oxidase (SOX); the cytosol: aminoacid oxidases (AAO), cyclooxygenease (COX), lipid oxygenase (LOX), xanthine oxidase (XO) and $O2 \cdot^-$ dismutases (SOD1).

THE INTRACELLULAR TARGETS OF ROS OXIDATION

ROS are highly reactive and oxidize either reversibly or irreversibly specific intracellular targets potentially altering their function. Virtually, all reducing groups present in the biological macromolecules could be targeted by ROS. Indeed, ROS (in particular $OH^\cdot$) can react with DNA and generate DNA mutations, a process involved in the first steps of carcinogenesis. ROS also target lipids, such as unsaturated fatty acids (present in the phospholipids composing cellular membranes) and proteins (in particular cysteine and proline residues). The damaging effects of ROS vary considerably among tissues and physical/pathological conditions depending on age and environmental factors such as diet. Given the potential harm that a non-regulated ROS accumulation could provoke to the cellular components, several systems have evolved to decrease intracellular ROS levels. These are generally called "scavenging" mechanisms since they are preferential ROS reducing agents (superoxide dismutases, catalase) or anti-oxidants (NADH, GSH and ascorbate) that maintain ROS levels within a physiological range and annihilate their harmful effects. Thus, in every cellular compartment, ROS concentration depends on the balance between production and scavenging. However, the antioxidant shield seems to control ROS concentration rather than eliminate them completely; thereby intracellular ROS levels are sufficient to target important cellular molecules [120,134].

In particular, it has been demonstrated that several proteins regulating intracellular signal transduction pathways or gene transcription are controlled by ROS, in particular H_2O_2 (Figure3). ROS reaction with specific amino acid residues within a protein can induce either small or vast conformational changes resulting in a drastic alteration of protein function. This can be regarded as a specific mechanism through which ROS regulate different intracellular signaling pathways.

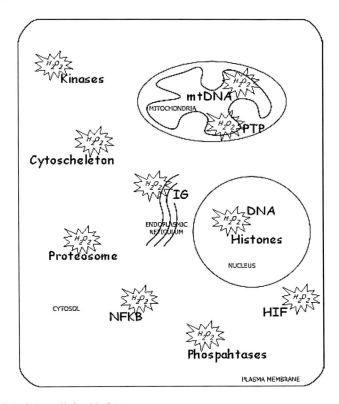

Figure 3. The multiple intracellular H2O2 targets.

Indeed, among the proteins modified by ROS, protein tyrosine phosphatases (PTPs) are a major target of ROS direct oxidation. Together with another family of enzymes with opposing function, protein tyrosine kinases (PTKs), PTPs regulate cellular levels of proteins phosphorylated on their tyrosine residues. Phosphorylation of specific tyrosine residues is one of the most important mechanisms involved in growth factors, cytokines and hormones signaling [24, 25]. PTP superfamily consists of classical tyrosine-specific phosphatases, dual specificity phosphatases, cdc25 phosphatases, and low molecular weight protein tyrosine phosphatase (LMW-PTP) [24, 25]. The catalytic site of PTPs is characterized by a conserved cysteine residue vulnerable to oxidation [20, 23, 32]. Different kinds of PTPs have been recognized to be reversibly or irreversibly oxidized and inactivated by ROS [32] that are thus able to potentiate the phosphorylation-based signaling cascades [120].

Another crucial target of ROS oxidation is the transcription factor hypoxia-inducible factor 1 (HIF-1), the main regulator of the expression of hundreds of genes in response to hypoxia [28, 29, 112]. HIF-1 consists of the O_2-dependent HIF-1α subunit and the O_2-

independent HIF-1β subunit [113]. Under normal oxygen pressure, HIF-1α is short-lived since newly synthesized protein is rapidly degraded through oxygen dependent pathways [59, 84, 113]. When oxygen pressure decreases, HIF-1α is stabilized and can translocate to the nucleus where it dimerizes with HIF-1β and starts transcription of target genes [84, 113].

Many regulatory macromolecules are targeted by H_2O_2: actin, myosin, tubulin (cytoskeleton); different kinases (Kinases); several serine/threonine and tyrosine phosphatases (Phosphatases); proteosome; the mitochondrial permeability transition pore (PTP); mitochondrial and nuclear DNA (DNA); telomeres;. histones; transcription factors such as HIF-1α or NFKB.

It has been proven on one hand that exogenous administration of H_2O_2 triggers HIF-1α stabilization under normoxia and on the other hand that specific inhibition of ROS production by NADPH oxidase blocks HIF response [49]. Recent evidence also links mitochondrial ROS and hypoxic response in human cells [18] as well as in yeast [53]. Indeed, exposure to low oxygen inhibits mitochondrial respiration while increasing ROS production through ETC [18, 52]. The consequent accumulation of ROS in the cytoplasm stabilizes HIF thus triggering the expression of HIF responsive genes [106]. Indeed, Rho^0 cells, deficient in mitochondrial functions, fail to activate the HIF pathway in response to hypoxia [18] and inhibitors of mitochondrial ROS generation abolish the cellular response to hypoxia [82]. Finally, it has been shown that mitochondrial ROS are sufficient to stabilize HIF and to induce the expression of hypoxia-responsive genes.Another example of ROS regulation of intracellular signaling pathways through the oxidation of key enzymes is represented by p38 mitogen-activated protein kinase (MAPK), a member of the complex superfamily of MAP serine/threonine protein kinases, also known as stress-activated kinases. P38 MAPK phosphorylates downstream targets directly regulating gene expression or is involved in other signaling pathways (e.g., NF-ĸB, insulin, cytokine, arachidonate) and in a large number of cellular processes including inflammation and immunity, cell growth and apoptosis, and tissue-specific stress responses. Indeed, p38 MAPK is a redox-sensitive MAPK that is activated in response to both endogenous and exogenous H_2O_2 in a variety of cells [109, 132, 131].

The list of important regulatory proteins targeted by ROS is growing daily and includes many others involved in a variety of different cellular processes: kinases and phosphatases as those described above; cytoskeleton components such as actin, myosin, tubulin; the proteosome; the mitochondrial permeability transition pore (PTP) and several other mitochondrial enzymes; transcription factors other than HIF-1 such as NF-kB and nuclear proteins such as histones [92].

ROS SIGNALING IN DIFFERENT CELLULAR CONTEXTS

In different organisms ROS can regulate different molecular pathways thus modulating specific cellular functions.

In fungi, intracellular ROS accumulation is implicated in processes like development of sexual fruiting bodies, ascospore germination as well as hyphal defense and growth (for review see [124]). In yeast, two major ROS regulated pathways were discovered, which are induced by increased ROS concentration. In. *Saccaromyces pombe* moderate H_2O_2 levels potentiate the Pap1 pathway while higher ROS levels induce the Sty1 pathway involved in surviving [105,135].

ROS are also implicated in signal transduction pathways and cell death in plants. Recent studies have implicated H_2O_2 as an endogenous component of phytohormone abscisic acid signaling in Arabidopsis (*Arabidopsis thaliana*) guard cells, which induces stomatal closure via activation of plasma membrane calcium channels [95]. Inhibition of seed germination and root elongation through the abscisic pathway is impaired in atrbohD/F (double mutants of NADPH oxidase catalytic subunits), which function through ROS production [71]. It was shown as well that activity of NADPH-oxidase is important for growth of root hairs [14] and for leaf elongation. [108]. Finally, plants also use ROS for defence from biotic stress. In response to pathogen attack, plants undergo an oxidative burst which is believed to be similar to that observed in animal immune responses involving phagocytes [63].

In *Caenorhabditis elegans* intracellular redox balance influences germline and vulval development. It was also demonstrated that *Caenorhabditis elegans* produce ROS as a mechanism of defense from pathogens [19].

In mammals, ROS spikes provoke different effects in terminally differentiated cells or in proliferative tissues. Not all the populations of differentiated cells in the body are subject to cell turn-over. Some cell types, generated during embryogenesis, are retained throughout adult life without dividing and replacing. Together with nerve cells and lens cells, muscle heart cells are permanent cells.

Cardiomyocyte are mononucleated cells and they are joined end to end by special structures called intercalated discs, they connect by an actin-myosin sliding filament mechanism, about 3 billion times in an average human life-span.

Myocardial infarction (essentially ischaemic/hypoxic injury to heart muscle) is a major cause of death and thrombolytic therapy is now widely used to dissolve blood clots and promote reperfusion. If ischaemia or hypoxia is insufficiently long to injure the heart irreversibly, the tissue can be salvaged by reperfusing it with blood. In this situation reperfusion is a beneficial process, however paradoxically such reperfusion can exacerbate the damage occurring during the ischaemic period [121]. Reperfusion injury is accompanied by enzyme release and morphological changes characteristic of necrosis [54]. The extent of damage can be visualised as an area of necrotic tissue known as the infarct whose area can be determined to provide a quantitative measure of injury. Quantification of damage may also be provided by measuring the release of intracellular proteins such as lactate dehydrogenase or troponin. In addition to the necrotic cell death that represents the major damage to the reperfused heart there is also evidence that some myocytes around the periphery of the infarct die by apoptosis [45] and [2].

Reperfusion is characterized by a burst of ROS production [66] mostly formed by complex 1 and complex 3 of the mitochondrial respiratory chain [6, 119, 144]. ROS together with elevated calcium concentration play a critical role in the transition from reversible to irreversible reperfusion injury, and mitochondria are the major target of these agents. In particular, they lead to the opening of the mitochondrial permeability transition pore, a major player in reperfusion injury [34, 54, 119]. Hence ROS are strongly implicated in the pathogenesis of postischemic myocardial stunning, necrosis, apoptosis and vascular dysfunction. To the contrary short periods of ischemic stress followed by reperfusion on the myocardium can sometimes induce adaptation that results in decreased sensitivity to a subsequent ischaemic insult [66] suggesting that ROS and also reactive nitrogen species, like NO, are important mediators of the signaling cascade responsible of cardioprotection during preconditioning. Hence cardiomyocyte represents a specific cell type where ROS can exert a double opposite effect.

Neurons are another example of postmitotic cells. In neurons, ROS are important determinants of cell death [80]. Indeed, it was shown that in many neurodegenerative diseases cell death is associated with ROS accumulation [1, 30, 56, 65, 115, 122,]. Redox balance in neurons has been demonstrated to be regulated by specific neuronal metabolite as in the case of neurotransmitters. The excitatory neurotransmitter glutamate is a major contributor to pathological cell death within the nervous system (so called glutamate toxicity) and is performed with ROS participation [30, 90]. One of two forms of glutamate toxicity is non-receptor-mediated oxidative glutamate toxicity [90]. Oxidative glutamate toxicity is initiated by high concentrations of extracellular glutamate that prevent cysteine uptake into the cells, followed by the depletion of intracellular cysteine and the loss of glutathione (GSH). With a diminishing supply of GSH, there is an accumulation of ROS that ultimately triggers massive apoptosis.

ROS mediated neuronal apoptosis has been also linked with physiological development of the central nervous system. In brain development, neuronal precursors proceed through the cell cycle to produce larger numbers of neurons than are needed, and excess neurons are eliminated by selective apoptosis in the early stages of life [68]. Mammalian brain neurons do not proliferate after the differentiation and stay maintained in a quiescent G0 state and no longer cycle [68]. Reentry in to the cell cycle, which precedes to cell death, is required for removal of many kinds of neurons [37]. That is why, even though some postmitotic neurons retain the capacity to respond to growth factors, results in reentering into the cell cycle and subsequent cell death. Likewise, overexpression of oncogenes results in apoptosis via cell cycle reentry rather than proliferation [41, 47]. It was shown that reentry of neurons to cell cycle in some cases is stimulated by ROS upregulation and later outcomes in apoptosis. For instance, mutation of apoptosis inducing gene (AIF) results in an increase of intracellular H_2O_2 associated with apoptosis of different kind of neurons, which die upon reentering the cell cycle (for review see [68]).

In fibroblasts, the most common type of cells of connected tissues, ROS exert a positive effect on growth. Fibroblasts secrete proteins of extracellular matrix and are activated (in terms of proliferation and migration) upon tissue damage and participate in wound healing. Induction of cellular proliferation starts upon stimulation of cell with various growth factors. ROS are involved in modulation of these signaling pathways. Often, stimulation of growth factor receptors with their ligands results in a burst of intracellular ROS in a variety of cell types [143]. Production of low levels of O_2^- and H_2O_2 was reported in response to EGF, VEGF, bFGF, and PDGF [3, 4, 16, 20, 125], which can facilitate proliferation of fibroblasts upon these GF stimulations. Treatment with ROS was able to increase proliferation *in vitro* of hamster, rat, mouse, and human fibroblasts. ROS are involved in wound healing like signals triggering fibroblast proliferation for subsequent scar formation. It was demonstrated that in wounds, high levels of lactate were produced, which has been suggested to stimulate proliferation of fibroblasts through the regulation of intracellular redox balance [136]. Secretion of some extracellular proteins like collagen by fibroblasts, can be also mediated through intracellular oxidative signals and ROS production [21, 117].

In adipocytes, ROS accumulation apparently leads to consequences in accordance with specific functions which adipose tissue executes in the organism

Primary function of adipose tissue is regulation of energy metabolism through storage of energy as triglycerides in numerous deposits of white tissue and dissipation of energy through non-shivering and diet-induced thermogenesis by brown adipose tissue. Adipose tissue is a potent endocrine organ, which specifically secrets dozens of hormones regulating metabolism, such as adiponectin, leptin, resistin, etc. and is involved in the onset of metabolic disorders [58] and longevity regulation [9].

Functional adipose cells arise through the differentiation of pre-adipocyte. In order to differentiate, pre-adipocytes stop proliferating and undergo growth arrest, which usually happens through contact inhibition. Treatment of adipocytes at the confluent stage of *in vitro* with differentiation cocktail (chief component of which is insulin), triggers expression of adipocyte differentiation transcription factors (PPARg, C/EBP, ADD1/SREBP-1, or CREB) that drive the cells to become mature adipocytes characterized by huge trygliceride deposition. Proliferation and differentiation of adipocyte as well as glucose and fatty acid uptake, lipogenesis and lipolysis in adipocytes are strictly regulated by insulin [79, 142].

ROS are tightly implicated in insulin signaling in adipocytes. The stimulation of an insulin receptor, results in a generation of H_2O_2 through membrane-bound NADPH oxidase [69, 70]. Also, a mitochondrial respiratory chain was shown to be an insulin-sensitive source of H_2O_2 [101,102]. Treatment of adipocytes with ROS mimics some of the insulin actions like activation of glucose transport, lipogenesis, inhibition of lipolysis, stimulation of glucose C1-oxidation, and glucose incorporation into glycogen [36, 73, 77, 85, 89, 90]. Moreover, it was shown that an increase in the intracellular level of ROS through the activation of amine oxidases in the cytosol stimulates differentiation of the adipose like cells lines 3T3, F442A, and 3T3-L1 [39, 46, 87, 91]. Indirect evidence of involvement of ROS in adipocyte differentiation has been also reported by using antioxidants such as α – lipoic acid and n-acetyl cysteine that were able to block differentiation and lipid accumulation of fat cells [26].

One mechanism suggested to explain the effect of ROS on insulin-mediated differentiation program involves phosphatases inhibition. Indeed, H_2O_2 inhibits phophatases involved in the insulin signal transduction like PTP1B, LMWPTP, TC 45, and PTEN [15, 24, 43, 81, 86], thus potentiating the insulin signal transduction cascade.

It is interesting to note that even though H_2O_2 has the same targets in different types of cells, the final result of its action depends on cell type. In fact, while in adipocytes H_2O_2 induces differentiation and inhibits proliferation in other contests, like fibroblast, it is a potent enhancer of growth [10]. It was shown that ROS produced in mitochondria act like anti-growth signal acts like anti-proliferative signals in 3T3-L1 adipocytes and on the contrary the decrease in ROS level (through uncoupling) slightly increases the adipocyte proliferation rate [13].

Another cell type where ROS influences a complex process of differentiation is the endothelial cells (EC). EC are the epithelium cells, which line blood vessels of the entire circulatory system. One of the crucial functions is angiogenesis, which enables wound healing, growth, and development of the organism. ROS are directly involved in the execution by EC of this function.

Angiogenesis is the process of new vessels forming from already pre-existing ones. Upon stimulation EC secretes proteases, which digest extracellular matrixes and allow cells to permeate the basement membrane, proliferate, migrate, and form tubular structures which become new formed capillaries.

Angiogenesis is stimulated by hypoxia. ROS produced in hypoxic conditions have been linked to the activation of HIF which stimulates the production of factors triggering angiogenesis [44, 104, 127, 132, 140]. The molecular mechanism of HIF stimulated angiogenesis implicates VEGF activation, growth factor with a profound stimulatory effect on the EC migration, proliferation and tube formation both *in vitro* and *in vivo* [38, 40, 74, 88, 93, 94, 96, 97, 98, 100, 128]. It was shown that in some kinds of endothelial cells in basal conditions there is no expression of VEGF which is however stimulated upon response to hypoxia, where 28-base pair element in the 5' promoter that mediates hypoxia-inducible transcription has been identified (74). Thus, ROS through HIF can potentiate VEGF function.

A role for ROS in tumor angiogenesis has also been reported. The rapidly proliferating cancer cells create tumor mass with low oxygen supply, and for the prominent development of tumor, growing out of new formed vessels is necessary. Cancer cells have been reported to have increased levels of ROS that are involved in the neo-angiogenesis required by the tumor [75, 123]. Apparently a genetic program that regulates ROS intracellular levels and the angiogenic property of cancer cells exist and oncogenes like Myc and Ras take part in this [139]. It has been shown that the transcription factor JunD reduces tumor angiogenesis by limiting intracellular ROS production. The accumulation of H_2O_2 in JunD-/- cells reduces the activity of HIF prolyl hydroxylases (PHDs) that target hypoxia-inducible factors-alpha for degradation [48].

ROS enhance different steps of angiogenesis like the migration, proliferation, and tube formation of endothelial cells. It has been shown that exogenous administration of low doses of H_2O_2 stimulates migration and proliferation of endothelial cells and also stimulates tube formation as a marker of angiogenesis [116,141]. Likewise, treatment of EC with a wide spectrum of antioxidants decreases the process of angiogenesis [22]. Main growth factors regulating angiogenesis (EGF, FGF, PDGF, and VEGF) are well known to produce ROS as important mediators upon activation of their receptors. H_2O_2 production in endothelial cells through NADPH oxidase upon angiopoietin treatment was also demonstrated which stimulated cell migration *in vitro* and tube formation *in vivo* [67]. At the molecular level, the involvement of ets-1, NF-kB, and c-Jun transcriptional factors has been demonstrated during ROS stimulated angiogensis. H_2O_2 stimulates expression of ets-1 [142] which is known to be involved in the angiogenesis regulation [62]. NF-kB, c-Jun regulate angiogenesis in EC and administration of antisense sequence of NF-kappaB blocks, completely, H_2O_2 stimulated angiogenesis while antisense sequence of c-Jun blocks it partially [116].

Hence, like in other cell types, H_2O_2 potentiates signals from growth factors in endothelial cells, resulting in the regulation of specific EC functions, angiogenesis.

The role of ROS on tissue change and plasticity becomes evident through the effects of ROS on stem cells [51,126].

Population of stem cells is unique in the organism in terms of simultaneous ability of self-renewal, i.e. to the maintenance of the stem cell pool, and to multi-lineage differentiation, property which allows them to give origin to different kinds of cells, repopulate, and restore damaged organs. Stem cell division results in the production of one daughter cell, which preserves stemness, and another daughter cell committed to differentiation. Different programs of cell fate suppose the presence of different molecular mechanisms which direct cells to the execution of these programs. Changes in intracellular ROS amount between stem cell and differentiated cell could be the parameters in which two of the daughter stem cells differ between themselves. Accumulation of some level of oxidants would lead to a genetic regulation able to drive cellular differentiation or self renewal in an appropriate manner. In fact, as it was reported for some kinds of progenitor cells, like for oligodendrocyte-type-2 astrocyte progenitor cells [118], population of embryonic rat cortical cells [130], HSC [50], that ROS accumulation is associated with the differentiation process. Indirect evidence of the role of ROS in stem cell differentiation has been reported, indicating differentiation degree correlates with the intracellular oxidized state [33, 35, 78, 110]. On the contrary, cells characterized by a reduced state have higher self-renewal potential [64]. Indeed, accumulation of ROS does not impair differentiation in some kinds of stem cells; however, it decreases their self-renewal capacity [61]. Strikingly, such discrimination mechanisms between stem and progenitor cells not only exist in nature, but also in some cases allows to researchers to divide cell populations into more and less differentiated ones [118]. In fact, ROS accumulation is connected with differentiation of stem cells, which has been investigated in studies on cardiac differentiation of embryonic stem cells [12]. It was shown that ROS produced through NADPH oxidase lead to expression of a variety cardiac-specific genes and TF like alpha-actin, beta-MHC, MLC2a, MLC2v, ANP, GATA-4, Nkx-2.5, MEF2C, and DTEF-1 [110,111].

In adult stem cells, increased intracellular levels of O_2^- resulted in osteogenic cell growth and maturation of mesenchymal stem cells [138]. Equally, ROS increase caused by hypoxia increases lipogenesis in differentiating MSC and inhibits Oct4 expression, a marker of undifferentiated cell states [42, 107]. In our experiments, differentiation of mouse MSC under hypoxic conditions both into adipo- and osteolineages was much more successful than in normoxia (manuscript in preparation). ROS also activated quiescent neural progenitor cells resulting in their amplification and the subsequent differentiation [89, 143]. Up to now few mechanisms have been described to explain the effect of ROS in stem cells, mainly in hematopoietic cells. It was found that the amount of ROS in the hematopoietic stem cell, was regulated by transcriptional factors of the FOXO family through the regulation of expression of genes involved in ROS regulation [129] and a central role in the maintenance of the stem cell pool belongs to stress induced p38 MAPK.

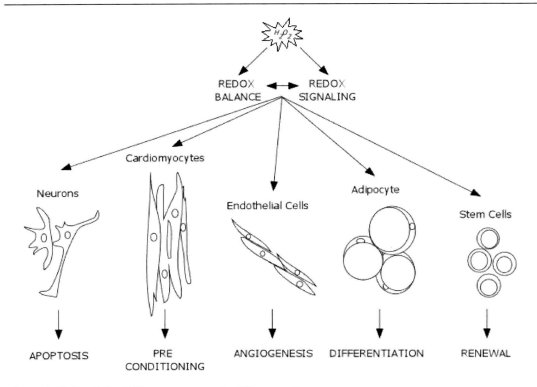

Figure 4. H2O2 elicits different responses in different cell contests.

SPECIFICITY OF ROS SENSITIVE PATHWAYS

ROS have been traditionally regarded as by-products of aerobic metabolism, and mitochondrial respiration is considered to be the major intracellular source of accidental ROS production.

Indirectly altered redox balance or specific oxidative alterations of signaling molecules induced by H_2O_2 accumulation trigger different cellular responses depending on the cell type.

However ROS are involved in the regulation of specific cellular processes that differ according the cellular contest. So, the reason for their specificity appears puzzling. The major obstacle to studying the role of H_2O_2 in biology has been the lack of tools that allow the direct determination of ROS concentration in the different cellular compartments. ROS are in general, difficult to be studied due to their relative instability and small size. In fact, ROS are mostly detected because of their consequences through the utilization of oxidative sensitive dies thereby ROS peaks pointed to specific targets appearing out of the resolution of the method. That's why up to now we are continuing to confuse the effect of ROS on overall redox balance with a specific signaling function. A second consideration must be taken about the molecular species involved. Not all ROS are equally implicated in signaling functions. H_2O_2, for example, is membrane-permeable and -diffusible, less-reactive and longer-lived than $\cdot OH$ or $O_2 \cdot^-$, and, as such, best suited for intra- and even inter-cellular signaling. Then the reversibility of ROS modification, the requisite of any kind of regulative signaling process, appears to also be a controversial issue. Indeed, the majority of oxidative modifications induced by ROS are irreversible and only the oxidized thiols of some cysteine residues present in specific peptide contests are fully reversible. In general redox signaling is being recognized to involve those cysteines which are located in an environment promoting dissociation of thiols. In contrast oxidative stress involves oxidation of a wide variety of residues and molecules [56].

Nevertheless, in spite of the doubts, due to specific oxidation events or to broad oxidative stress, ROS are key regulator of cellular processes. Specific responses, depending on cell contest, in fact are triggered both by a generic stress effect of ROS and by the specific oxidation of well recognized molecular targets. It appears therefore that the variety of cell types express different ROS sensitive pathways that sensitize them to the main response that ROS can elicit. Basically, the cell contest provides the specificity to both ROS accumulation and response.

In this view, the mechanisms of ROS production should be co-evolved with the sensor mechanisms. For example, the mitochondrial apoptosis triggered by the opening of mitochondrial permeability transition, pore induced by ROS, might be evolved together with the mechanism that controls mitochondrial ROS production; or the response of endothelial cells to ischemia, or proliferating cells to growth factors, could likely be the result of the adaptation of the pathways that control gene expression programs involved respectively in angiogenesis and growth with the burst of ROS that originates from the alteration of metabolism due to hypoxia or from the activation of specific plasma membrane oxidases.

Finally the specificity of ROS signaling would reside entirely in the cell contest rather than in the property of the ROS molecule or target.

CONCLUSION

The appearance of photosynthesis around two million years ago, resulted in the production and enrichment of the atmosphere with molecular oxygen. It is suggested that at that time first aerobic organisms appeared and started to use O_2 reduction as the driving force for energy production. Partially reduced O_2 appeared in living cells first probably as an unspecific by-product of the aerobic metabolism, and was later intentionally produced by specific enzymatic systems.

ROS reacted with surrounding molecules, changing their native structure and often damaging them. However, such a long time of joint evolution of the cell with ROS resulted not only in the production of ROS defense mechanisms inside the cell like antioxidants and ROS scavenging enzymes, but also in the development of ROS sensitive pathways and even specific ROS generating enzymes which became active part of cellular life.

REFERENCES

[1]   Ames, B.N., Shigenaga, M.K., Hagen, T.M. (1993) Oxidants, antioxidants, and the
        degenerative diseases of aging. *Proc Natl Acad Sci U S A.* 90, 7915-22.

[2]   Anversa, P., Cheng, W., Liu, Y., Leri, A., Redaelli, G., Kajstura, J. (1998) Apoptosis
        and myocardial infarction, *Basic Res. Cardiol.* 93, 8–12.

[3]   Bae, Y.S., Kang, S.W., Seo, M.S., Baines, I.C., Tekle, E., Chock, P.B., Rhee, S.G.
        (1997) Epidermal growth factor (EGF)-induced generation of hydrogen peroxide.
        Role in EGF receptor-mediated tyrosine phosphorylation. *J. Biol. Chem.* 272, 217–
        221.

[4]   Bae, Y.S., Sung, J.Y., Kim, O.S., Kim, Y.J., Hur, K.C., Kazlauskas, A., Rhee, S.G.
        (2000). Platelet-derived growth factor-induced H(2)O(2) production requires the
        activation of phosphatidylinositol 3-kinase. *J. Biol. Chem.* 275, 10527–10531.

[5]   Balaban, R. S., Nemoto, S., and Finkel, T. (2005) Mitochondria, oxidants, and
        ageing. *Cell* 120, 483–495.

[6]   Becker, L.B. (2004) New concepts in reactive oxygen species and cardiovascular
        reperfusion physiology, *Cardiovasc. Res.* 61, 461–470.

[7]   Bevan, A.P., Burgess, J.W., Yale, J.F., Drake, P.G., Lachance, D., Baquiran, G.,
        Shaver, A., Posner, B.I. (1995) In vivo insulin mimetic effects of pV compounds: role
        for tissue targeting in determining potency. *Am. J. Physiol.* 268, E60-6.

[8]   Bevan, A.P., Drake, P.G., Yale, J.F., Shaver, A., Posner, B.I. (1995) Peroxovanadium
        compounds: biological actions and mechanism of insulin-mimesis. *Mol. Cell
        Biochem.* 153, 49-58.

[9]   Bluher, M., Kahn, B.B., Kahn, C.R. (2003) Extended longevity in mice lacking the
        insulin receptor in adipose tissue. *Science.* 299, 572-4.

[10]   Brivanlou, A. H. and Darnell, J. E., Jr. (2002) Signal transduction and the control of
        gene expression. *Science.* 295, 813–818.

[11]   Brunelle, J.K., Bell E.L., Quesada, N.M., Vercauteren, K., Tiranti, V., Zeviani, M.,
        Scarpulla, R.C., Chandel, N.S. (2005) Oxygen sensing requires mitochondrial ROS
        but not oxidative phosphorylation. *Cell Metab.* 6, 409-14.

[12]   Buggisch, M., Ateghang, B., Ruhe, C., Strobel, C., Lange, S., Wartenberg, M., Sauer,
        H. (2007) Stimulation of ES-cell-derived cardiomyogenesis and neonatal cardiac cell
        proliferation by reactive oxygen species and NADPH oxidase. *J Cell Sci.* 120, 885-
        94.

[13]   Carriere, A., Fernandez, Y., Rigoulet, M., Penicaud, L., Casteilla, L. (2003) Inhibition
        of preadipocyte proliferation by mitochondrial reactive oxygen species. *FEBS Lett.*
        550, 163-7.

[14]   Carol, R.J and Dolan, L. (2006) The role of reactive oxygen species in cell growth:
        lessons from root hairs. *J. Exp. Bot.* 57, 1829-1834.

[15]   Caselli, A., Marzocchini, R., Camici, G., Manao, G., Moneti, G., Pieraccini, G.,
        Ramponi, G. (1998) The inactivation mechanism of low molecular weight
        phosphotyrosine-protein phosphatase by H2O2. *J. Biol. Chem.* 273, 32554-60.

[16] Catarzi, S., Biagioni, C., Giannoni, E., Favilli, F., Marcucci, T., Iantomasi, T., Vincenzini, M.T. (2005) Redox regulation of platelet-derived-growth-factor-receptor: role of NADPH-oxidase and c-Src tyrosine kinase. *Biochim. Biophys. Acta.* 1745, 66-75.

[17] Chance, B., Sies, H. and Boveris, A. (1979) Hydroperoxide metabolism in mammalian organs. *Physiol. Rev.* 59, 527–605.

[18] Chandel, N.S., McClintock, D.S., Feliciano, C.E., Wood, T.M., Melendez, J.A., Rodriguez, A.M., Schumacker, P.T. (2000) Reactive oxygen species generated at mitochondrial complex III stabilize hypoxia-inducible factor-1alpha during hypoxia: a mechanism of O2 sensing. *J. Biol. Chem.* 2000 275, 25130-8.

[19] Chavez, V., Mohri-Shiomi, A., Maadani, A., Vega, L.A., Garsin, D.A. (2007) Oxidative Stress Enzymes Are Required for DAF-16-Mediated Immunity Due to Generation of Reactive Oxygen Species by Caenorhabditis elegans. *Genetics* 176, 1567-1577.

[20] Chen, C.H., Cheng, T.H., Lin, H., Shih, N.L., Chen, Y.L., Chen, Y.S., Cheng, C.F., Lian, W.S., Meng, T.C., Chiu, W.T., Chen, J.J. (2006) Reactive oxygen species generation is involved in epidermal growth factor receptor transactivation through the transient oxidization of Src homology 2-containing tyrosine phosphatase in endothelin-1 signaling pathway in rat cardiac fibroblasts. *Mol. Pharmacol.* 69, 1347-55.

[21] Chen, K., Chen, J., Li, D., Zhang, X., Mehta, J.L. (2004) Angiotensin II regulation of collagen type I expression in cardiac fibroblasts: modulation by PPAR-gamma ligand pioglitazone. *Hypertension.* 44, 655-61.

[22] Chen, Y.H., lin, S.J., Chen, Y.L., Liu, P.L., Chen, J.W. (2006) Anti-inflammatory effects of different drugs/agents with antioxidant property on endothelial expression of adhesion molecules.*Cardiovasc. Hematol. Disord. Drug Targets.* 6, 279-304.

[23] Cheng-Hsien, C., Yung-Ho, H., Yuh-Mou, S., Chun-Cheng, H., Horng-Mo, L., Huei-Mei, H., Tso-Hsiao, C., (2006) Src homology 2-containing phosphotyrosine phosphatase regulates endothelin-1-induced epidermal growth factor receptor transactivation in rat renal tubular cell NRK-52E. *Pflugers Arch.* 452, 16-24.

[24] Chiarugi, P., Cirri, P., Marra, F., Raugei, G., Camici, G., Manao, G., Ramponi, G. (1997) LMW-PTP is a negative regulator of insulin-mediated mitotic and metabolic signaling. *Biochem. Biophys. Res. Commun.* 238, 676-82.

[25] Chiarugi, P., Cirri, P., Marra, F., Raugei, G., Fiaschi, T., Camici, G., Manao, G., Romanelli, R. G., Ramponi, G. (1998) The Src and signal transducers and activators of transcription pathways as specific targets for low molecular weight phosphotyrosine-protein phosphatase in platelet-derived growth factor signaling. *J. Biol. Chem.* 273, 6776-6785

[26] Cho KJ, Moon HE, Moini H, Packer L, Yoon DY, Chung AS. (2003). Alpha-lipoic acid inhibits adipocyte differentiation by regulating pro-adipogenic transcription factors via mitogen-activated protein kinase pathways. *J. Biol. Chem. 278*, 34823-33.

[27]   Cho, Y.M., Kwon, S., Pak, Y.K., Seol, H.W., Choi, Y.M., Park do, J., Park, K.S., Lee, H.K. (2006) Dynamic changes in mitochondrial biogenesis and antioxidant enzymes during the spontaneous differentiation of human embryonic stem cells. *Stem Cells.* 24, 2110-9.

[28]   Compernolle, V., Brusselmans, K., Franco, D., Moorman, A., Dewerchin, M., Collen, D., and Carmeliet, P. 2003. Cardia bifida, defective heart development and abnormal neural crest migration in embryos lacking hypoxia-inducible factor-1 . *Cardiovasc. Res.* 60, 569-579.

[29]   Covello, K.L., Kehler, J., Yu, H., Gordan, J.D., Arsham, A.M., Hu, C.J., Labosky, P.A., Simon, M.C., Keith, B. (2006) HIF-2alpha regulates Oct-4: effects of hypoxia on stem cell function, embryonic development, and tumor growth. *Genes.Dev.* 20, 557-70.

[30]   Coyle, J.T. and   Puttfarcken, P. (1993) Oxidative stress, glutamate, and neurodegenerative disorders. *Science.* 262, 689-95.

[31]   Czech, M.P., Lawrence, Jr, J.C., Lynn, W.S. (1974) Evidence for the involvement of sulfhydryl oxidation in the regulation of fat cell hexose transport by insulin. *Proc. Natl. Acad. Sci. U.S.A.* 71, 4173-4177.

[32]   den Hertog, J., Groen, A., van der Wijk, T. (2005) Redox regulation of protein-tyrosine phosphatases. *Arch. Biochem. Biophys.* 434,11–15.

[33]   Dernbach, E., Urbich, C., Brandes, R.P., Hofmann, W.K., Zeiher, A.M., Dimmeler, S. (2004) Antioxidative stress-associated genes in circulating progenitor cells: evidence for enhanced resistance against oxidative stress. *Blood.*104, 3591-7.

[34]   DiLisa, F. and   Bernardi, P. (2006) Mitochondria and ischemia–reperfusion injury of the heart: fixing a hole, *Cardiovasc. Res.* 70, 191–199.

[35]   D'Ippolito, G., Diabira, S., Howard, G.A., Roos, B.A., Schiller, P.C. (2006) Low oxygen tension inhibits osteogenic differentiation and enhances stemness of human MIAMI cells. *Bone.* 39, 513-22.

[36]   Drake, P.G., Bevan, A.P., Burgess, J.W., Bergeron, J.J., Posner, B.I. (1996) A role for tyrosine phosphorylation in both activation and inhibition of the insulin receptor tyrosine kinase in vivo. *Endocrinology.* 137, 4960-8.

[37]   ElShamy, W.M., Fridvall, L.K., Ernfors, P. (1998) Growth arrest failure, G1 restriction point override, and S phase death of sensory precursor cells in the absence of neurotrophin-3. *Neuron.* 21, 1003–1015.

[38]   Ema, M., Taya, S., Yokotani, N., Sogawa, K., Matsuda, Y., and Fujii-Kuriyama, Y. 1997. A novel bHLH-PAS factor with close sequence similarity to hypoxia-inducible factor 1   regulates the VEGF expression and is potentially involved in lung and vascular development. *Proc. Nat. Acad. Sci.* 94, 4273-4278.

[39]   Enrique-Tarancon, G., Marti, L., Morin, N., Lizcano, J.M., Unzeta, M., Sevilla, L., Camps, M., Palacin, M., Testar, X., Carpene, C., Zorzano, A. (1998) Role of semicarbazide-sensitive amine oxidase on glucose transport and GLUT4 recruitment to the cell surface in adipose cells. *J. Biol. Chem.* 273, 8025-32.

[40]   Ergun, S., Kilik, N., Ziegeler, G., Hansen, A., Nollau, P., Gotze, J., Wurmbach, J.H., Horst, A., Weil, J., Fernando, M., Wagener, C. (2000) CEA-related cell adhesion molecule 1: a potent angiogenic factor and a major effector of vascular endothelial growth factor. *Mol. Cell* 5, 311–320.

[41]   Feddersen, R.M., Ehlenfeldt, R., Yunis, W.S., Clark, H.B., Orr, H.T. (1992) Disrupted cerebellar cortical development and progressive degeneration of Purkinje cells in SV40 T antigen transgenic mice. *Neuron.* 9, 955–966.

[42]   Fink, T., Abildtrup, L., Fogd, K., Abdallah, B.M., Kassem, M., Ebbesen, P., Zachar, V. (2004) Induction of adipocyte-like phenotype in human mesenchymal stem cells by hypoxia. *Stem. Cells.* 22, 1346-55.

[43]   Finkel, T. (1998) Oxygen radicals and signaling. *Curr. Opin. Cell Biol.* 10, 248–253.

[44]   Flamme, I., Frohlich, T., von Reutern, M., Kappel, A., Damert, A., and Risau, W. 1997. HRF, a putative basic helix-loop-helix-PAS-domain transcription factor is closely related to hypoxia-inducible factor-1 and developmentally expressed in blood vessels. *Mech. Dev.* 63, 51-60.

[45]   Fliss, H. and Gattinger, D. (1996) Apoptosis in ischemic and reperfused rat myocardium, *Circ. Res.* 79, 949–956.

[46]   Fontana, E., Boucher, J., Marti, L., Lizcano, J.M., Testar, X., Zorzano, A., Carpene, C. (2001) Amine oxidase substrates mimic several of the insulin effects on adipocyte differentiation in 3T3 F442A cells. *Biochem. J.* 356, 769-77.

[47]   Frade, J.M. (2000) Unscheduled re-entry into the cell cycle induced by NGF precedes cell death in nascent retinal neurones. *J. Cell Sci.* 113, 1139–1148.

[48]   Gerald, D., Berra, E., Frapart, Y.M., Chan, D.A., Giaccia, A.J., Mansuy, D., Pouysségur, J., Yaniv, M., Mechta-Grigoriou, F. (2004) JunD reduces tumor angiogenesis by protecting cells from oxidative stress. *Cell.* 118, 781-94.

[49]   Gleadle, J.M., Ebert, B.L., Ratcliffe, P.J. (1995) Diphenylene iodonium inhibits the induction of erythropoietin and other mammalian genes by hypoxia. Implications for the mechanism of oxygen sensing. *Eur. J. Biochem.* 234, 92-9.

[50]   Gupta R, Karpatkin S, Basch RS. (2006) Hematopoiesis and stem cell renewal in long-term bone marrow cultures containing catalase. *Blood.* 107,1837-46.

[51]   Gustafsson, M.V., Zheng, X., Pereira, T., Gradin, K., Jin, S., Lundkvist, J., Ruas, J.L., Poellinger, L., Lendahl, U., Bondesson, M. (2005) Hypoxia requires notch signaling to maintain the undifferentiated cell state. *Dev. Cell.* 9, 617-28.

[52]   Guzy, R.D., Hoyos, B., Robin, E., Chen, H., Liu, L., Mansfield, K.D., Simon, M.C., Hammerling, U., Schumacker, P.T. (2005) Mitochondrial complex III is required for hypoxia-induced ROS production and cellular oxygen sensing. *Cell. Metab.* 6, 401-8.

[53]   Guzy, R.D., Mack, M.M., Schumacker, P.T. (2007) Mitochondrial Complex III Is Required for Hypoxia-Induced ROS Production and Gene Transcription in Yeast. *Antioxid. Redox. Signal.* 9, 1317-28.

[54]   Halestrap, A.P.,Clarke, S.J., Khaliulin, I. (2007) The role of mitochondria in protection of the heart by preconditioning. *Biochim Biophys Acta.* 1767, 1007-1031.

[55]   Halliwell, B. (1984) Chloroplast metabolism. Oxford University Press, Oxford.

[56]   Halliwell, B. (1992) Reactive oxygen species and the central nervous system. *J. Neurochem* 59, 1609-1623.

[57]   Halliwell, B. and Gutteridge, J. M. C. (1998) Free Radicals in Biology and Medicine
        Oxford University Press, Oxford.

[58]   Havel, P.J. (2004) Update on adipocyte hormones: regulation of energy balance and
        carbohydrate/lipid metabolism. *Diabetes.* 53, S143-51.

[59]   Huang, L.E., Arany, Z., Livingston, D.M., Bunn, H.F. (1996) Activation of hypoxia-
        inducible transcription factor depends primarily upon redox-sensitive stabilization of
        its alpha subunit. *J. Biol. Chem.* 271, 32253-9.

[60]   Ito, K., Hirao, A., Arai, F., Matsuoka, S., Takubo, K., Hamaguchi, I., Nomiyama, K.,
        Hosokawa, K., Sakurada, K., Nakagata, N., Ikeda, Y., Mak, T.W., Suda, T. (2004)
        Regulation of oxidative stress by ATM is required for self-renewal of haematopoietic
        stem cells. *Nature.* 431, 997-1002.

[61]   Ito, K., Hirao, A., Arai, F., Takubo, K., Matsuoka, S., Miyamoto, K., Ohmura, M.,
        Naka, K., Hosokawa, K., Ikeda, Y., Suda, T. (2006) Reactive oxygen species act
        through p38 MAPK to limit the lifespan of hematopoietic stem cells. *Nat Med.*
        12,446-51.

[62]   Iwasaka, C., Tanaka, K., Abe, M., Sato, Y. (1996) Ets-1 regulates angiogenesis by
        inducing the expression of urokinase-type plasminogen activator and matrix
        metalloproteinase-1 and the migration of vascular endothelial cells. *J. Cell. Physiol.*
        169, 522-31.

[63]   Jabs, T., Tschope, M., Colling, C., Hahlbrock, K., Scheel, D. (!997) Elicitor-
        stimulated ion fluxes and O2- from the oxidative burst are essential components in
        triggering defense gene activation and phytoalexin synthesis in parsley. *Proc. Natl.
        Acad. Sci. USA.* 94, 4800-4805.

[64]   Jang, Y.Y., Sharkis, S.J. (2007) A low level of reactive oxygen species selects for
        primitive hematopoietic stem cells that may reside in the low-oxygenic niche. *Blood .*
        In press.

[65]   Jenner, P. (1994) Oxidative damage in neurodegenerative disease. *Lancet* 344, 796-
        798.

[66]   Kevin, L.G. Camara, A.K.S. Riess, M.L. Novalija E., Stowe, D.F. (2003) Ischemic
        preconditioning alters real-time measure of O-2 radicals in intact hearts with ischemia
        and reperfusion, *Am. J. Physiol.* 284, H566–H574.

[67]   Kim, Y.M., Kim, K.E., Koh, G.Y., Ho, Y.S., Lee, K.J. (2006) Hydrogen peroxide
        produced by angiopoietin-1 mediates angiogenesis. *Cancer Res.* 66, 6167-74.

[68]   Klein, J.A. and   Ackerman, S.L. (2003) Oxidative stress, cell cycle, and
        neurodegeneration. *J. Clin. Invest.* 111. 785-93.

[69]   Krieger-Brauer, H.I., Kather, H. (1992) Human fat cells possess a plasma membrane-
        bound H2O2-generating system that is activated by insulin via a mechanism
        bypassing the receptor kinase. *J. Clin. Invest.* 89, 1006-13.

[70]   Krieger-Brauer, H.I., Kather, H. (1995) The stimulus-sensitive H2O2-generating
        system present in human fat-cell plasma membranes is multireceptor-linked and under
        antagonistic control by hormones and cytokines. *Biochem. J.* 307, 543-8.

[71]   Kwak, J.M., Mori, I.C., Pei, Z.M., Leonhardt, N., Torres, M.A., Dangl, J.L., Bloom, R.E., Bodde, S., Jones, J,D., Schroeder, J.L. (2003) NADPH oxidase AtrbohD and AtrbohF genes function in ROS-dependent ABA signaling in Arabidopsis. *EMBO J.* 22, 2623-2633.

[72]   Lawrence, J. C., Larner, J. (1978) Activation of glycogen synthase in rat adipocytes by insulin and glucose involves increased glucose transport and phosphorylation. *J. Biol. Chem.* 253, 2104-2113.

[73]   Leaman, D. W., Leung, S., Li, X., Stark, G. R. (1996) Regulation of STAT-dependent pathways by growth factors and cytokines. *FASEB J.* 10, 1578–1588.

[74]   Levy, A.P., Levy, N.S., Wegner, S., Goldberg, M.A. (1995) Transcriptional regulation of the rat vascular endothelial growth factor gene by hypoxia. *J. Biol. Chem.* 270,13333–13340. .

[75]   Lim, S.D., Sun, C., Lambeth, J.D., Marshall, F., Amin, M., Chung, L., Petros, J.A., Arnold, R.S. (2005) Increased Nox1 and hydrogen peroxide in prostate cancer. *Prostate.* 62, 200-7.

[76]   Lin, Q., Lee, Y.J., Yun, Z. Differentiation arrest by hypoxia. *J. Biol. Chem.* 2006 Oct 13;281(41):30678-83.

[77]   Little, S.A., de Haen, C. (1980) Effects of hydrogen peroxide on basal and hormone-stimulated lipolysis in perifused rat fat cells in relation to the mechanism of action of insulin. *J. Biol. Chem.* 255, 10888-95.

[78]   Lonergan, T., Brenner, C., Bavister, B. (2006) Differentiation-related changes in mitochondrial properties as indicators of stem cell competence. *J. Cell Physiol.* 208, 149-53.

[79]   MacDougald, O. A., Cornelius, P., Liu, R. and Lane, M. D. (1995) Insulin regulates the transcription of the CAAT/enhancer binding protein (C/EBP) a, b, and d genes in fully-differentiated 3T3-L1 adipocytes. *J. Biol. Chem.* 270, 647-654.

[80]   Madhavan, L., Ourednik, V., Ourednik, J. (2006) Increased "vigilance" of antioxidant mechanisms in neural stem cells potentiates their capability to resist oxidative stress. *Int J. Radiat. Biol.* 82, 640-7.

[81]   Mahadev, K., Zilbering, A., Zhu, L., Goldstein, B.J. (2001) Insulin-stimulated hydrogen peroxide reversibly inhibits protein-tyrosine phosphatase 1b in vivo and enhances the early insulin action cascade. *J. Biol. Chem.* 276, 21938-42.

[82]   Majander, A., Finel, M., Wikstrom, M. (1994) Diphenyleneiodonium inhibits reduction of iron-sulfur clusters in the mitochondrial NADH-ubiquinone oxidoreductase (Complex I). *J. Biol. Chem.* 269, 21037-42.

[83]   Marti, L., Morin, N., Enrique-Tarancon, G., Prevot, D., Lafontan, M., Testar, X., Zorzano, A., Carpene, C. (1998) Tyramine and vanadate synergistically stimulate glucose transport in rat adipocytes by amine oxidase-dependent generation of hydrogen peroxide *J. Pharmacol. Exp. Ther.* 285, 342-9.

[84]   Maxwell, P. H. (2005) Hypoxia-inducible factor as a physiological regulator. *Exp. Physiol.* 90, 791–797.

[85]   May, J. M. and de Haen, C. (1979) The insulin-like effect of hydrogen peroxide on pathways of lipid synthesis in rat adipocytes. *J. Biol. Chem.* 254, 9017-9021

[86]   Meng, T.C., Buckley, D.A., Galic, S., Tiganis, T., Tonks, N.K. (2004) Regulation of insulin signaling through reversible oxidation of the protein-tyrosine phosphatases TC45 and PTP1B. *J. Biol. Chem.* 279, 37716-25.

[87]   Mercier, N., Moldes, M., El Hadri, K., Feve, B. (2001) Semicarbazide-sensitive amine oxidase activation promotes adipose conversion of 3T3-L1 cells. *Biochem. J.* 358, 335-42.

[88]   Mesri, E.A., Federoff, H.J., Brownlee, M. (1995) Expression of vascular endothelial growth factor from a defective herpes simplex virus type 1 amplicon vector induces angiogenesis in mice. *Circ. Res.* 76, 161–167.

[89]   Morrison, S.J., Csete, M., Groves, A.K., Melega, W., Wold, B., Anderson, D.J. (2000) Culture in reduced levels of oxygen promotes clonogenic sympathoadrenal differentiation by isolated neural crest stem cells.*J. Neurosci.* 20, 7370-7376.

[90]   Murphy. T.H., Miyamoto, M., Sastre, A., Schnaar, R.L., Coyle, J.T. (1989) Glutamate toxicity in a neuronal cell line involves inhibition of cystine transport leading to oxidative stress. *Neuron.* 2, 1547-58.

[91]   Moldes, M., Fe' ve, B., Pairault, J. (1999) Molecular cloning of a major mRNA species in murine 3T3 adipocyte lineage : differentiation-dependent expression, regulation, and identification as semicarbazide-sensitive amine oxidase. *J. Biol. Chem.* 274, 9515-9523.

[92]   Murillo, M.M., Carmona-Cuenca, I., Del Castillo, G., Ortiz, C., Roncero, C., Sanchez, A., Fernandez, M., Fabregat, I. (2007) Activation of NADPH oxidase by transforming growth factor-beta in hepatocytes mediates up-regulation of epidermal growth factor receptor ligands through a nuclear factor-kappaB-dependent mechanism. *Biochem. J.* 405, 251-9.

[93]   Nagy, J.A., Vasile, E., Feng, D., Sundberg, C., Brown, L.F., Detmar, M.J., Lawitts, J.A., Benjamin, L., Tan, X., Manseau, E.J., Dvorak, A.M., Dvorak, H.F. (2002) Vascular permeability factor/vascular endothelial growth factor induces lymphangiogenesis as well as angiogenesis. *J. Exp. Med.* 196, 1497–1506.

[94]   Nicosia, R.F., Nicosia, S.V., Smith, M. (1994) Vascular endothelial growth factor, platelet-derived growth factor, and insulin-like growth factor-1 promote rat aortic angiogenesis in vitro. *Am. J. Pathol.* 145, 1023-1029.

[95]   Pei, Z.M., Murata, Y., Benning, G., Thomine, S., Klusener, B., Alle, G.J., Grill, E., Schroeder, J.L. (2000) Calcium channels activated by hydrogen peroxide mediate abscisic acid signalling in guard cells. *Nature* 406, 731-734.

[96]   Pepper, M.S., Ferrara, N., Orci, L., Montesano, R. (1992) Potent synergism between vascular endothelial growth factor and basic fibroblast growth factor in the induction of angiogenesis in vitro. *Biochem Biophys Res Commun* 189, 824–831.

[97]   Pepper, M.S., Wasi, S., Ferrara, N., Orci, L., Montesano, R. (1994) In vitro angiogenic and proteolytic properties of bovine lymphatic endothelial cells. *Exp. Cell. Res.* 210, 298–305.

[98]   Phillips, G.D., Stone, A.M., Jones, B.D., Schultz, J.C., Whitehead, R.A., Knighton, D.R. (1994) Vascular endothelial growth factor (rhVEGF165) stimulates direct angiogenesis in the rabbit cornea. *In Vivo* 8, 961–965.

[99]   Piccoli, C., D'Aprile, A., Ripoli, M., Scrima, R., Lecce, L., Boffoli, D., Tabilio, A.,
         Capitanio, N., Grayson, W.L., Zhao, F., Bunnell, B., Ma, T. (2007) Bone-marrow
         derived hematopoietic stem/progenitor cells express multiple isoforms of NADPH
         oxidase and produce constitutively reactive oxygen species. *Biochem. Biophys. Res.
         Commun.* 353, 965-72.

[100]   Plouet, J., Schilling, J., Gospodarowicz, D. (1989) Isolation and characterization of a
         newly identified endothelial cell mitogen produced by AtT20 cells. *EMBO J.* 8,
         3801–3808.

[101]   Pomytkin, I.A., Kolesova, O.E. (2002) Key role of succinate dehydrogenase in
         insulin-induced inactivation of protein tyrosine phosphatases. *Bull Exp Biol Med.*
         133, 568-70.

[102]   Pomytkin, I.A. and Kolesova, O.E. (2003) Effect of insulin on the rate of hydrogen
         peroxide generation in mitochondria. *Bull. Exp. Biol. Med.* 135, 541-2.

[103]   Posner, B.I., Faure, R., Burgess, J.W., Bevan, A.P., Lachance, D., Zhang-Sun, G.,
         Fantus, I.G., Ng, J.B., Hall, D.A., Lum, B.S. (1994) Peroxovanadium compounds. A
         new class of potent phosphotyrosine phosphatase inhibitors which are insulin
         mimetics. *J. Biol. Chem.* 269, 4596-604.

[104]   Pugh, C.W., Tan, C.C., Jones, R.W., Ratcliffe, P.J. (1991) Functional analysis of an
         oxygen-regulated transcriptional enhancer lying 3' to the mouse erythropoietin gene.
         Proc. Nat. Acad. Sci. 88, 10553-10557.

[105]   Quinn, J., Findlay, V.J., Dawson , K., Millar, J.B., Jones, N., Morgan, B.A., Toone,
         W.M. (2002) Distinct regulatory proteins control the graded transcriptional response
         to increasing H(2)O(2) levels in fission yeast Schizosaccharomyces pombe. *Mol. Biol.
         Cell.* 13, 805-816.

[106]   Riva, C., Donadieu, E., Magnan, J., Lavieille, J.P. (2007) Age-related hearing loss in
         CD/1 mice is associated to ROS formation and HIF target proteins up-regulation in
         the cochlea. *Exp. Gerontol.* 42, 327-336.

[107]   Ren, H., Cao, Y., Zhao, Q., Li, J., Zhou, C., Liao, L., Jia, M., Zhao, Q., Cai, H., Han,
         Z.C., Yang, R., Chen, G., Zhao, R.C. (2006) Proliferation and differentiation of bone
         marrow stromal cells under hypoxic conditions. *Biochem. Biophys. Res. Commun.*
         347, 12-21.

[108]   Rodriguez, A.A., grunberg, K.A., Taleisnik, E.L. (2002) Reactive oxygen species in
         the elongation zone of maize leaves are necessary for leaf extension. *Plant Physiol.*
         129, 1627-1632.

[109]   Rosenberger, J., Petrovics, G., Buzas, B. (2001) Oxidative stress induces proorphanin
         FQ and proenkephalin gene expression in astrocytes through p38- and ERK-MAP
         kinases and NF-kappaB. *J. Neurochem.* 79, 35-44.

[110]   Sauer, H., Neukirchen, W., Rahimi, G., Grunheck, F., Hescheler, J., Wartenberg, M.
         (2004) Involvement of reactive oxygen species in cardiotrophin-1-induced
         proliferation of cardiomyocytes differentiated from murine embryonic stem cells.*Exp.
         Cell. Res.* 294, 313-24.

[111]   Sauer, H., Rahimi, G., Hescheler, J., Wartenberg, M. (2000) Role of reactive oxygen
         species and phosphatidylinositol 3-kinase in cardiomyocyte differentiation of
         embryonic stem cells. *FEBS Lett.* 476, 218-23.

[112] Semenza, G.L. (2000) HIF-1 and human disease: One highly involved factor. *Genes and Dev.* 14, 1983-1991.

[113] Semenza, G. L. (2004) Hydroxylation of HIF-1: oxygen sensing at the molecular level. *Physiology (Bethesda)* 19, 176–182.

[114] Schapira, A.H.V. (1996) Entering the powerhouse. Odyssey 2, 8.

[115] Shigenaga, M.K., Hagen, T.M., Ames, B.N. (1994) Oxidative damage and mitochondrial decay in aging. *Proc. Natl .Acad. Sci. U S A.* 91, 10771-8.

[116] Shono, T., Ono, M., Izumi, H., Jimi, S.I., Matsushima, K., Okamoto, T., Kohno, K., Kuwano, M. (1996) Involvement of the transcription factor NF-kappaB in tubular morphogenesis of human microvascular endothelial cells by oxidative stress. *Mol. Cell Biol.* 16, 4231-9.

[117] Siwik, D.A., Pagano, p.J., Colucci, W.S. (2001) Oxidative stress regulates collagen synthesis and matrix metalloproteinase activity in cardiac fibroblasts. *Am. J. Physiol. Cell Physiol.* 280, C53-60.

[118] Smith, J., Ladi, E., Mayer-Proschel, M., Noble, M. (2000) Redox state is a central modulator of the balance between self-renewal and differentiation in a dividing glial precursor cell. *Proc Natl Acad Sci U S A.* 97, 10032-7.

[119] Solaini, G. and Harris, D.A. (2005) Biochemical dysfunction in heart mitochondria exposed to ischaemia and reperfusion, *Biochem. J.* 390, 377–394.

[120] Stone, J. R. and Yang, S. (2006) Hydrogen peroxide: a signaling messenger. *Antioxid. Redox Signal.* 8, 243–270.

[121] Sun, J.Z., Tang, X.L., Park, S.W., Qiu, Y., Turrens, J.F., Bolli, R. (1996) Evidence for an essential role of ROS in the genesis of late preconditioning against myocardial stunning in conscious pigs. *J.Clin.Invest.* 97, 562-576.

[122] Suzuki, K., Nakamura, M., Hatanaka, Y., Kayanoki, Y., Tatsumi, H., Taniguchi, N. (1997) Induction of apoptotic cell death in human endothelial cells treated with snake venom: implication of intracellular reactive oxygen species and protective effects of glutathione and superoxide dismutases. *J. Biochem. (Tokyo).* 122, 1260-4.

[123] Szatrowski, T.P. and Nathan, C.F. (1991) Production of large amounts of hydrogen peroxide by human tumor cells. *Cancer Res.* 51, 794-8.

[124] Takemodo, D., Tanaka, A., Scott, B. (2007) NADPH oxidases in fungi: Diverse roles of reactive oxygen species in fungal cellular differentiation. *Fungal Genet Biol.* In press.

[125] Thannickal, V. J., Fanburg, B. L. (1995) Activation of an H_2O_2-generating NADH oxidase in human lung fibroblasts by transforming growth factor beta 1. *J. Biol. Chem.* 270, 30334-30338.

[126] Thompson, J.G., McNaughton, C., Gasparrini, B., McGowan, L.T., Tervit, H.R. (2000) Effect of inhibitors and uncouplers of oxidative phosphorylation during compaction and blastulation of bovine embryos cultured in vitro. *J Reprod Fertil.* 118, 47-55.

[127] Tian, H., McKnight, S.L., and Russell, D.W. 1997. Endothelial PAS domain protein 1 (EPAS1), a transcription factor selectively expressed in endothelial cells. *Genes and Dev.* 11, 72-82.

[128]   Tolentino, M.J., Miller, J.W., Gragoudas, E.S., Chatzistefanou, K., Ferrara, N., Adamis, A.P. (1996) Vascular endothelial growth factor is sufficient to produce iris neovascularization and neovascular glaucoma in a nonhuman primate. *Arch. Ophthalmol* 114, 964–970.

[129]   Tothova, Z., Kollipara, R., Huntly, B.J., Lee, B.H., Castrillon, D.H., Cullen, D.E., McDowell, E.P., Lazo-Kallanian, S., Williams, I.R., Sears, C., Armstrong, S.A., Passegue, E., DePinho, R.A., Gilliland, D.G. (2007) FoxOs are critical mediators of hematopoietic stem cell resistance to physiologic oxidative stress. *Cell.* 128, 325-339.

[130]   Tsatmali, M., Walcott, E.C., Crossin, K.L. (2005) Newborn neurons acquire high levels of reactive oxygen species and increased mitochondrial proteins upon differentiation from progenitors. *Brain Res.* 1040, 137-50.

[131]   Usatyuk, P.V., Vepa, S., Watkins, T., He, D., Parinandi, N.L., Natarajan, V. (2003) Redox regulation of reactive oxygen species-induced p38 MAP kinase activation and barrier dysfunction in lung microvascular endothelial cells. *Antioxid. Redox. Signal.* 5, 723-730.

[132]   Ushio-Fukai, M., Alexander, R.W., Akers, M., Griendling, K.K. (1998) p38 MAP kinase is a critical component of the redox-sensitive signaling pathways by angiotensin II: role in vascular smooth muscle cell hypertrophy. *J Biol Chem.* 273,15022–15029.

[133]   Ushio-Fukai, M., Zuo, L., Ikeda, S., Tojo, T., Patrushev, N.A., Alexander, R.W. (2005) cAbl Tyrosine Kinase Mediates Reactive Oxygen Species– and Caveolin-Dependent AT$_1$ Receptor Signaling in Vascular Smooth Muscle_*Circulation Research.* 97, 829-836.

[134]   Valko, M., Leibfritz, D., Moncol, J., Cronin, M.T., Mazur, M., Telser, J. (2007) Free radicals and antioxidants in normal physiological functions and human disease. *Int. J. Biochem Cell Biol.* 39, 44-84.

[135]   Vivancos, A.P., Castillo, E.A., Jones, N., Ayte, J., Hidalgo, E. (2004) Activation of the redox sensor Pap1 by hydrogen peroxide requires modulation of the intracellular oxidant concentration. *Mol. Microbiol.* 52, 1427-1435.

[136]   Wagner, S., Hussain, M.Z., Hunt, T.K., Bacic, B., Becker, H.D. (2004) Stimulation of fibroblast proliferation by lactate-mediated oxidants. *Wound Repair Regen.* 12, 368-73.

[137]   Walsh, D.A. (2007) Pathophysiological mechanisms of angiogenesis. *Adv. Clin. Chem.* 44, 187-221.

[138]   Wang, F.S., Wang, C.J., Sheen-Chen, S.M., Kuo, Y.R., Chen, R.F., Yang, K.D. (2002) Superoxide mediates shock wave induction of ERK-dependent osteogenic transcription factor (CBFA1) and mesenchymal cell differentiation toward osteoprogenitors. *J Biol Chem.* 277, 10931-7.

[139]   Watnick, R.S., Cheng, Y.N., Rangarajan, A., Ince, T.A., Weinberg, R.A. (2003) Ras modulates Myc activity to repress thrombospondin-1 expression and increase tumor angiogenesis. Cancer Cell. 3, 219-231.

[140]   Wiesener, M., Turley, H., Allen, W., William, C., Eckardt, K., Talks, K., Wood, S., Gatter, K., Harris, A., Pugh, C., Ratcliffe, P.J., Maxwell, P.H. (1998) Induction of endothelial PAS domain protein-1 by hypoxia: Characterization and comparison with hypoxia-inducible factor-1α. *Blood.* 92, 2260-2268.

[141]   Yasuda, M., Ohzeki, Y., Shimizu, S., Naito, S., Ohtsuru, A., Yamamoto, T., Kuroiwa, Y. (1999) Stimulation of in vitro angiogenesis by hydrogen peroxide and the relation with ETS-1 in endothelial cells. *Life Sci.* 64, 249-58.

[142]   Zhang, B., Berger, J., Zhou, G., Elbrecht, A., Biswas, S., White-Carrington, S., Szalkowski, D., Moller, D. E. (1996) Insulin- and mitogen-activated protein kinasemediated phosphorylation and activation of peroxisome proliferator-activated receptor c. *J. Biol. Chem.* 271, 31771-31774.

[143]   Zhao, T., Zhang, CP., Zhu, L.L., Jin, B., Huang, X., Fan, M. (2007) Hypoxia promotes the differentiation of neural stem cells into dopaminergic neurons. *Sheng Li Xue Bao.* 59, 273-7.

[144]   Zweier, J.L. and Talukder, M.A.H.. (2006) The role of oxidants and free radicals in reperfusion injury, *Cardiovasc. Res.* 70, 181–190.

In: Progress in Cell Growth Process Research
Editor: Takumi Hayashi, pp. 89-118

ISBN 978-1-60456-325-2
© 2008 Nova Science Publishers, Inc.

Chapter 3

IMPROVED PROLIFERATION OF NORMAL SOMATIC CELLS BY TREATMENT OF CONDITIONED MEDIA DERIVED FROM HYBRID CELLS

M. Q. Islam[1, 2, 3*]

[1]CellAmp Laboratories, Westmansgatan 29, Wahlbecks Industrial Park,
S-582 16 Linköping, Sweden
[2]Laboratory of Cancer Genetics, Laboratory Medicine Center (LMC), University
Hospital Linköping, S-581 85 Linköping, Sweden
[3]Institution of Clinical and Experimental Medicine, (Formerly Department of
Biomedicine and Surgery), Faculty of Health Sciences, Linköping University,
S-581 85 Linköping, Sweden

ABSTRACT

Generally, normal diploid somatic cells cultivated in standard growth media supplemented with ordinary fetal bovine serum do not replicate indefinitely. However, under similar culture conditions transformed cells with abnormal chromosome complements replicate indefinitely. Interestingly, embryonic stem cells contain diploid karyotype yet they have unlimited proliferation potential if maintained in appropriate culture conditions. Although normal somatic stem cells also contain diploid chromosomes, they are unable to proliferate indefinitely in vitro. In contrast to embryonic stem cells, somatic stem cells can potentially be used in autologous cell transplantation but their restricted proliferation limits their successful application in clinical settings. Therefore, improvement of proliferation of somatic stem cells is not only desirable for clinical but also for research applications. We have recently developed

[*]Correspondence: M. Quamrul Islam, Ph.D., CellAmp Laboratories, Westmansgatan 29, Wahlbecks Industrial Park, S-582 16 Linköping, Sweden, Tel: +46 13 273110 e-mail: quis@cellamplabs.com.

a two-step cell culture protocol to improve the proliferation of various types of normal somatic cells derived from diverse mammalian species. In the first step of the method, immortal hybrid cells are generated containing polyploid chromosomes derived from normal cells by fusing normal somatic cells with a hypo-diploid immortal murine cell line GM05267 using polyethylene glycol. In the second step, conditioned media are collected from the proliferating hybrid cells and subsequent cultivation of normal parental somatic cells in the presence of this conditioned media to generate long-term growing somatic cell lines containing diploid chromosomes. In the present article, the background of the discovery of a two-step cell culture protocol will be presented along with an update of recent findings to demonstrate that this method has general applicability. The generation of hybrid cells using the specific murine cell line can be used in the generation of hybrids with tissue specific cell types and can be used to produce tissue specific growth-factors to improve the proliferation of tissue specific somatic cells, including adult stem cells.

Keywords: somatic cell, embryonic stem cell, adult stem cell, autologous transplantation, senescence, immortality, conditioned media, method.

INTRODUCTION

Somatic Cell Culture Methodology and Cellular Senescence

Normal somatic cells replicate for a limited number of times *in vitro* before entering a non-dividing state called replicative senescence (Hayflick 1965). Distinguishing features of senescent cells are a flattened morphology and an inability to synthesize DNA in response to serum growth factor stimuli (Goldstein 1990). Senescent cells remain viable for extended periods of time if adequate nutrients are supplied through regular changes of medium. Different types of replicative senescence have been described. They include (i) replicative senescence, thought to be caused by telomere shortening, (ii) premature senescence, assumed to be induced by activation of certain oncogenes, and (iii) stress-induced senescence, suggested to be induced by inadequate culturing conditions (Serrano and Blasco 2001; Wright and Shay 2001; Lloyd 2002; Ben-Porath and Weinberg 2005). It has been suggested that replicative senescence in normal cells is a natural safeguard against unrestrained cell proliferation to prevent neoplastic transformation (Wynford-Thomas 1999; Campisi 2001; Lynch 2006; Zhang 2007). However, a unified theory to explain replicative senescence is still lacking (Rubin 1997; Rubin 2002; Blagosklonny 2003; Blagosklonny 2006).

Normal somatic cells are commonly cultivated using standard cell culture media supplemented with fetal bovine serum. In this condition most of the normal somatic cell types proliferate for a limited number of times (Hayflick 1965). Conversely, under similar culture conditions tumor and transformed cells carrying abnormal genomes are able to divide indefinitely (Duncan et al. 2000; Drayton and Peters 2002; Yaswen and Stampfer 2002). This observation suggests that normal somatic cells perhaps overcome their limited proliferation by disrupting normal growth regulatory functions through permanent damage of genetic materials (Hahn and Weinberg 2002). Interestingly, there are instances where normal somatic cells under appropriate cell culture conditions can proliferate extensively (Loo et al. 1987;

Mathon et al. 2001; Ramirez et al. 2001; Tang et al. 2001). This may indicate that normal cells grown under optimized culture conditions can proliferate in a manner similar to immortal cells. It is commonly believed that normal cells experience various types of culture shocks that induce cell cycle arrest and consequent cessation of replication (Ben-Porath and Weinberg 2005).

Genetic Manipulation of Somatic Cells to Improve Proliferation

Normal somatic cells can be transformed into cell lines of indefinite proliferation by transferring specific genes, although no consensus has yet been reached on the number of genetic events required for the transformation of a normal cell (Hahn and Weinberg 2002; Akagi et al. 2003). Nevertheless, cell lines with indefinite proliferative capacity can be generated from normal somatic cells by forced expression of the catalytic component of human telomerase (hTERT) (Drayton and Peters 2002; Harley 2002; Newbold 2002). It should be remembered that normal human somatic cells are more resistant to immortalization than their rodent counterparts (Itahana et al. 2004; Smith and Kipling 2004; Campisi 2005).

Fusion of normal somatic cells with embryonic stem (ES) cells can generate hybrid cells with indefinite proliferation and the resulting hybrid stem cells display many features of ES cells including improved self-renewal and pluripotency (Ambrosi and Rasmussen 2005; Alberio et al. 2006). This indicates that the ES cell genome has the ability to reprogram the somatic cell genome into a state similar to that of the embryo. However, the continuous presence of ES cell genome in the hybrid cells is necessary to maintain ES cell phenotypes. These hybrid stem cells often retain near-diploid chromosomes (Matveeva et al. 1998; Medvinsky and Smith 2003; Matveeva et al. 2005). Because of rapid loss of chromosomes hybrid stem cells suffer from limitations in expression of cellular factors necessary for generative purposes. Instead of transferring the entire cell genome by cell-cell fusion, attempts have been made to convert somatic cells directly into ES-like cells by the introduction of a selected set of genes (Takahashi and Yamanaka 2006; Okita et al. 2007; Wernig et al. 2007). However, the induced pluripotent stem (iPS) cells produce both benign (teratomas) and malignant tumors upon sub-cutaneous transplantation (Okita et al. 2007). Although direct conversion of somatic cells into embryonic cells by gene transfer has many advantages, their clinical application may not be possible because of tumor related problems.

Epigenetic Reprogramming of Somatic Cells to Improve Proliferation

The nuclei of somatic cells can be reprogrammed by the cytoplasmic factors of enucleated oocytes, a technique commonly known as somatic cell nuclear transfer (SCNT), to generate diploid embryonic stem cells (Chen et al. 2003). However, the success of somatic nuclei reprogramming by SCNT method is limited because of technical problems and scarcity of oocytes (Hall et al. 2006). An alternative of SCNT technique has been developed to reprogram somatic cells for long-term proliferation by temporary cell-cell contact without the transfer of any genetic or cytoplasmic factors and this epigenetic reprogramming technique can be applied to generate patient-specific stem cells (Islam et al. 2007a). A two-step cell culture protocol has been developed to improve the proliferation of normal somatic cells by replicative reprogramming (Islam et al. 2006b; Islam et al. 2007b). In the first step of the method, immortal hybrid cells are generated containing polyploid somatic cell chromosomes by fusing normal somatic cells with the immortal murine cell line GM05267. In the second step, conditioned media (CM) are collected from the highly proliferating hybrid cells and normal somatic cells are cultivated in the presence of this hybrid cell-derived CM. Continuous treatment of normal somatic cells by hybrid cell CM produces cell lines with diploid chromosomes (Islam et al. 2006b). In the present article, details of the discovery of two-step cell culture protocol will be presented along with an update of recent results to demonstrate that this method has general applicability.

BACKGROUND OF THE GENERATION OF IMMORTALIZED HYBRID CELLS WITH UNIQUE PROPERTIES

Methodology to Generate Hybrid Cells

Spontaneous fusion of cells *in vitro* and generation of hybrid cells was first discovered in early sixties (Barski et al. 1961; Barski and Cornefert 1962). Subsequently, it was found that hybrid cells can be produced by treating mixed cells with inactivated virus or polyethylene glycol (PEG). Since that time, cell hybridization has become an important research tool in many areas of biology (Ruddle and Creagan 1975; Puck and Kao 1982; Duelli and Lazebnik 2003).

Hybrid cells can be produced routinely by co-culture of two types of adherent cells with short time exposure to PEG (Islam and Islam 1994; Islam and Islam 2000). Essential steps to generate PEG-mediated induced hybrid cells are presented in Figure 1. In brief, after individual trypsinization of two types of monolayer cells, equal numbers of cells (1×10^6 cells from each parent) are mixed in a tube and the mixed cells are plated in a 60 mm culture dish. Incubation for three to four hours allows the attachment and spreading of cells. Twenty to thirty minutes prior to PEG treatment, serum-free medium containing 100 µg/ml of phytohemagglutinin p (PHA-P) is added to increase contact between cells. After removing the medium, the mixed cell layer is briefly treated with 45% PEG for 60 seconds and then washed several times with serum free media. 24 hours later, the fused cells are removed by trypsinization, suspended in selective medium and plated onto 100 mm culture dishes. Hybrid cells are enriched by preferential killing of non-fused parental cells using selective medium. Colonies of hybrid cells are isolated using cloning rings and can be propagated as clonal cell lines by transferring them into individual culture flasks.

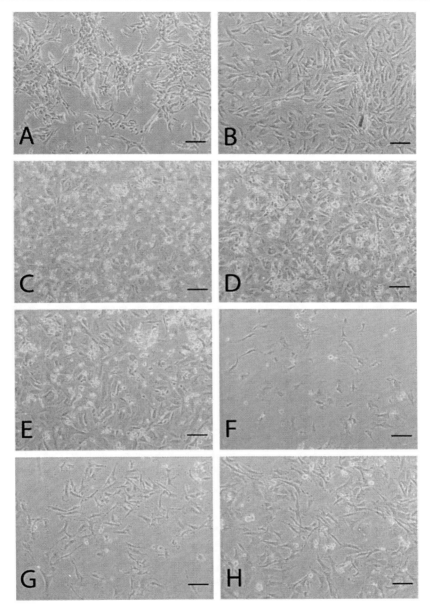

Figure 1. Fusion of co-cultured monolayer cells to generate hybrid cells by polyethylene glycol (PEG) treatment. Sub-confluent culture of the murine F7 cells (HAT-sensitive and neomycin-resistant) (A), sub-confluent culture of normal bovine nucleus pulposus (BNP) cells (HAT-resistant and neomycin-sensitive) at passage 2 (B), co-culture of F7 and BNP cells for 3 hours followed by 30 minutes treatment of phytohemagglutinin-P increases contacts between cells prior to PEG treatment (C), co-cultured cells treated with PEG for 1 minute and subsequent recovery of PEG-treated cells for 30 minutes at 37°C (D), further recovery of PEG-treated cells after changing media followed by overnight incubation at 37°C (E), cultivation of PEG-treated cells in the presence of HAT and G418 for 5 days eliminate all non-fused parental cells and allow the replication of only recombinant hybrid cells (F), cultivation of enriched recombinant cells for additional for 5 days in the presence of HAT-G418 allow their further proliferation (G), and generation of large number of highly proliferative bovine-murine hybrid cells after 15 days growth in selective media (H). *Bars* 100 μm.

Immortal Murine Cell Line GM05267 as a Universal Fusion Partner to Generate Hybrids

The murine kidney-derived immortal fibroblast cell line GM05267 (obtained from the National Institutes of General Medical Sciences (NIGMS), Camden, NJ, USA) and its derivatives are appropriate parents to generate hybrid cells. The GM05267 cells are deficient for the enzyme hypoxanthine-phosphoribosyl-transferase (HPRT-), resulting their inability to replicate in presence of hypoxanthine-aminopterin-thymidine (HAT) (Szybalska and Szybalski 1962; Migeon et al. 1981). Mutation of HPRT gene in the GM05267 cells is useful for the enrichment of recombinant hybrid cells by eliminating the non-fused mutant cells from the fusion mixture using HAT medium (Szybalski and W 1992). A neomycin-resistance gene was introduced into the GM05267 cell line to make it a universal fusion partner. Introduction of neomycin-resistant gene into HPRT-deficient cells allows preferential elimination of neomycin-sensitive cells of other fusing partner by growing the PEG-treated cells in presence of G418. Recombinant hybrid cells between neomycin-resistant GM05267 cells and any type of neomycin-sensitive cells containing HPRT+ gene can be isolated by the growing fused cells in the presence of HAT and G418 through elimination of all non-recombinant parental cells. The neomycin-resistant gene was introduced into the GM05267 cell line by calcium phosphate precipitation method (Islam and Islam 2000). In order to introduce neomycin-resistant gene into the GM05267 cell line plasmid DNA containing pSV2neo was mixed with calcium chloride and BES-buffered-saline, and the mixture was added to the monolayer of GM05267 cells. The culture dish was allowed to stand for 30 min at room temperature and then transferred into an incubator at 37°C with 5% CO_2. After overnight incubation, medium was removed and the cells were fed with fresh DMEM medium containing G418. Cells were maintained in culture with twice weekly media replenishment. After three weeks, G418-resistant cells were transferred to a culture flask for further multiplication. The resulting cell line was designated GM05267-Neo[R].

GM05267-Neo[R] cells were grown and sub-cultured for several passages in appropriate culture media with concomitant observation of their growth properties. Sub-cloning and subsequent selective rounds of culturing gave rise to a number of cell lines which displayed unique growth characteristics. One of the cell lines established by such selection was GM05267-Neo[R]-F-7 (hereafter F7) (Islam et al. 2006b; Islam et al. 2007b).

Fusion of F7 Cells with Normal Cells Generates Hybrid Cells with Accelerated Growth

The immortal murine F7 cells (HAT-sensitive and G418-resistant) and normal porcine fibroblasts (HAT-resistant and G418-sensitive) of the strains AG08114 and AG12077 (NIA, Aging Cell Culture Repository, Coriell Institute for Medical Research, Camden, NJ, USA) were trypsinized and equal numbers of murine cells and porcine cells were mixed in centrifuge tubes and seeded into 60 mm tissue culture dishes. After 4-6 hours, cell fusion was induced by PEG. The fused cells were trypsinized after 24 hours incubation, suspended in medium containing G418 plus HAT, and plated into larger culture dishes. After 7–10 days, hybrid colonies were isolated by cloning rings and subsequently clonal cell lines were established (Islam et al. 2007b).

The parental murine cell line F7 contained approximately 36 autosomes and one X chromosome. The porcine parental cell strains, namely AG08114 and AG12077, contained a normal karyotype with 38 chromosomes. Hybrid cells between F7 cells and porcine fibroblasts were expected to contain 78 chromosomes. Surprisingly, cytogenetic analysis of hybrid cell lines showed near-tetraploid porcine and near-diploid murine chromosomes (hereafter 2:1 hybrids). The numbers of porcine chromosomes retained by the hybrid lines ranged from 67 to 103 and murine chromosomes from 24 to 31 (Islam et al. 2007b). Since the porcine cells contained mostly diploid chromosomes, it is likely that the porcine tetraploid chromosomes of 2:1 hybrids resulted either from fusion of a tetraploid porcine cell with a F7 cell or from three-way fusion between two diploid porcine cells with one F7 cell.

Selective Growth Advantage of 2:1 Hybrid Cells over Porcine Parental Cells

The consistent presence of 2:1 porcine-murine chromosomes in all clonally derived hybrid cell lines indicates a selective advantage for this chromosome combination. If this assumption is correct, then instead of clonal cell lines, isolation of pooled hybrid cells would show a 2:1 combination of porcine-murine chromosomes in the majority of the metaphase cells. To test this hypothesis, we performed a competitive proliferation assay (CPA). Essentially the CPA is performed on a mass population cells after fusion of two cell types. Selection is applied against the murine (HAT-sensitive) immortal cells (half-selection) but not against the porcine (G418-sensitive) fibroblast cells (Islam et al. 2007b). One would logically expect that a mixture of hybrid cells and porcine fibroblasts be found in such mass cultured cells. However, if the hybrid cells and fibroblast cells have different growth rates, then the faster growing cells would be expected to overgrow the culture. After fusion of F7 cells with porcine fibroblasts and subsequent elimination F7 cells by HAT selection, a mixture of porcine fibroblasts and hybrid cells was expected. Cytogenetic analyses of the HAT-selected mass cell populations showed that 95% of the metaphase cells contained 2:1 porcine-murine chromosome combination. This indicates that the 2:1 hybrid cells had a selective advantage for growth over the porcine parental fibroblast cells and hybrid cells of other chromosome combinations. Fusion of the uncloned original GM05267 cell line with porcine fibroblasts and subsequent CPA analysis of the HAT-selected mixed population of cells showed mostly metaphases containing 2:1 porcine-murine chromosomes (Islam et al. 2007b), indicating that the original GM05267 cell line also contained cells able to generate 2:1 hybrid cells.

Production of Growth Stimulatory Factors by 2:1 Porcine-Murine Hybrids

Immortal F7 fibroblasts have high replication rates whilst normal porcine fibroblasts have poor replication rates. The hybrid cells acquired combinations of the two parents producing fibroblastic cell morphology with high replication rates. The hybrid cells grew like immortal cells. They lacked contact inhibited growth and continued proliferation in the post confluent conditions. High mitotic activity in the hybrid cells at high densities with slightly acidic media led us to assume that they secrete growth promoting factors into the CM. To test this hypothesis, CM was collected from different cultures, filtered, and then diluted by mixing 20% CM with 80% fresh media (hereafter diluted CM). The diluted CM was then added to the non-replicating porcine fibroblasts to test whether the CM contained any growth promoting activity.

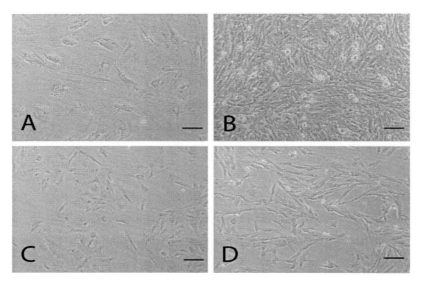

Figure 2. Generation of immortal porcine-murine hybrid cells by fusion of porcine fibroblasts with murine F7 cells and collection of conditioned media (CM) of porcine-murine hybrid cells and subsequent treatment of non-replicating porcine fibroblasts with CM induce replication. Fusion of non-replicating normal porcine fibroblasts (A) with murine F7 cells produces immortal hybrid cells (B), collection of CM from highly replicating hybrid cells and treatment of non-replicating porcine cells (C) induce replication (D), indicating the CM of hybrid cells contain bioactive factors that stimulate replication of previously non-replicating cells. *Bars* 100 μm.

Addition of diluted CM was sufficient to convert the non-replicating fibroblasts into a replicating state indicating that the CM of the 2:1 hybrid cells contained factors capable of promoting growth (Figure 2). The biological activity of CM could be maintained up to 6 months by storing them in the refrigerator at 4°C (Islam et al. 2007b) and even longer time by freezing at -70°C.

GM05267-Derived Cells with a Specific Karyotype Generate 2:1 Hybrids

To investigate whether cell morphology and growth of the immortal murine cells had any effect in the generation of 2:1 hybrid, two sub-lines (VJ-1 and VJ-4) were isolated from the original GM05267 cell line with slower growth and flatter morphology than the F7 cells (Figure 3). After transferring a hygromycin resistant gene into these cell lines (VJ-1-HR and VJ-4-HR), the modified cell lines were fused with the normal porcine fibroblast cells.

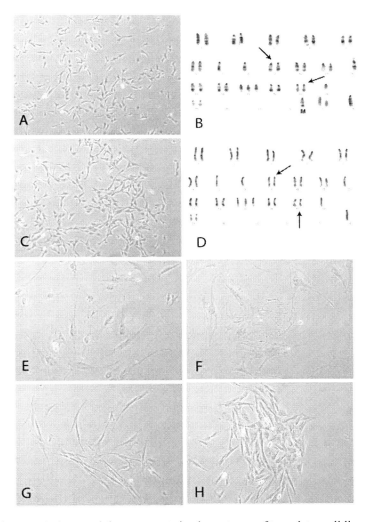

Figure 3. Cellular morphology and the representative karyotypes of two sister cell lines of the F7 cell line, containing two copies each of chromosomes 9 and 17 (compared to the karyotype of the F7 cells containing single copy of these chromosomes), and the derived hybrid cells without improved growth generated by fusing the two cell lines with normal porcine fibroblasts. Morphology of the VJ-1-HR cell line (A), a representative karyotype of the VJ-1HR cell line (B), morphology of VJ-4-HR cell line (C), a representative karyotype of the VJ-4HR cell line (D), fusion of the VJ-1-HR and VJ-4-HR with normal porcine fibroblast produced hybrid cells without accelerated growth(E-H), indicating that the two extra chromosomes present in the VJ-1 and VJ-4 lines (indicated by arrows) suppress the growth of hybrid cells. *Bars* 100 μm.

The fused cells were then divided equally and one part was grown in HAT medium containing hygromycin and the other part was grown in HAT medium without hygromycin. Contrary to the accelerated growth of the 2:1 hybrid cells, the double resistant (HAT and hygromycin resistant) cell colonies were slow growing and some of them failed to proliferate after a few division (Figure 3). Karyotype analyses of the VJ-1-HR and VJ-4-HR cell lines showed that they contained two copies each of chromosomes 9 and 17 (Figure 3), instead of single copy of these chromosomes in the F7 cell line and the original GM05267 cell line. These results indicate that these chromosomes may carry genes which suppress growth of hybrid cells, implying that the accelerated growth of 2:1 hybrid cells is associated with the losses of chromosomes 9 and 17 from the majority of the GM05267 cells and complete loss from all F7 cells.

To test whether the generation of 2:1 hybrids was limited to the fusion of F7 cells with normal porcine fibroblast cells, an immortal porcine fibroblast cell line AG12077-IM was fused with the F7 cell line. After CPA, it was found that the mass population of HAT-selected cells contained immortal porcine fibroblast cells without accelerated growth (Islam et al. 2007b). This result was surprising because interactions of immortal porcine fibroblast genome and immortal murine genome were expected to produce hybrid cells of accelerated growth because of additive effects of two immortal genomes. Karyotype analysis of the immortal porcine cell line AG012077 showed an abnormal karyotype with many missing copies of chromosomes as well as marker chromosomes. This may indicate that porcine cells with a normal karyotype can generate 2:1 hybrid cells with accelerated growth upon fusion with GM05267-derived immortal cells containing a specific karyotype. It has been demonstrated that morphologically aged and non-cycling normal cells are easier to reprogram during animal cloning than the more rapidly cycling immortal cells (Kasinathan et al. 2001; Gao et al. 2003). Interestingly, the fusion of F7 murine cells with normal porcine cells containing a complete genome, but not with immortal cells containing a deleted genome, and aged phenotype produce hybrid cells with accelerated growth. This result may suggest that in reprogramming the genetic information of the donor cells is more important than the aging status of the cells (Campbell et al. 1996; Zakhartchenko et al. 1999; Shi et al. 2003).

Telomerase Independent Mechanism of Growth Activation of 2:1 Hybrids

Transfer of human telomerase gene (hTERT) into normal cells extends their life spans (Harley 2002). To determine whether the hTERT had any role on the growth behavior of hybrid cells, the immortal porcine cell line AG12077-IM with an introduced hTERT gene was fused with the F7 cells. The CPA of mass cultured cells failed to show the phenotype of activated growth indicating that growth activation is unlikely to be controlled directly by telomerase. Since the fusion of senescent porcine cells with the F7 cells produced hybrid cells of accelerated growth the immortal porcine cell line AG12077-IM cell line was induced for ageing by depriving cells of new growth medium for several weeks. The non-replicating AG12077-IM cells were then fused with F7 cells and the resulting hybrid cells failed to show accelerated growth (Islam et al. 2007b). This result indicates that the cell aging may not play any direct role in the growth activation phenotype of hybrid cells.

GENERAL APPLICABILITY OF THE TWO-STEP PROTOCOL

Generation of Pig Mesenchymal Stem Cell Hybrids

Our two-step protocol to induce proliferation of the non-replicative somatic cells has successfully been applied to pig mesenchymal stem (MS) cells. It should be noted that MS cells divide for only 30-40 population doublings *in vitro* before becoming senescent (Sethe et al. 2006). Fusion of normal porcine MS cells and immortal murine F7 cells produced immortal hybrid cells containing polyploid porcine chromosomes. The CM derived from these hybrid cells can induce proliferation of various types of non-replicating cells (see below).

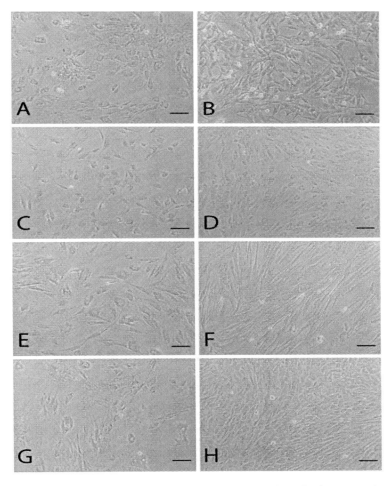

Figure 4. Generation of hybrid cells with accelerated growth by fusion of primary porcine mesenchymal stem (MS) cells and murine F7 cells. Non-replicating porcine MS cells (A) fused with F7 cells generated porcine-murine immortal hybrid cells with accelerated growth (B), collection of CM from hybrid cells and treatment of non-replicating porcine MS cells (D) with CM induced replication (F, H) of previously non-replicating cells, but not in those non-replicating cells which were not treated with CM of porcine MS hybrid cells (C, E, G). *Bars* 100 µm.

Cytogenetic analysis of clonal hybrid cell lines showed that most of them retained polyploid porcine chromosomes (Islam et al. 2006b). These hybrid cell lines also contained approximately 22 murine chromosomes indicating that about 13 chromosomes were lost from the F7 cell parent following fusion. Compared to the murine chromosomes, retention of porcine chromosomes by the porcine MS cell hybrids was extremely high with an average of 72 chromosomes ranging from 56 to 119. The mean numbers of combine porcine and murine chromosomes in the hybrids was about 94 ranging from 85 to 128 (Islam et al. 2006b). This result reconfirms the findings of normal porcine fibroblast cells that the fusion of normal porcine cells with murine F7 cells consistently produces hybrid cells containing polyploid porcine chromosomes (Islam et al. 2007b).

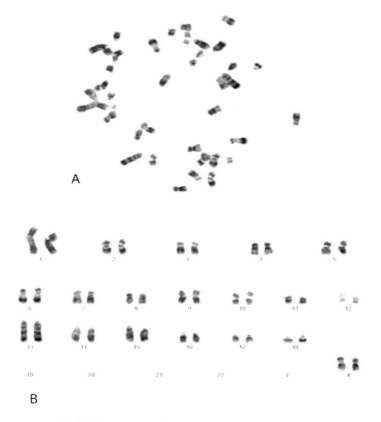

Figure 5. Maintenance of diploid karyotype of normal porcine MS cells grown in the presence of CM of porcine MS hybrid cells during their long-time proliferation, a representative metaphase cell containing 38 chromosomes (A) and karyotype of the same cell showing normal diploid chromosomes (B).

Like the parental porcine MS cells, hybrid cells showed fibroblastic morphology and large cell size. Many hybrid cell lines had exceeded 200 population doublings and they grew like immortal cells. Interestingly, the hybrid cells lack contact inhibition and they continue to divide even in post-confluence conditions producing multiple cell layers, contrary to the monolayer of parental porcine MS cells. Similar to the porcine fibroblast-derived hybrid cells (Islam et al. 2007), porcine MS-derived hybrid cells also contained bioactive factors in the

CM capable of inducing proliferation of both early passage and late passage porcine MS cells (Islam et al. 2006b). The porcine MS cells cultivated in the presence of diluted CM of MS-derived hybrid cells showed the morphology of freshly isolated porcine MS cells with high mitotic activity compared to same cells grown in the absence of CM (Figure 4). These results demonstrate that the hybrid cells between porcine MS cells and murine F7 cells produce diffusible factors in the CM which can increase the proliferation of porcine MS cells. The diploid karyotype of porcine MS cells did not alter even after prolonged culture in the presence of CM (Figure 5).

No Obstacle to Induce Proliferation of Non-Replicating Cells Derived from Diverse Mammalian Species by CM of Porcine MS Cell Hybrids

Treatment with diluted CM derived from porcine MS cell hybrids induced replication in non-replicating fibroblast-like cells derived from porcine chondrocytes (Figure 6), indicating that there is no major barrier to induce replication of cells of closely related tissue by the CM of hybrid cells derived from cells of another tissue of the same species.

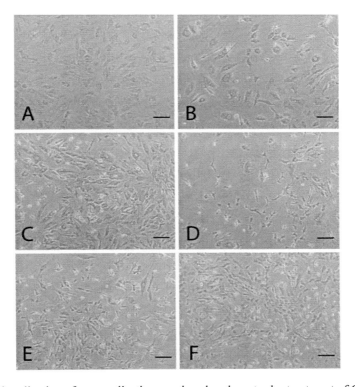

Figure 6. Induced replication of non-replicating porcine chondrocytes by treatment of CM derived from porcine MS cell hybrids. Non-replicating fibroblast-like porcine chondrocytes (A), passaging of the same cells with culture medium containing no CM failed to induce replication (B), induced replication of non-replicating porcine chondrocytes by treatment of CM derived from porcine MS cell hybrids (C-F), indicating that CM of hybrid cells generated from one type of porcine cell (mesenchymal stem cells) can induce proliferation of another type of porcine cell (fibroblast-like chondrocytes). *Bars* 100 μm.

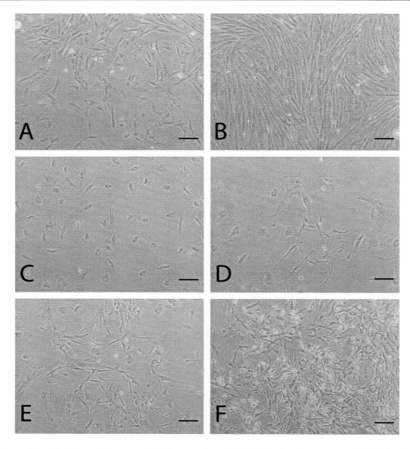

Figure 7. Induced replication of non-replicating canine fibroblasts by treatment of CM derived from porcine MS cell hybrids. Sub-confluent culture of newly established primary canine fibroblast at passage 0 (A), same culture at confluence (B), replication of the canine cells completely ceased after passage 2 (C), induced replication of rare non-replicating canine cells by CM of porcine MS cell hybrids (D), retention of original CM resulted two types of induced replication of the non-replicating cells, primary-induced replication by the direct action of CM and secondary-induced replication of the non-replicating cells by combined effects of CM and contact-mediated signals of primary-induced replicated cells (E), prolonged retention of original CM in the same flask ultimately converted all non-replicating canine cells into highly replicating form producing multiple layers of transformed-like cells (F). Two major conclusions can be made from these results that the CM of hybrid cells derived from one tissue is able to induce replication of non-replicating cells of different tissue and species, and the growth promoting signals of induced-replicated cells can be transmitted to their non-replicating counterparts by direct cell-cell contact. *Bars* 100 µm.

To exclude the species barrier to induce replication of cells of other species, non-replicating canine fibroblasts were treated with diluted CM of porcine MS cell hybrids. The result showed that a few canine cells (ranged from 0.007 to 0.01%) were directly induced to replicate producing colonies of replicating cells in the background of mostly non-replicating cells within 2-3 weeks of addition of cross-species CM. However, prolonged retention of the original CM induced replication of remaining non-replicating canine cells by direct contact of replicating cells. Ultimately, every single non-replicating canine cell was induced to replicate if the original CM was not changed indicating that the induced replicated canine cells are able transmit their growth promoting signals to their non-replicative counterparts by direct contact. This result is consistent with contact-mediated epigenetic reprogramming of non-replicating somatic cells for long-term proliferation by co-culture of non-replicating cells and immortal murine cells (Islam et al. 2007b). Prolonged retention of the original CM in the same culture flask (until the culture became confluent) induced rapid replication and morphological transformation of canine cells. With the increase of numbers of replicating cells, they aligned with each other producing multiple cell layers, contrary to the monolayer culture of the original canine fibroblasts (Figure 7). The transformed canine cells can be passaged by 1:4 split ratios in the presence of 20% own CM mixed with 80% fresh media for many generations without any visible sign of reduction of replication rates.

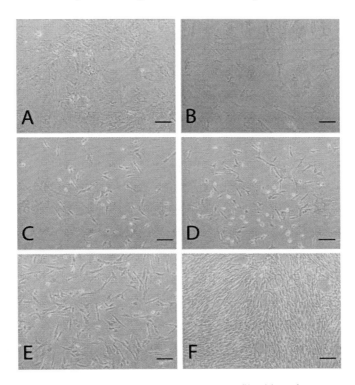

Figure 8. Induced replication of non-replicating Syrian hamster fibroblasts by treatment of CM derived from porcine MS cell hybrids. Confluent culture of newly established primary Syrian hamster fibroblast cells at passage 0 (A), same cell after two passages ceased replication completely (B), induced replication of non-replicating cells by treatment of CM derived from porcine MS cell hybrids (C), retention of the original CM in the same culture flask induced replication of both replicating and non-replicating cells (D, E), and prolonged retention of CM induced replication of more non-replicating cells and ultimately cells of the entire flask were transformed producing multi-layer culture (F). These results suggest that CM of hybrid cells derived from one species can induce replication of cells of another species and the induced replicated cells can relay their growth promoting signals to their non-replicating counterparts by direct cell-cell contact. *Bars* 100 μm.

Similar to the canine cells, non-replicating fibroblasts of Syrian hamster were treated with CM of porcine MS cell hybrids. The result of the cross-species CM treatment showed that only rare non-replicating Syrian hamster cells, similar to canine cells, were directly activated for replication. However, retention of the original CM for 3-4 weeks induced replication of remaining non-replicating Syrian hamster cells by direct contact of replicating cells. Similar to canine cells, morphological transformation of Syrian hamster cells also occurred within 4-6 weeks if the original CM was not replaced. The induced replicated Syrian hamster cells produced multiple cell layers in post-confluence conditions, contrary to the monolayer culture of non-replicating hamster fibroblasts (Figure 8).

Taken together, these results indicate that the induced replicated cells continuously produce growth stimulatory factors in the CM and that these diffusible factors appear capable of inducing replication in a concentration dependent manner. The transformed hamster cells can be maintained at high replicating state if passaged in identical fashion as the transformed canine cells. This may indicate that the induced transformation of non-replicating cells is a conditional phenotype which requires appropriate culture conditions to maintain.

Unlike other normal somatic cells, cultivation of chondrocyte-like cells obtained from the nucleus pulposus (NP) of bovine intervertibral discs with standard culture medium did not limit replication. Modestly replicating bovine cells were treated with CM derived from porcine MS cell hybrids to test whether they could be transformed to produce highly replicating multi-layer cells. Although the replication of bovine NP cells could be improved by the treatment of CM derived from porcine MS cell hybrids, the induced replicated NP cells were still sensitive to contact inhibition and they produced strictly monolayer cultures (Figure 9).

This result may indicate that the genome of non-replicating cell exists in a permissive state allowing the activation of a growth promoting signalling pathway in response to external cues. In contrast, genome of replicating cell probably stays in a non-permissive condition to alter the existing growth signalling pathway in response to external cues. This is probably why the partially transformed bovine cells grow as monolayer (Figure 9), contrary to the fully transformed canine and Syrian hamster cells which grow as multiple cell layers (Figure 7 and Figure 8). It is possible that two types of transformed cells employ different signalling pathways for their replications. In contrast to normal somatic stem cells, adult epiblast-like pluripotent stem cells reported to grow like immortal cells with no sign of cellular senescence (Young and Black 2004; Young et al. 2004). Also, these epiblast-like pluripotent stem cells do not follow the contact inhibited growth and continue to replicate at high densities producing multiple cell layers at confluence. In this respect, it would be interesting to know whether our induced transformed somatic cells derived from different species also express pluripotent stem cell markers. Generation of pluripotent stem cells directly from somatic cells without genetic manipulations has enormous value both in biology and in medicine.

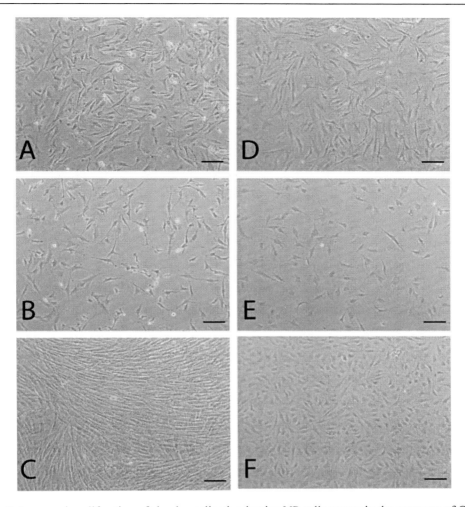

Figure 9. Improved proliferation of slowly replicating bovine NP cells grown in the presence of CM derived from porcine MS cell hybrids (A-C), in contrast to the NP cells grown in the absence of CM (D-F). Bovine NP cells at passage 10 grown in the presence of CM of porcine MS cell hybrids for 6 days showed morphological alteration and improved proliferation (A), passaging of the improved proliferating NP cells in the medium containing hybrid cell CM maintained proliferation (B), retention of the original CM-containing medium in the same flask produced confluent culture with high cell density of fibroblast-like thin cells (C), sub-confluent culture of bovine NP cells at passage 10 grown in standard medium without CM showing distinct morphological features of non-replicating cells (D), passage of the same cells in standard medium in the absence of CM showing no visible mitotic cell (E), retention of cells in the same medium stopped cell proliferation completely producing strictly a monolayer culture (F). Note distinct morphology of transformed bovine NP cells by CM of porcine MS cell hybrids (C) compared to the transformed counterparts of canine and Syrian hamster fibroblast cells in Figure 7F and Figure 8F, respectively. *Bars* 100 μm.

Generation of Murine Mesenchymal Stem Cell Hybrids

To extend the findings of our two-step protocol, the murine MS cell line 4D was fused with the F7 cells to generate hybrid cells. Since the F7 cell line contained approximately 36 chromosomes including one X chromosome and the murine MS cell line 4D contained 80 chromosomes including two copies of X and one to two copies of Y, fusion between F7 and 4D cells would be expected to produce hybrid cells containing approximately 115 chromosomes. Cytogenetic analysis of the isolated hybrid cell lines revealed that they contained chromosome numbers ranging from 88 to 117, close to the expected chromosome numbers of hybrid cells. The presence of distinct sex chromosomes from both 4D and F7 parents in the metaphases of all cell lines confirmed that they were truly hybrid cells. Morphologically, the F7 parental cells were smaller in size with high proliferation and the 4D cells were flat with slow proliferation. The hybrid cells had flattened morphology with high proliferation rates similar to immortal cells. Culture of post-mitotic murine fibroblasts in the presence of diluted CM of hybrid cells reinitiates mitotic activities (Islam et al. 2006a) showing that the CM of murine MS cell hybrids can be used to induce replication of other types of murine cells.

Hybrid Cells Generated by Fusion of Cells Derived from Diverse Mammalian Species

Immortalization of limited proliferation primary somatic cells by fusion with F7 cells and improvement of proliferation of other cells through treatment of hybrid cell-derived CM is not limited to porcine fibroblasts (Islam et al. 2007b), porcine mesenchymal stem cells (Islam et al. 2006b), and murine mesenchymal stem cells (Islam et al. 2006a), somatic cells of other species including fibroblasts of Chimpanzee, human, equine, Syrian hamster, canine, rat, and murine, and nucleus pulposus cells of bovine have been immortalized by fusing with F7 cells. The resulting hybrid cells grew like immortal cells with high proliferation (Figure 10 and Figure 11). These hybrid cell lines could serve as common resource to produce CM which has potential applications to improve the proliferation of normal somatic cells with limited replication derived from same species or different species.

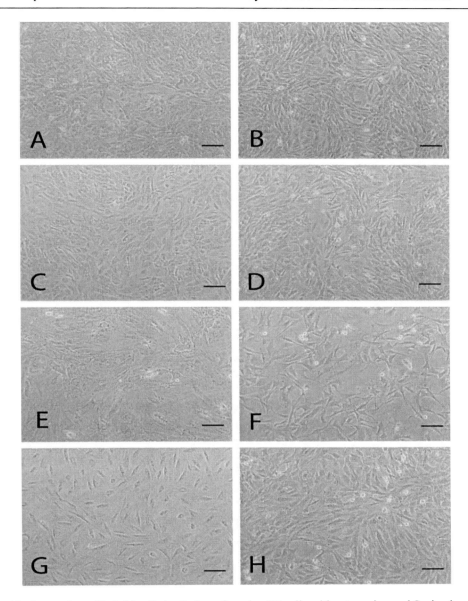

Figure 10. Generation of hybrid cells by fusion of murine F7 cells with rat, canine and Syrian hamster somatic cells. Rat fibroblast cells (A), rat fibroblast hybrid cells (B), rat sub-cutaneous fat cells (C), rat sub-cutaneous fat cell hybrids (D), Syrian hamster fibroblasts (E), Syrian hamster fibroblast hybrid cells (F), canine fibroblast cells (G), and canine fibroblast hybrid cells (H). Note the improved proliferation in all types of hybrid cells. The CM of generated hybrid cells has potential application to improve proliferation of cells derived from same species and/or different species. *Bars* 100 μm.

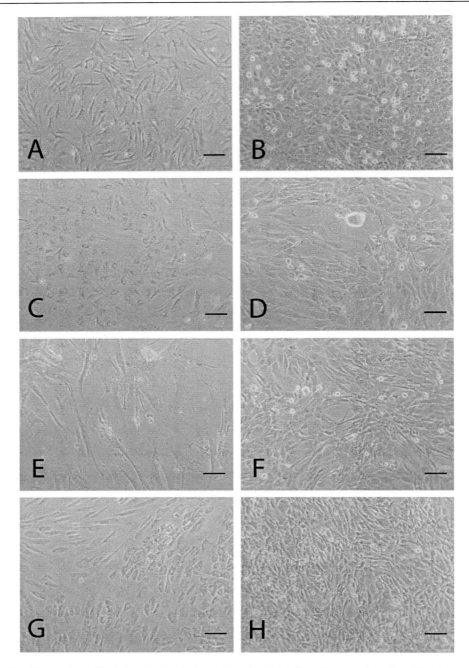

Figure 11. Generation of hybrid cells by fusion of murine F7 cells with somatic cells of bovine, equine, Chimpanzee and human. Bovine NP cells (A), bovine NP cell hybrids (B), equine sub-cutaneous fat cells (C), equine sub-cutaneous fat cell hybrids (D), Chimpanzee fibroblasts (E), Chimpanzee fibroblast hybrid cells (F), human fibroblasts (G), and human fibroblast hybrid cells (H). Note the improved proliferation in all types of hybrid cells. The CM of generated hybrid cells has potential application to improve proliferation of other cells. *Bars* 100 μm.

POSSIBLE MECHANISM OF ACCELERATED GROWTH OF IMMORTALIZED HYBRID CELLS

Chromosome content of hybrid cells and expression of tissue specific phenotypes

One unique feature of hybrid cells generated by the fusion of cells of two different species is the partial loss of chromosomes of one species against the complete chromosome background of another species. In such inter-species hybrid cells preferential loss of chromosomes from one parent is useful for chromosomal mapping of mammalian genes. In order to assign genes to specific porcine chromosomes, we earlier generated immortal porcine-murine hybrid cells by fusing the immortal murine cell line GM05267-Hyg^R, a sister cell line of F7, containing near-tetraploid chromosome complements with normal diploid pig fibroblasts (Gao and Islam 2001). These hybrid cells retained hypo-diploid porcine and near tetraploid murine chromosomes (1:2 hybrids), in contrast to the hybrid cells generated by fusion of F7 cells containing hypo-diploid chromosomes with diploid normal porcine fibroblasts, where only 2:1 porcine-murine hybrid cells were observed (Islam et al. 2007b). These results demonstrate that the composition of porcine and murine chromosomes in two series of hybrids is opposite, although both series of hybrid cell lines were generated by fusing two immortal cell lines of a common origin. It should be noted that the F7 is a unique cell line containing many single copy chromosomes including chromosomes 9 and 17. Fusion of F7 cells with different types of primary cells derived from various species consistently produce hybrid cells with activated growth. On the contrary, fusion of GM05267-derived independent cell lines, carrying disomy of chromosomes 9 and 17, with normal cells produce hybrid cells of neither activated growth nor tetraploid normal cell genome. This observation led to the conclusion that the activated growth phenotype is mediated by epigenetic reprogramming of normal cell genome through a direct involvement of F7 genome containing a specific karyotype.

It has been claimed that the fusion between normal cells with limited proliferation and immortal cells with unlimited proliferation produces hybrid cells of limited proliferation, implying that the phenotype of limited proliferation is dominant over unlimited proliferation (Pereira-Smith and Smith 1983; Tominaga et al. 2002). This conclusion predicts that hybrid cells containing normal cell derived polyploid chromosomes would not proliferative long in culture. However, the 2:1 porcine-murine hybrids not only have indefinite proliferation but are highly replicative. Other investigators have also produced hybrid cells with indefinite proliferation by fusion of immortal embryonal carcinoma cells with different types of normal somatic cells (Takagi 1997). These results support the notion that fusion between immortal cells and normal cells can produce hybrid cells of unlimited proliferation. It has been argued that the lack of expression of senescent phenotypes in these hybrids is due to rapid loss of many of the chromosomes of normal cells (Ran and Pereira-Smith 2000). The results of our 2:1 hybrids containing large numbers of normal cell porcine chromosomes with no sign of replicative senescence contradict this hypothesis. Our result suggests that the cellular senescence is not a genetically controlled trait and that this phenotype may have an epigenetic basis (Neumeister et al. 2002; Atkinson and Keith 2007).

Somatic cell genetic studies indicate that the phenotype of hybrid cells is determined by relative contribution of two parental genomes. For example, the expression of genes of two parental genomes is commonly reset where extinction of previously active genes and expression of previously silent genes occurs. It should be noted that hybrid cells generated by fusion of two differentiated cell types representing diploid (2N) genome from each parent (1:1 hybrid) express only the house keeping genes by completely repressing the tissue specific genes. On the contrary, hybrid cells representing tetraploid (4N) genome from one parent and 2N genome from the other (2:1 or 1:2) generally maintain the phenotypes of 4N parent (Gourdeau and Fournier 1990; Massa et al. 2000). This means that the ratio of two parental genomes of hybrid cells is important for the expression of differentiated cellular traits (Gourdeau and Fournier 1990). It is known that normal cells produce various types of growth factors and cytokines, which are beneficial for cell proliferation and cell survival (Le Pillouer-Prost 2003; Li et al. 2005). Normal MS cells also produce various growth factors and cytokines (Majumdar et al. 1998; Deans and Moseley 2000; Majumdar et al. 2000; Dormady et al. 2001; Minguell et al. 2001). Since the 2:1 hybrid cells contain 4N genome from normal porcine cells, it is expected that they express phenotypes of porcine cells. In fact, the 2:1 hybrid cells secrete diffusible growth stimulatory factors into the CM which not only can enhance their own proliferation but proliferation of non-replicating various types of normal cells (Islam et al. 2006b). On the contrary, the 2:1 hybrids, containing excessive chromosomes derived from porcine fibroblasts of limited proliferation, have an unlimited proliferation, a phenotype of F7 cells which is represented by a very small genome size. This may indicate that the F7 cell line containing a small genome has the unusual property of reprogramming a large sized genome derived from normal cells. It seems that the 2:1 porcine-murine hybrid cell system is yet another example of an abnormal growth phenotype associated with cellular reprogramming (Young et al. 1998).

Has the Accelerated Growth of 2:1 Hybrid Cells an Epigenetic Basis?

It should be noted that the murine F7 cell line contains single copies of several chromosomes including 6, 7, 8, 9, 12, 17 and 18 (Islam et al. 2006b). Except for chromosome 8, these mouse chromosomes carry imprinted genes where one of the two alleles is functional (Morison and Reeve 1998). Since the GM05267-derived F7 cells have high proliferation rates, it is possible that one or more paternally expressed growth promoting genes have been retained and the antagonistically acting maternally expressed growth inhibitory genes have been lost from the GM05267 cell line and its derivatives. This might have caused the constitutive activation of a growth promoting pathway because of dosage differences between the growth promoting and the growth inhibitory genes, as predicted from the conflict theory for imprinted genes (Haig and Graham 1991). In this respect the IGF signalling pathway, a pathway known to be involved in regulating cellular growth, may be of importance (Efstratiadis 1998). It should be noted that in cultured somatic cells expression of both IGF-I and IGF-II is affected by cell density and other growth limiting factors (Kutoh et al. 1995; Wang and Adamo 2000; Baqir and Smith 2003). Coincidentally, the 2:1 porcine-murine hybrid cells show an elevated mitotic activity at high cell densities and in acidic media.

Considering the reciprocal imprinting of IGF-II and its antagonist IGF-IIR (Hernandez et al. 2003), it is possible that the single copy of chromosome 7 of F7 cell line may represent the functional paternal allele of IGF-II and the single copy of chromosome 17 of the F7 cell line may represent the non-functional paternal allele of IGF-IIR, because of losses of respective "maternal" chromosomes. This assumption predicts that due to lack of murine IGF-IIR product in the 2:1 hybrid cells the murine IGF-II could join with the porcine IGF-IIR and this may block the porcine-derived growth inhibitory functions. This hypothetical inter-species interaction of gene products in the 2:1 porcine-murine hybrids may activate growth promoting signals constitutively in a dosage dependent manner, where the growth inhibitory function may be permanently paralysed (Young et al. 2001). However, this model does not exclude the possibility of generation of inter-species hybrid cells with activated growth by fusion of two diploid cells, so long as there is sufficient evolutionary conservation between two species of the interacting genes so that the inter-species gene products are able to perform normal biochemical functions similar to the single species products. In such diploid-diploid hybrid cells activated growth would still be possible due to the presence of an active copy of mouse IGF-II gene derived from the F7 cell line by overriding the growth inhibitory signals of the fusing diploid cell partner through the extra dose of the IGF-II gene. At the moment, however, we can not exclude the possibility that the abnormal growth phenotype of the 2:1 hybrid cell is controlled by other genes and by more complex mechanisms (Lewis and Redrup 2005).

CONCLUSION

An ideal source of cells for cell replacement therapies should fulfill two important criteria. Firstly it must have unlimited capacity for proliferation and secondly be capable of producing all types of cells required for tissue regeneration. ES cells fulfill these requirements (Hyslop et al. 2005). However, their therapeutic use has several potential problems: (i) since they derive from embryos, ethical and legal questions have been raised over the use of these cells in both research and therapy (de Wert and Mummery 2003; Bobbert 2006), (ii) ES cells derived from one individual embryo can not be used for cell replacement in other individuals because of the potential for immune rejection (Bradley et al. 2002), and (iii) transplantation of ES cells even in immune suppressed animals, can induce the formation of undifferentiated tumors in the three germ layers (Thomson and Odorico 2000). Such problems could be overcome by using autologous adult stem cells (Czyz et al. 2003; Raff 2003). To date, various types of adult stem cells have been isolated from almost all organ types (Young and Black 2004). Although adult stem cells have the potential to produce cells of multiple lineage their application in cell-based therapies has thus far been limited possibly due to their restricted proliferation potential (Hassan and El-Sheemy 2004; Javazon et al. 2004; Lee et al. 2004; Orlic 2005; Minguell and Erices 2006; Sethe et al. 2006). In this respect, any improvement to the proliferative capacity of adult stem cells would be desirable in order to generate large numbers of adult stem cells both for research and therapeutic applications.

Interestingly, a new method has recently been developed to induce somatic cells into ES-like cells, called induced pluripotent stem (iPS) cells, by a simple recipe of transferring a selected set of four genes (Takahashi and Yamanaka 2006; Okita et al. 2007; Wernig et al. 2007). Using this technique, it is possible convert somatic cells into patient specific iPS cells for therapeutic application. However, one disadvantage of iPS cells is the requirement of transfer of the c-Myc protooncogene into somatic cells for achieving long-term proliferation and sustaining ES-cell phenotypes.Therefore, it is no surprise that the iPS cells are prone to neoplastic transformation and this attribute of iPS cells is a serious obstacle for their clinical applications (Okita et al. 2007). Naturally, more research will be needed to overcome the tumor problems of iPS cells before using them in clinical settings. In this respect, any method to generate long-term growing cell lines by replicative reprogramming of somatic cells without any transfer of genes will be advantageous. We have demonstrated that somatic cells can be reprogrammed for improved proliferation by culturing them in the presence of CM derived from hybrid cells generated by fusion of normal somatic cells with murine F7 cells (Islam et al. 2006b; Islam et al. 2007b). This simple method does not require any transfer of genetic material to convert somatic cells into immortal-like cells. Unlike transformed tumor cells, improved proliferation of somatic cells by the treatment of hybrid cell-derived CM and their cultivation for extended period in CM does not alter diploid karyotype. Importantly, the immortal-like growth of replicative reprogrammed cells is a conditional phenotype whose expression is dependent on the supply of CM in the culture media. This may indicate that the phenotype of cellular senescence is expressed because of lack of appropriate growth factors in the culture medium and it is possible that the CM of hybrid cells supply the missing factors which prevent senescence. If this is the case, then the genetic basis of cellular senescence is questionable.

The two-step cell culture protocol, immortalization of somatic stem cells of limited proliferation by fusion with F7 cells and improvement of proliferation of somatic cells by treatment of CM derived from hybrid cells, allows unlimited replication of limited proliferation somatic stem cells. Replicative reprogramming of somatic cells by the described cell culture method has many potential applications both in biology and medicine. Production of unlimited numbers of somatic stem cells with improved proliferation would be useful for conducting *in vitro* experiments to determine their biological properties and *in vivo* testing to know their value for autologous cell-based therapies.

ACKNOWLEDGEMENTS

The author gratefully acknowledges contributions of all co-workers who were directly or indirectly involved in this study. The author wishes to give special thanks to the following collaborators: Jochen Ringe, Tissue Engineering Laboratory, Department of Rheumatology, Charité-University Medicine Berlin, Berlin, Germany, for providing porcine chondrocytes; Elisabet Roman Granath, ATG Hästklinik, Mantorp, Sweden, for providing equine fat cells, and Chris A. Sharp, Charles Salt Centre for Human Metabolism, Robert Jones and Agnes Hunt Orthopaedic and District Hospital NHS Trust, Gobowen, United Kingdom, for providing bovine NP cells, careful reading of the manuscript and suggesting linguistic changes to improve the quality of presentation.

REFERENCES

Akagi T, Sasai K, Hanafusa H (2003) Refractory nature of normal human diploid fibroblasts with respect to oncogene-mediated transformation. *Proc. Natl. Acad. Sci. U S A* 100:13567-13572.

Alberio R, Campbell KH, Johnson AD (2006) Reprogramming somatic cells into stem cells. *Reproduction* 132:709-720.

Ambrosi DJ, Rasmussen TP (2005) Reprogramming mediated by stem cell fusion. *J. Cell. Mol. Med.* 9:320-330.

Atkinson SP, Keith WN (2007) Epigenetic control of cellular senescence in disease: opportunities for therapeutic intervention. *Expert Rev. Mol. Med.* 9:1-26

Baqir S, Smith LC (2003) Growth restricted in vitro culture conditions alter the imprinted gene expression patterns of mouse embryonic stem cells. *Cloning Stem Cells* 5:199-212

Barski G, Cornefert F (1962) Characteristics of "hybrid"-type clonal cell lines obtained from mixed cultures in vitro. *J. Natl. Cancer Inst.* 28:801-821.

Barski G, Sorieul S, Cornefert F (1961) "Hybrid" type cells in combined cultures of two different mammalian cell strains. *J. Natl. Cancer Inst.* 26:1269-1291.

Ben-Porath I, Weinberg RA (2005) The signals and pathways activating cellular senescence. *Int. J. Biochem. Cell Biol.* 37:961-976.

Blagosklonny MV (2003) Cell senescence and hypermitogenic arrest. *EMBO Rep.* 4:358-362.

Blagosklonny MV (2006) Cell senescence: hypertrophic arrest beyond the restriction point. *J. Cell Physiol.* 209:592-597.

Bobbert M (2006) Ethical questions concerning research on human embryos, embryonic stem cells and chimeras. *Biotechnol. J.* 1:1352-1369.

Bradley JA, Bolton EM, Pedersen RA (2002) Stem cell medicine encounters the immune system. *Nat. Rev. Immunol.* 2:859-871.

Campbell KH, Loi P, Otaegui PJ, Wilmut I (1996) Cell cycle co-ordination in embryo cloning by nuclear transfer. *Rev. Reprod.* 1:40-46.

Campisi J (2001) Cellular senescence as a tumor-suppressor mechanism. *Trends Cell Biol.* 11:S27-31.

Campisi J (2005) Senescent cells, tumor suppression, and organismal aging: good citizens, bad neighbors. *Cell* 120:513-522.

Chen Y, He ZX, Liu A, Wang K, Mao WW, Chu JX, Lu Y, Fang ZF, Shi YT, Yang QZ, Chen da Y, Wang MK, Li JS, Huang SL, Kong XY, Shi YZ, Wang ZQ, Xia JH, Long ZG, Xue ZG, Ding WX, Sheng HZ (2003) Embryonic stem cells generated by nuclear transfer of human somatic nuclei into rabbit oocytes. *Cell Res.* 13:251-263.

Czyz J, Wiese C, Rolletschek A, Blyszczuk P, Cross M, Wobus AM (2003) Potential of embryonic and adult stem cells in vitro. *Biol. Chem.* 384:1391-1409.

de Wert G, Mummery C (2003) Human embryonic stem cells: research, ethics and policy. *Hum. Reprod.* 18:672-682.

Deans RJ, Moseley AB (2000) Mesenchymal stem cells: biology and potential clinical uses. *Exp. Hematol.* 28:875-884.

Dormady SP, Bashayan O, Dougherty R, Zhang XM, Basch RS (2001) Immortalized multipotential mesenchymal cells and the hematopoietic microenvironment. *J. Hematother. Stem. Cell Res*. 10:125-140.

Drayton S, Peters G (2002) Immortalisation and transformation revisited. *Curr. Opin. Genet. Dev.* 12:98-104.

Duelli D, Lazebnik Y (2003) Cell fusion: a hidden enemy? *Cancer* Cell 3:445-448.

Duncan EL, Wadhwa R, Kaul SC (2000) Senescence and immortalization of human cells. *Biogerontology* 1:103-121.

Efstratiadis A (1998) Genetics of mouse growth. *Int. J. Dev. Biol.* 42:955-976.

Gao S, McGarry M, Ferrier T, Pallante B, Priddle H, Gasparrini B, Fletcher J, Harkness L, De Sousa P, McWhir J, Wilmut I (2003) Effect of cell confluence on production of cloned mice using an inbred embryonic stem cell line. *Biol. Reprod.* 68:595-603.

Gao X, Islam MQ (2001) A gene on pig chromosome 14 suppresses cellular anchorage independence of the mouse cell line GM05267. *Cytogenet. Cell Genet.* 94:62-66.

Goldstein S (1990) Replicative senescence: the human fibroblast comes of age. *Science* 249:1129-1133.

Gourdeau H, Fournier RE (1990) Genetic analysis of mammalian cell differentiation. Annu. Rev. Cell Biol. 6:69-94.

Hahn WC, Weinberg RA (2002) Rules for making human tumor cells. *N. Engl. J. Med.* 347:1593-1603.

Haig D, Graham C (1991) Genomic imprinting and the strange case of the insulin-like growth factor II receptor. *Cell* 64:1045-1046.

Hall VJ, Stojkovic P, Stojkovic M (2006) Using therapeutic cloning to fight human disease: a conundrum or reality? *Stem Cells* 24:1628-1637.

Harley CB (2002) Telomerase is not an oncogene. *Oncogene* 21:494-502.

Hassan HT, El-Sheemy M (2004) Adult bone-marrow stem cells and their potential in medicine. *J. R. Soc. Med.* 97:465-471.

Hayflick L (1965) The Limited in Vitro Lifetime of Human Diploid Cell Strains. *Exp. Cell Res.* 37:614-636.

Hernandez L, Kozlov S, Piras G, Stewart CL (2003) Paternal and maternal genomes confer opposite effects on proliferation, cell-cycle length, senescence, and tumor formation. *Proc. Natl. Acad. Sci. U S A* 100:13344-13349.

Hyslop LA, Armstrong L, Stojkovic M, Lako M (2005) Human embryonic stem cells: biology and clinical implications. *Expert Rev. Mol. Med.* 7:1-21.

Islam, MQ, Meirelles, L da S, Nardi, NB, Magnusson, P, Islam, K. (2006a) Polyethylene glycol-mediated fusion of mouse mesenchymal stem cells with mouse fibroblasts generates hybrid cells with improved proliferation and altered differentiation. *Stem. Cells Dev.* 15:905-919.

Islam K, Islam MQ (1994) Assignment of TK1 encoding thymidine kinase to Syrian hamster chromosome 9 by microcell-mediated chromosome transfer. *Cytogenet. Cell Genet.* 66:177-180.

Islam MQ, Islam K (2000) Suppressor genes for malignant and anchorage-independent phenotypes located on human chromosome 9 have no dosage effects. *Cytogenet. Cell Genet.* 88:103-109.

Islam MQ, Islam K, Sharp CA (2007a) Epigenetic reprogramming of nonreplicating somatic cells for long-term proliferation by temporary cell-cell contact. *Stem Cells Dev.* 16:253-268.

Islam MQ, Panduri V, Islam K (2007b) Generation of somatic cell hybrids for the production of biologically active factors that stimulate proliferation of other cells. *Cell Prolif.* 40:91-105.

Islam MQ, Ringe J, Reichmann E, Migotti R, Sittinger M, da SML, Nardi NB, Magnusson P, Islam K (2006b) Functional characterization of cell hybrids generated by induced fusion of primary porcine mesenchymal stem cells with an immortal murine cell line. *Cell Tissue Res.* 326:123-137.

Itahana K, Campisi J, Dimri GP (2004) Mechanisms of cellular senescence in human and mouse cells. *Biogerontology* 5:1-10.

Javazon EH, Beggs KJ, Flake AW (2004) Mesenchymal stem cells: paradoxes of passaging. *Exp. Hematol.* 32:414-425.

Kasinathan P, Knott JG, Moreira PN, Burnside AS, Jerry DJ, Robl JM (2001) Effect of fibroblast donor cell age and cell cycle on development of bovine nuclear transfer embryos in vitro. *Biol Reprod.* 64:1487-1493.

Kutoh E, Schwander J, Margot JB (1995) Cell-density-dependent modulation of the rat insulin-like-growth-factor-binding protein 2 and its gene. *Eur. J. Biochem.* 234:557-562.

Le Pillouer-Prost A (2003) Fibroblasts: what's new in cellular biology? *J. Cosmet. Laser Ther.* 5:232-238.

Lee MS, Lill M, Makkar RR (2004) Stem cell transplantation in myocardial infarction. *Rev. Cardiovasc. Med.* 5:82-98.

Lewis A, Redrup L (2005) Genetic imprinting: conflict at the Callipyge locus. *Curr. Biol.* 15:R291-294.

Li H, Zou X, Baatrup A, Lind M, Bunger C (2005) Cytokine profiles in conditioned media from cultured human intervertebral disc tissue. Implications of their effect on bone marrow stem cell metabolism. *Acta Orthop.* 76:115-121.

Lloyd AC (2002) Limits to lifespan. *Nat. Cell Biol.* 4:E25-27.

Loo DT, Fuquay JI, Rawson CL, Barnes DW (1987) Extended culture of mouse embryo cells without senescence: inhibition by serum. *Science* 236:200-202.

Lynch MD (2006) How does cellular senescence prevent cancer? *DNA Cell Biol.* 25:69-78.

Majumdar MK, Thiede MA, Haynesworth SE, Bruder SP, Gerson SL (2000) Human marrow-derived mesenchymal stem cells (MSCs) express hematopoietic cytokines and support long-term hematopoiesis when differentiated toward stromal and osteogenic lineages. *J. Hematother. Stem Cell Res.* 9:841-848.

Majumdar MK, Thiede MA, Mosca JD, Moorman M, Gerson SL (1998) Phenotypic and functional comparison of cultures of marrow-derived mesenchymal stem cells (MSCs) and stromal cells. *J. Cell Physiol.* 176:57-66.

Massa S, Junker S, Matthias P (2000) Molecular mechanisms of extinction: old findings and new ideas. *Int. J. Biochem. Cell Biol.* 32:23-40.

Mathon NF, Malcolm DS, Harrisingh MC, Cheng L, Lloyd AC (2001) Lack of replicative senescence in normal rodent glia. *Science* 291:872-875.

Matveeva NM, Pristyazhnyuk IE, Temirova SA, Menzorov AG, Vasilkova A, Shilov AG, Smith A, Serov OL (2005) Unequal segregation of parental chromosomes in embryonic stem cell hybrids. *Mol. Reprod. Dev.* 71:305-314.

Matveeva NM, Shilov AG, Kaftanovskaya EM, Maximovsky LP, Zhelezova AI, Golubitsa AN, Bayborodin SI, Fokina MM, Serov OL (1998) In vitro and in vivo study of pluripotency in intraspecific hybrid cells obtained by fusion of murine embryonic stem cells with splenocytes. *Mol. Reprod. Dev.* 50:128-138.

Medvinsky A, Smith A (2003) Stem cells: Fusion brings down barriers. Nature 422:823-825.

Migeon BR, Brown TR, Axelman J, Migeon CJ (1981) Studies of the locus for androgen receptor: localization on the human X chromosome and evidence for homology with the Tfm locus in the mouse. *Proc. Natl. Acad. Sci. U S A* 78:6339-6343.

Minguell JJ, Erices A (2006) Mesenchymal stem cells and the treatment of cardiac disease. *Exp. Biol. Med.* (Maywood) 231:39-49.

Minguell JJ, Erices A, Conget P (2001) Mesenchymal stem cells. *Exp. Biol. Med.* (Maywood) 226:507-520.

Morison IM, Reeve AE (1998) A catalogue of imprinted genes and parent-of-origin effects in humans and animals. *Hum. Mol. Genet.* 7:1599-1609.

Neumeister P, Albanese C, Balent B, Greally J, Pestell RG (2002) Senescence and epigenetic dysregulation in cancer. *Int. J. Biochem. Cell Biol.* 34:1475-1490.

Newbold RF (2002) The significance of telomerase activation and cellular immortalization in human cancer. *Mutagenesis* 17:539-550.

Okita K, Ichisaka T, Yamanaka S (2007) Generation of germline-competent induced pluripotent stem cells. *Nature.*

Orlic D (2005) BM stem cells and cardiac repair: where do we stand in 2004? *Cytotherapy* 7:3-15.

Pereira-Smith OM, Smith JR (1983) Evidence for the recessive nature of cellular immortality. *Science* 221:964-966.

Puck TT, Kao FT (1982) Somatic cell genetics and its application to medicine. *Annu. Rev. Genet.* 16:225-271.

Raff M (2003) Adult stem cell plasticity: fact or artifact? *Annu. Rev. Cell Dev. Biol.* 19:1-22.

Ramirez RD, Morales CP, Herbert BS, Rohde JM, Passons C, Shay JW, Wright WE (2001) Putative telomere-independent mechanisms of replicative aging reflect inadequate growth conditions. *Genes. Dev.* 15:398-403.

Ran Q, Pereira-Smith OM (2000) Genetic approaches to the study of replicative senescence. *Exp. Gerontol.* 35:7-13.

Rubin H (1997) Cell aging in vivo and in vitro. *Mech. Ageing Dev.* 98:1-35.

Rubin H (2002) Promise and problems in relating cellular senescence in vitro to aging in vivo. *Arch. Gerontol. Geriatr.* 34:275-286.

Ruddle FH, Creagan RP (1975) Parasexual approaches to the genetics of man. *Annu. Rev. Genet.* 9:407-486

Serrano M, Blasco MA (2001) Putting the stress on senescence. *Curr. Opin. Cell Biol.* 13:748-753.

Sethe S, Scutt A, Stolzing A (2006) Aging of mesenchymal stem cells. *Ageing Res. Rev.* 5:91-116.

Shi W, Hoeflich A, Flaswinkel H, Stojkovic M, Wolf E, Zakhartchenko V (2003) Induction of a senescent-like phenotype does not confer the ability of bovine immortal cells to support the development of nuclear transfer embryos. *Biol. Reprod.* 69:301-309.

Smith SK, Kipling D (2004) The role of replicative senescence in cancer and human ageing: utility (or otherwise) of murine models. *Cytogenet. Genome. Res.* 105:455-463.

Szybalska EH, Szybalski W (1962) Genetics of human cell line. IV. DNA-mediated heritable transformation of a biochemical trait. *Proc. Natl. Acad. Sci. U S A* 48:2026-2034.

Szybalski, W (1992) Use of the HPRT gene and the HAT selection technique in DNA-mediated transformation of mammalian cells: First step toward developing hybridoma techniques and gene therapy. *BioEssays* 14:495-500.

Takagi N (1997) Mouse embryonal carcinoma cell-somatic cell hybrids as experimental tools for the study of cell differentiation and X chromosome activity. *Cancer Genet. Cytogenet.* 93:48-55.

Takahashi K, Yamanaka S (2006) Induction of pluripotent stem cells from mouse embryonic and adult fibroblast cultures by defined factors. *Cell* 126:663-676.

Tang DG, Tokumoto YM, Apperly JA, Lloyd AC, Raff MC (2001) Lack of replicative senescence in cultured rat oligodendrocyte precursor cells. *Science* 291:868-871.

Thomson JA, Odorico JS (2000) Human embryonic stem cell and embryonic germ cell lines. *Trends Biotechnol.* 18:53-57.

Tominaga K, Olgun A, Smith JR, Pereira-Smith OM (2002) Genetics of cellular senescence. *Mech. Ageing Dev.* 123:927-936.

Wang L, Adamo ML (2000) Cell density influences insulin-like growth factor I gene expression in a cell type-specific manner. *Endocrinology* 141:2481-2489

Wernig M, Meissner A, Foreman R, Brambrink T, Ku M, Hochedlinger K, Bernstein BE, Jaenisch R (2007) In vitro reprogramming of fibroblasts into a pluripotent ES-cell-like state. *Nature.*

Wright WE, Shay JW (2001) Cellular senescence as a tumor-protection mechanism: the essential role of counting. *Curr. Opin. Genet .Dev.* 11:98-103.

Wynford-Thomas D (1999) Cellular senescence and cancer. *J. Pathol.* 187:100-111.

Yaswen P, Stampfer MR (2002) Molecular changes accompanying senescence and immortalization of cultured human mammary epithelial cells. Int. *J. Biochem. Cell Biol.* 34:1382-1394.

Young HE, Black AC, Jr. (2004) Adult stem cells. *Anat. Rec. A Discov. Mol. Cell Evol. Biol* .276:75-102.

Young HE, Duplaa C, Yost MJ, Henson NL, Floyd JA, Detmer K, Thompson AJ, Powell SW, Gamblin TC, Kizziah K, Holland BJ, Boev A, Van De Water JM, Godbee DC, Jackson S, Rimando M, Edwards CR, Wu E, Cawley C, Edwards PD, Macgregor A, Bozof R, Thompson TM, Petro GJ, Jr., Shelton HM, McCampbell BL, Mills JC, Flynt FL, Steele TA, Kearney M, Kirincich-Greathead A, Hardy W, Young PR, Amin AV, Williams RS, Horton MM, McGuinn S, Hawkins KC, Ericson K, Terracio L, Moreau C, Hixson D, Tobin BW, Hudson J, Bowyer FP, 3rd, Black AC, Jr. (2004) Clonogenic analysis reveals reserve stem cells in postnatal mammals. II. Pluripotent epiblastic-like stem cells. *Anat. Rec. A Discov. Mol. Cell Evol. Biol.* 277:178-203.

Young LE, Fernandes K, McEvoy TG, Butterwith SC, Gutierrez CG, Carolan C, Broadbent PJ, Robinson JJ, Wilmut I, Sinclair KD (2001) Epigenetic change in IGF2R is associated with fetal overgrowth after sheep embryo culture. *Nat. Genet.* 27:153-154.

Young LE, Sinclair KD, Wilmut I (1998) Large offspring syndrome in cattle and sheep. *Rev. Reprod.* 3:155-163.

Zakhartchenko V, Alberio R, Stojkovic M, Prelle K, Schernthaner W, Stojkovic P, Wenigerkind H, Wanke R, Duchler M, Steinborn R, Mueller M, Brem G, Wolf E (1999) Adult cloning in cattle: potential of nuclei from a permanent cell line and from primary cultures. *Mol. Reprod .Dev* .54:264-272.

Zhang H (2007) Molecular signaling and genetic pathways of senescence: Its role in tumorigenesis and aging. *J. Cell Physiol.* 210:567-574.

In: Progress in Cell Growth Process Research
Editor: Takumi Hayashi, pp. 119-134

ISBN 978-1-60456-325-2
© 2008 Nova Science Publishers, Inc.

Chapter 4

CELL PROLIFERATION AND DIFFERENTIATION IN THE ADULT HIPPOCAMPUS

Katsuya Uchida[2]

Laboratory of Information Biology, Graduate School of Information Sciences,
Tohoku University. Aramaki aza Aoba 6-3-09, Aoba-ku, Sendai 980-8579, Japan

ABSTRACT

Embryonic stem cells that derive from the inner cell mass of the blastocyst induce a variety of tissues and form the central nervous system. The cells that differentiate into neural progenitor cells exist on the ventricular zone of the embryonic brain and produce neuronal and glial cells during the developmental period. Although neurogenesis—the generation of new neuronal cells—has been thought to terminate after the embryonic stage, it has recently been found that neural progenitor cells exist in parts of the adult brain, namely the subventricular zone and the dentate gyrus of the hippocampus. Furthermore, it has been suggested that glial fibrillary acidic protein (GFAP)-positive cells are capable of trans-differentiating to give rise to neural progenitor cells in the adult brain. In the processes of cell growth, neural progenitor cells derived from GFAP-positive cells express a variety of cell-specific markers such as nestin, polysialylated neural cell adhesion molecule (PSA-NCAM), and others. In addition, the proliferation rate of neural progenitor cells and expression level of cell markers during cell growth is altered by various conditions such as increases in mitotic activity related to exercise, environmental enrichment, and ischemic insult, whereas decreases in cell proliferation are related to aging and stress. This chapter describes recent research on the function of neural plasticity–related molecules and discusses their role in adult neurogenesis.

2 Tel: +81-22-7954764 ,Fax: +81-22-7954765 , E-mail: uchida@bio.is.tohoku.ac.jp.

INTRODUCTION

In the 1960s, Altman et al. [1] showed for the first time that "undifferentiated cells" exist in the dentate gyrus of the hippocampus and subventricular zone of the adult brain. However, the finding that neural progenitor cells exist in the adult brain attracted little attention of neuroscientists at the time. With progress in neurogenesis research, however, investigators have found that neural progenitor cells reside in the adult dentate gyrus of the hippocampus at the border zone between the granule cell layer and the hilus (CA4), namely the subgranular zone. Further, newly generated cells in this area gradually move into the granule cell layer over a few weeks and finally differentiate into neurons [2]. Mature neurons in the granular layer later receive synaptic input [3] and project functional connections to the CA3 region [4]. In the 1990s, Eriksson et al. [5] published the surprising demonstration that neurogenesis occurs in the adult human hippocampus. Since that discovery, the study of adult neurogenesis has continued to accelerate from the standpoint of regenerative medicine, especially with regard to therapy for spinal cord injury, stroke, and Parkinson's disease. However, all newly born cells do not become functional neurons; a portion of young cells in the subgranular zone die during cell growth [6, 7]. To gain a better understanding of cell proliferation and differentiation in the adult brain, and to make progress in regenerative medicine, it will be necessary to identify factors that regulate cell proliferation and modulate cell survival.

NEURAL DEVELOPMENT

During development, pluripotent embryonic stem cells generate somatic stem cells, which form the endoderm, mesoderm and ectoderm. Under the influence of the organizer, a portion of the ectoderm differentiates into neuroectodermal cells and forms the neural tube. The inner layer of the neural tube later becomes the ventricular zone of the embryonic brain, and neural progenitor cells also reside along this inner layer. Therefore the neuroepithelial cells, as neural progenitor cells, of the inner layer of the neural tube and the ventricular zone have a marked proliferative capacity and produce a great variety of neurons in the fetal brain. In the developing brain, neuroepithelial cells in the ventricular zone of the fetal brain generate not only immature neurons but also radial glia and Cajal-Retzius cells, which are indispensable for the correct stratification of the neocortex. In short, radial glia function as precursor cells and act as a guidance structure leading new neurons from the ventricular zone to their appropriate position, whereas the Cajal-Retzius cells secrete reelin, a protein necessary for normal formation of the six-layered neocortex [8]. Under the coordinate action of these players, brain morphogenesis progresses. However, the proliferative activity of the ventricular zone that produces these cells gradually declines with development of the brain, and the niches are finally limited to two regions: the subventricular zone and dentate gyrus of the hippocampus.

After completion of neuronal stratification, radial glial cells in the neocortex disappear and transform into astrocytes [9, 10]. However in adult brain, radial glial cells are still found in the dentate gyrus of the hippocampus and subventricular zone. Radial glial cells in the dentate gyrus express GFAP, an astrocyte marker, and vimentin (marker of mesenchymal cells and radial glia) [11]. The somas that express these markers are located in the border zone of the granule cell layer, the subgranular zone, whereas glial protrusions extend to the molecular layer of the dentate gyrus [11]. Furthermore, radial glia lie adjacent to cells expressing PSA-NCAM, a marker of immature neurons [11, 12], and contact between axons from these neurons and radial glial protrusions is widely observed in the molecular layer of the dentate gyrus. This situation is similar to the location of newly generated neurons and glial cells in the fetal ventricular zone: correspondingly new neurons migrate vertically from the ventricular surface to the pial surface along glial protrusions. Therefore, the existence of radial glia in the dentate gyrus of the adult hippocampus strongly implies that new neurons continue to be generated throughout life. In fact, the rodent dentate gyrus generates a large number of dividing cells; for example, rats generate 9000 cells per day [13]. Although the majority of newly generated cells die within a few weeks [6], surviving cells certainly receive synaptic input [3] and project functional connections to CA3 [4]. Thus the existence of newly generated neurons is important in brain functions such as learning and memory.

THE ORIGIN OF NEURAL STEM CELLS IN THE ADULT BRAIN

In 1999, two groups reported the origin of neural stem cells in the subventricular zone. Johansson et al. [14] found that ependymal cells are neural stem cells, while Doetsch et al. [15] found that GFAP-positive astrocytes in the subventricular zone are neural stem cells named "type B cells". In fact, Doetsch et al. [16] showed that after anti-mitotic treatment neural progenitor cells (type A cells) and transiently amplifying progenitor cells (type C cells) are eliminated but GFAP-positive B cells remain. Two days after anti-mitotic treatment, type C cells regenerate from type B cells, and finally the type A cells regenerate within two weeks. These results suggest that neural stem cells are astrocytes in the subventricular zone. However, the ependymal cell is certainly important in adult neurogenesis because Noggin produced by ependymal cells antagonizes bone morphogenic protein (BMP) signaling in type B cells, promoting neurogenesis [17].

On the other hand, Seri et al. [18] found that astrocytes give rise to new neurons in the adult hippocampus. The GFAP-positive astrocytes in the subgranular zone of the dentate gyrus also express vimentin (a marker of radial glia) [11] and nestin (an intermediate filament and marker of neural stem cells) [19]. These radial glia-like stem cells are named "type-1 cells". Some type-1 cells become type-2 cells, which express nestin but not GFAP. The type-2 cell has two subtypes, discriminated by doublecortin (DCX), a microtubule-associated protein; the DCX-negative type 2 cell is named "type-2 a", and the DCX-positive type 2 cell is named "type-2 b". Because DCX is a marker for migrating neuronal cells [20], type 2b cells are considered more immature neurons compared with type 2a. Type 2b cells later become nestin-negative "type-3 cells", and newly generated cells finally express markers of mature neurons, such as NeuN and calbindin. Therefore, it is commonly assumed that GFAP-positive, radial glia-like cells in the adult hippocampus are neural stem cells.

MOLECULAR MECHANISMS
UNDERLYING NEURAL STEM CELL FUNCTION

During the developmental period neural stem cells (also known as neuroepithelial cells or neural progenitor cells) generate neurons, astrocytes and oligodendrocytes. Neural stem cell lineage is controlled by various factors, including transcription factors, growth factors, and others. Until now, it was thought that neuronal differentiation of neural stem cells is induced by brain-derived neurotrophic factor (BDNF) [21, 22] and neurotrophin-3 (NT-3) [21, 23], whereas glial differentiation is promoted by ciliary neurotrophic factor (CNTF) [24], cytokines [25, 26] and thyroid hormone [27] in vitro.

Regarding molecular mechanisms of cell differentiation, activation of Notch is important in cell differentiation of neural stem cells. In the 1910s, T. H. Morgan's laboratory discovered the *Drosophila melanogaster* fruit fly mutant *Notch*, which had wing notches [28]. Following the discovery of the invertebrate *Notch*, this gene was also identified in vertebrates, and studies have revealed that signaling via the Notch receptor and its ligands inhibits cell differentiation of neural stem cells and maintains an undifferentiated state [29, 30]. Although many reports have elucidated Notch signaling during development, little is known about the function of Notch in the adult hippocampus. Recently, Tanigaki et al. [31] found that Notch provides a CNTF-independent instructive signal for glial differentiation in adult hippocampus-derived progenitor cells.

On the other hand, BMPs, members of the transforming growth factor superfamily, are also important in determining cell fate [32]. BMPs function as inhibitory factors for neurogenesis [33] and divert cell fate to the glial lineage [34]. For consideration of neurogenesis, we should pay attention to the existence of BMP antagonists in the adult brain. The endogenous BMP antagonist, Noggin, is expressed in the subventricular zone [35] and dentate gyrus of the adult brain [36]. In fact, Noggin inhibits BMP effects and induces neurogenesis [35, 37]. The time points during which developmental stage–related molecules are still expressed in these regions provide evidence that the adult brain retains the capacity to generate new neurons.

The transcription factor Pax6 is also important in developmental processes. Indeed, the Pax6 mutant *Small eye* displays various abnormalities including cytoarchitectonic abnormalities, failure of cell migration, and a cell adhesion abnormality [38]. Gotz et al. [39] found that these abnormalities result from distorted morphogenesis attributed to radial glial alterations. Further, Pax6 regulates the proneural gene *Neurogenin2* (*Ngn2*) [40]. *Ngn2* encodes a basic helix-loop-helix transcription factor and has been shown to promote cell cycle arrest and neuronal differentiation of neuroepithelial cells by opposing BMPs [41,42, 43]. Therefore, Pax6 is probably essential for neuronal differentiation in the fetal and adult brain. In fact, Makekawa et al. [44] found that Pax6 is important during cell growth in the postnatal hippocampus. The accumulation of additional findings will elucidate the importance of Pax6 in adult neurogenesis.

REGULATION OF NEUROGENESIS UNDER PHYSIOLOGICAL CONDITIONS

(I) Physical Activity

Exercise increases the cell proliferation and survival rate of newly generated neurons. Van Praag et al. found that exercise facilitates not only cell proliferation but also cell survival [45]. Although they confirmed the effect of other tasks (enriched environment and learning), exercise was most effective in generating new neurons. Many scientists have shown that voluntary running markedly increases the rate of cell proliferation up to 10 days after running begins. Therefore, running has a marked positive effect on neurogenesis.

What factors contribute to the positive effects of physical activity? Farmer et al. [46] showed that BDNF mRNA levels were significantly elevated in the dentate gyrus of runners. BDNF is involved in various aspect of brain function including long-term potentiation [47] and is essential for CNS development and neuronal survival throughout life [48]. Moreover, a recent report suggested that BDNF functions as a proliferation factor [49], and BDNF knock out mice show decreased neurogenesis [50,ref lee 2002]. It is therefore reasonable that exercise-induced BDNF expression stimulates neurogenesis during running.

On the other hand, voluntary running also helps to accumulate circulating insulin-like growth factor I (IGF-I) in the hippocampus [51]. Although IGF-I receptors are expressed in the hippocampus [52], little is known about IGF-I protein synthesis in this area. Therefore the influence of IGF-I on the hippocampus may depend on circulating IGF-I levels. Interestingly, Torres-Aleman's group have shown that expression of BDNF mRNA in the hippocampus is enhanced by intra-carotid injection of IGF-I without a running task [51], and exercise-induced positive effects on neurogenesis are attenuated by injection of an antibody against IGF-I [53]. These results suggest that (1) injection of IGF-I mimics exercise-induced BDNF expression and that BDNF expression is under the control of IGF-I, and (2) IGF-I is essential for the positive effects of physical activity on neurogenesis. In addition, O'kusky et al. found that IGF-I overexpression produces a persistent increase in the total number of neurons and synapses in the young adult dentate gyrus [54]. Taken together, these results suggest that cell proliferation and survival of newly generated neurons in the dentate gyrus are strongly dependent on the level of IGF-I in the brain.

Vascular endothelial growth factor (VEGF) functions as an angiogenic factor, although this growth factor also has neurotrophic and neuroprotective effects [55]. VEGF has several receptor subtypes [56], and VEGF receptor 2 (Flk1) is expressed in undifferentiated cells, such as hemocytoblasts and hemangioblasts [57]. Jin et al. [58] found that 5-bromodeoxyuridine (BrdU)-incorporating (dividing) cells express Flk1 and are also positive for DCX, whose expression overlaps with PSA-NCAM [59]. Therefore this result suggests that VEGF acts on immature neurons and functions as a survival-promoting factor. Here, we should pay attention to angiogenesis because newly generated neurons exist along blood vessels running along the inner edge of the granular cell layer in the dentate gyrus, and because vascular endothelial cells provide microenvironmental elements that support neurogenesis [60, 61]. Jin et al. [58] found that intracerebroventricular injection of VEGF stimulates BrdU incorporation into both neuronal and non-neuronal cells; BrdU incorporation is also observed in von Willebrand factor–positive vascular endothelial cells. To understand the effects of VEGF on neurogenesis, it is important to know whether angiogenesis with neurogenesis is observed in blood vessels lying adjacent to BrdU-positive, newly generated neurons in the subgranular zone. Recently, Pereira et al. [62] measured changes in cerebral blood volume in running animals with magnetic resonance imaging technology, and found that exercise increases dentate gyrus cerebral blood volume. Therefore, exercise-induced neurogenesis may promote angiogenesis. These results suggest that, at a minimum, physical exercise gives rise to angiogenesis in the dentate area. On the other hand, regarding the effects of physical activity on expression of VEGF, Fabel et al. [63] found that peripheral VEGF is necessary for the effects of running on adult hippocampal neurogenesis because peripheral blockade of VEGF abolished running-induced neurogenesis. This result is very similar to the increase in IGF-I levels with exercise and decrease with injection of anti-IGF-I. Therefore, expression of IGF-I and VEGF may correlate. If these factors independently act on exercise-induced neurogenesis, the effects of exercise on neurogenesis will not be completely inhibited by either anti-IGF-I or anti-VEGF alone. In fact, two reports suggest that IGF-I induces VEGF mRNA expression in vitro [64, 65]. As these studies have not been verified in vivo, this point requires further study.

(II) Effects of a Stimulating Environment

In the 1960-70s, it was reported that exposure to an enriched environment leads to increased brain weight and a change in acetylcholinesterase activity, thereby improving brain function [67, 67]. At that time, however, little was known about the effects of environmental enrichment on neurogenesis. Later, Kempermann et al. [68] found that living in an enriched environment increases neurogenesis.

Experimental animals are usually housed in simple cages. When animals are housed in an enriched environment, the hippocampus experiences a survival-promoting effect on newly generated cells. However, no changes are observed in the rate of cell proliferation compared with control animals [45, 68, 69]. Therefore, it appears that environmental enrichment induces expression of neurotrophic factors rather than mitogenic factors in the animal brain; alternately, environmental enrichment may inhibit spontaneous apoptosis. In fact, many reports suggest that exposure to an enriched environment leads to an increase in expression of neurotrophic factors in the dentate gyrus of the hippocampus. Similar to exercise, environmental enrichment induces BDNF expression in the hippocampus [70] and stimulates expression of nerve growth factor (NGF) and NT-3 [71, 72]. Without the function of these neurotrophic factors, neurons die by apoptosis. Thus, a state having increased survival rates without cell proliferation indicates that spontaneous apoptosis of newly generated neurons is inhibited by these neurotrophic factors.

REGULATION OF NEUROGENESIS UNDER PATHOLOGICAL CONDITIONS

(I) Developmental Disorders

One cause of mental retardation is thyroid deficiency [73]. Thyroid hormone regulates gene transcription functions in relation to various important aspects of brain development [74, 75, 76]. Several studies have indicated that thyroid hormone affects neuronal morphogenesis. Rami et al. [77] showed that thyroid hormone levels influence cell body volume as well as the number of dendritic branch points in hippocampal pyramidal neurons and dentate granule neurons. Gold et al. [78] demonstrated that hyperthyroidism cause a decrease in dendritic spine density in adult hippocampal CA1 pyramidal neurons. Regarding abnormalities of morphogenetic mechanisms, Montero-Pedrazuela et al. [79] hypothesized that an abnormality of microtubule assembly in the absence of thyroid hormone causes impaired outgrowth of the dendrite tree. Thus, Developmental disorders such as mental retardation are probably caused by thyroid hormone–related morphological changes.

On the other hand, thyroid hormone influences the number of immature neurons and their projections into the molecular layer of the dentate gyrus [79] and participates in cell proliferation and survival of newly generated neurons in the dentate gyrus. Uchida et al. [80] reported that the number of BrdU-positive cells in the subgranular zone of hypothyroid mutant mice was ~35% lower compared with wild type mice, and this decrease was reversed to basal levels in wild type mice by injection of triiodothyronine (T3). Further, Montero-Pedrazuela et al. [79] also showed that thyroid hormone influenced not only cell proliferation but also survival of hippocampal progenitor cells. These results suggest that thyroid hormone directly or indirectly influences expression of mitogenic and neurotrophic factors. Interestingly, Giordano et al. [81] found that expression of NGF and NT-3 mRNA in the hippocampus is upregulated by treatment with thyroxine (T4). Alvarez-Dolado et al. [82] also showed that hypothyroidism causes a decrease in the expression of NGF in the adult hippocampus, and injection of T3 into hypothyroid animals restores NGF expression to near basal levels. Because NGF and NT-3 (likewise BDNF) function as differentiation and survival factors [83, 84], a decrease in the survival of newborn cells in the absence of thyroid hormone may be attributed to downregulation of these factors.

(II) Ischemic Insult

Cerebral ischemia induces excess release of glutamate and an increase in the intracellular Ca^{2+} concentration in neurons, which provokes enzymatic processes leading to irreversible neuronal injury [85]. Ischemia usually brings about programmed cell death in the hippocampus CA1 region four days after ischemia [86], subsequently ischemic injury induces cell proliferation in the brain [87, 88, 89]. The proliferative activity of progenitor cells in the dentate gyrus of the hippocampus reaches the maximal twelve-fold increase 11 days after ischemia [87], whereas pyramidal neurons in the CA1 region do not regenerate later.

Regarding synaptic plasticity, expression of synapsin-I, a marker of synaptogenesis, is induced in the mossy fiber layer of the hippocampus after transient forebrain ischemia [90, 91]. However, expression of synapsin-I is probably unrelated to ischemia-induced neurogenesis because induction of synapsin-I is only observed four days after ischemia and because cell proliferation in the dentate gyrus begins nine days after ischemia. Thus, expression of synapsin-I suggests that the ischemic brain retains the capacity to remodel synapses, rather than synaptogenesis occurring only in newly generated neurons.

On the other hand, middle cerebral artery occlusion induces neurogenesis in the striatum; Arvidsson et al. [92] reported that significantly more newly generated neurons exist in the striatum ipsilateral to the occlusion compared with the contralateral striatum. In fact, they found that new neurons that had incorporated BrdU expressed neuronal markers. Expression of Meis2 and Pbx, markers of developing striatal cells, is observed within two weeks after ischemic insult, and DARPP32, a marker of mature striatal neurons, is later observed in the ipsilateral hemisphere. These results suggest that neuronal regeneration occurs at least in the striatum.

Regarding hippocampal neurogenesis after ischemic insult, interestingly, Nakatomi et al. [93] reported that damaged pyramidal CA1 neurons regenerate by treatment with both fibroblast growth factor and epidermal growth factor. Further, they found that regenerated pyramidal neurons are derived from the posterior periventricular area. These results suggest that the brain retains regenerative capacity if the appropriate environment is preserved in damaged regions.

(III) Stress

Stress activates the hypothalamic-pituitary-adrenal axis (HPA axis) and promotes secretion of adrenal steroids. Circulating glucocorticoids pass through the blood-brain barrier and act on neurons through specific receptors. Activation of the HPA axis may attenuate the rate of adult neurogenesis. Gould et al. [94, 95, 96] found that corticosterone regulates neural progenitor cell proliferation in the dentate gyrus of the adult rat; adrenalectomy markedly increases the number of [^{3}H]thymidine-labeled vimentin-positive cells. Because vimentin-positive radial glia function as neural progenitor cells, an increment in vimentin-positive cells after adrenalectomy raises the possibility that lack of circulating corticosterone enhances adult neurogenesis. In fact, Cameron et al. [97] showed that the rate of neurogenesis in the dentate gyrus depends on circulating corticosterone levels. Besides verified stress paradigms such as adrenalectomy, corticosterone supplementation, psychosocial stress [98] and the scent of a natural enemy [99] have also been reported to attenuate the rate of neurogenesis. Therefore, stress is considered an inhibitory factor for neurogenesis.

On the other hand, Alonso et al. [100] evaluated the importance of the HPA axis using receptor antagonists. Under various stress conditions, corticotropin-releasing factor (CRF) and vasopressin stimulate the release of adrenocorticotropin hormone (ACTH), which induces secretion of adrenal steroids. They showed that inhibition of CRF1 (a corticotropin-releasing factor receptor subtype) or V1b (a vasopressin receptor subtype) receptors with antagonists improves the inhibition of neurogenesis by chronic mild stress. Perhaps these results are attributable to inhibition of adrenal steroids. Because CRF1 and V1b receptors indeed exist in the hippocampus and the amygdala [101, 102], however, the effects of CRF1 and V1b blockade on neurogenesis may be partially attributable to direct action on the hippocampus. This point requires further study.

In general, exposure to chronic stress induces a depressive reaction, during which glucocorticoids induce atrophy of hippocampal CA3 pyramidal neurons, and neurogenesis is attenuated. Antidepressant treatment is highly effective in improving stress-induced suppression of neurogenesis [103, 104]. One class of antidepressants, selective serotonin reuptake inhibitors (SSRI), leads to activation of cyclic AMP response binding protein (CREB) [105]. Consequently, activation of CREB induces BDNF expression and ultimately improves neurogenesis and reduces neurodegeneration [106].

CONCLUSION

Adult neurogenesis studies have greatly advanced from Altman's initial report in the 1960's. Only recently have studies revealed that the rate of neurogenesis is not uniform and is influenced by physiological and pathological conditions. Further, studies indicate the involvement of a large number of regulatory factors in neurogenesis. It remains unclear, however, why adult neurogenesis is limited to two regions—the dentate gyrus and subventricular zone. What mechanisms guide newly generated cells to appropriate positions in the granule cell layer? These mechanistic details of adult neurogenesis remain unclear. Innovative new research techniques may be needed to settle these issues, just as major advances in the life sciences were accomplished by the advent of molecular biology. When these questions are resolved in the near future, neuronal regenerative technology may advance dramatically.

ACKNOWLEDGMENT

I thank Dr. K. Itoi (Division of Neuroendocrinology, Graduate School of Medicine, Tohoku University) and Ms. C. Anakubo (Department of Social Education, Faculty of Integrated Welfare, Tohoku Fukushi University) for advice on the manuscript.

REFERENCES

[1]   Altman J; Das GD. Autoradiographic and histological evidence of postnatal hippocampal neurogenesis in rats. *J. Comp. Neurol.*, 1965, 124, 319-335.

[2]   Kempermann G; Jessberger S; Steiner B; Kronenberg G. Milestones of neuronal development in the adult hippocampus. *Trends Neurosci.*, 2004, 27, 447-52.

[3]   Markakis EA; Gage FH. Adult-generated neurons in the dentate gyrus send axonal projections to field CA3 and are surrounded by synaptic vesicles. *J. Comp. Neurol.*, 1999, 406, 449–460.

[4]   van Praag H; Schinder AF; Christie BR; Toni N; Palmer TD; Gage FH. Functional neurogenesis in the adult hippocampus. *Nature*, 2002, 415, 1030–1034.

[5]   Eriksson PS; Perfilieva E; Björk-Eriksson T; Alborn AM; Nordborg C; Peterson DA; Gage FH. Neurogenesis in the adult human hippocampus. *Nat. Med.*, 1998, 4, 1313-1317.

[6]   Kempermann G; Kuhn HG; Gage FH. Genetic influence on neurogenesis in the dentate gyrus of adult mice. *Proc. Natl. Acad. Sci. U S A*, 1997, 94,10409-10414.

[7]   Biebl M; Cooper CM; Winkler J; Kuhn HG. Analysis of neurogenesis and programmed cell death reveals a self-renewing capacity in the adult rat brain. *Neurosci. Lett.*, 2000, 291,17-20.

[8]   D'Arcangelo G; Miao GG; Chen SC; Soares HD; Morgan JI; Curran T. A protein related to extracellular matrix proteins deleted in the mouse mutant reeler. *Nature*, 1995, 374, 719-723.

[9]   Schmechel DE; Rakic P. A Golgi study of radial glial cells in developing monkey telencephalon: morphogenesis and transformation into astrocytes. *Anat. Embryol*.(Berl), 1979, 156, 115-152.

[10]   Voigt T. Development of glial cells in the cerebral wall of ferrets: direct tracing of their transformation from radial glia into astrocytes. *J. Comp. Neurol.*, 1989, 289, 74-88.

[11]   Seki T; Arai Y. Temporal and spacial relationships between PSA-NCAM-expressing, newly generated granule cells, and radial glia-like cells in the adult dentate gyrus. *J. Comp. Neurol.*, 1999, 410, 503-513.

[12]   Seki T; Arai Y. Highly polysialylated neural cell adhesion molecule (NCAM-H) is expressed by newly generated granule cells in the dentate gyrus of the adult rat. *J. Neurosci.*, 1993, 13, 2351-2358.

[13]   Taupin P; Gage FH. Adult neurogenesis and neural stem cells of the central nervous system in mammals. *J. Neurosci. Res.*, 2002, 69, 745-749.

[14]   Johansson CB; Momma S; Clarke DL; Risling M; Lendahl U; Frisén J. Identification of a neural stem cell in the adult mammalian central nervous system. *Cell*, 1999, 96, 25-34.

[15]   Doetsch F; Caillé I; Lim DA; García-Verdugo JM; Alvarez-Buylla A. Subventricular zone astrocytes are neural stem cells in the adult mammalian brain. *Cell*, 1999, 97, 703-716.

[16]   Doetsch F; García-Verdugo JM; Alvarez-Buylla A. Regeneration of a germinal layer in the adult mammalian brain. *Proc. Natl. Acad. Sci. U S A*, 1999, 96, 11619-11624.

[17]   Lim DA; Tramontin AD; Trevejo JM; Herrera DG; García-Verdugo JM; Alvarez-Buylla A. Noggin antagonizes BMP signaling to create a niche for adult neurogenesis. *Neuron,* 2000, 28, 713-726.

[18]   Seri B; García-Verdugo JM; McEwen BS; Alvarez-Buylla A. Astrocytes give rise to new neurons in the adult mammalian hippocampus. *J. Neurosci.*, 2001, 21, 7153-7160.

[19] Wei LC; Shi M; Chen LW; Cao R; Zhang P; Chan YS. Nestin-containing cells express glial fibrillary acidic protein in the proliferative regions of central nervous system of postnatal developing and adult mice. *Brain. Res. Dev. Brain Res*, 2002, 139, 9-17.

[20] Meyer G; Perez-Garcia CG; Gleeson JG. Selective expression of doublecortin and LIS1 in developing human cortex suggests unique modes of neuronal movement. *Cereb. Cortex*, 2002, 12, 1225-1236.

[21] Takahashi J; Palmer TD; Gage FH. Retinoic acid and neurotrophins collaborate to regulate neurogenesis in adult-derived neural stem cell cultures. *J. Neurobiol.*, 1999, 38, 65-81.

[22] Schinstine M; Iacovitti L. 5-Azacytidine and BDNF enhance the maturation of neurons derived from EGF-generated neural stem cells. *Exp. Neurol.*, 1997, 144, 315-325.

[23] Pappas IS; Parnavelas JG. Neurotrophins and basic fibroblast growth factor induce the differentiation of calbindin-containing neurons in the cerebral cortex. *Exp. Neurol.*, 1997, 144, 302-314.

[24] Whittemore SR; Morassutti DJ; Walters WM; Liu RH; Magnuson DS. Mitogen and substrate differentially affect the lineage restriction of adult rat subventricular zone neural precursor cell populations. *Exp. Cell Res.*, 1999, 252, 75-95.

[25] Nakashima K; Taga T. Mechanisms underlying cytokine-mediated cell-fate regulation in the nervous system. *Mol. Neurobiol.*, 2002, 25, 233-244.

[26] Nakanishi M; Niidome T; Matsuda S; Akaike A; Kihara T; Sugimoto H. Microglia-derived interleukin-6 and leukaemia inhibitory factor promote astrocytic differentiation of neural stem/progenitor cells. *Eur. J. Neurosci.*, 2007, 25, 649-658.

[27] Johe KK; Hazel TG; Muller T; Dugich-Djordjevic MM; McKay RD. Single factors direct the differentiation of stem cells from the fetal and adult central nervous system. *Genes Dev.*, 1996, 10, 3129-3140.

[28] Morgan, TH. The theory of the gene. 1928, Yale University Press, 77-81.

[29] Artavanis-Tsakonas S; Rand MD; Lake RJ. Notch signaling: cell fate control and signal integration in development. *Science*, 1999, 284, 770-776.

[30] Chojnacki A; Shimazaki T; Gregg C; Weinmaster G; Weiss S. Glycoprotein 130 signaling regulates Notch1 expression and activation in the self-renewal of mammalian forebrain neural stem cells. *J. Neurosci.*, 2003, 23, 1730-1741.

[31] Tanigaki K; Nogaki F; Takahashi J; Tashiro K; Kurooka H; Honjo T. Notch1 and Notch3 instructively restrict bFGF-responsive multipotent neural progenitor cells to an astroglial fate. *Neuron,* 2001, 29, 45-55.

[32] Hall AK; Miller RH. Emerging roles for bone morphogenetic proteins in central nervous system glial biology. *J. Neurosci. Res.*, 2004, 76, 1-8.

[33] Shou J; Rim PC; Calof AL. BMPs inhibit neurogenesis by a mechanism involving degradation of a transcription factor. *Nat. Neurosci.*, 1999, 2, 339-345.

[34] Adachi T; Takanaga H; Kunimoto M; Asou H. Influence of LIF and BMP-2 on differentiation and development of glial cells in primary cultures of embryonic rat cerebral hemisphere. *J. Neurosci. Res.*, 2005, 79, 608-615.

[35]   Lim DA; Tramontin AD; Trevejo JM; Herrera DG; García-Verdugo JM; Alvarez-Buylla A. Noggin antagonizes BMP signaling to create a niche for adult neurogenesis. *Neuron,* 2000, 28, 713-726.

[36]   Fan X; Xu H; Cai W; Yang Z; Zhang J. Spatial and temporal patterns of expression of Noggin and BMP4 in embryonic and postnatal rat hippocampus. *Brain. Res. Dev. Brain Res.*, 2003, 146, 51-58.

[37]   Fan XT; Xu HW; Cai WQ; Yang H; Liu S. Antisense Noggin oligodeoxynucleotide administration decreases cell proliferation in the dentate gyrus of adult rats. *Neurosci. Lett,* 2004, 366, 107-111.

[38]   Stoykova A: Götz M: Gruss P: Price J. Pax6-dependent regulation of adhesive patterning, R-cadherin expression and boundary formation in developing forebrain. Development, 1997, 124, 3765-3777.

[39]   Götz M; Stoykova A; Gruss P. Pax6 controls radial glia differentiation in the cerebral cortex. *Neuron,* 1998, 21, 1031-1044.

[40]   Scardigli R; Bäumer N; Gruss P; Guillemot F; Le Roux I. Direct and concentration-dependent regulation of the proneural gene Neurogenin2 by Pax6. Development, 2003, 130, 3269-3281.

[41]   Mizuguchi R; Sugimori M; Takebayashi H; Kosako H; Nagao M; Yoshida S; Nabeshima Y; Shimamura K; Nakafuku M. Combinatorial roles of olig2 and neurogenin2 in the coordinated induction of pan-neuronal and subtype-specific properties of motoneurons. *Neuron,* 2001, 31, 757-771.

[42]   Novitch BG; Chen AI; Jessell TM. Coordinate regulation of motor neuron subtype identity and pan-neuronal properties by the bHLH repressor Olig2. Neuron, 2001, 31, 773-789.

[43]   Scardigli R; Schuurmans C; Gradwohl G; Guillemot F. Crossregulation between Neurogenin2 and pathways specifying neuronal identity in the spinal cord. Neuron, 2001, 31, 203-217.

[44]   Maekawa M; Takashima N; Arai Y; Nomura T; Inokuchi K; Yuasa S; Osumi N. Pax6 is required for production and maintenance of progenitor cells in postnatal hippocampal neurogenesis. *Genes Cells,* 2005, 10, 1001-1014.

[45]   van Praag H; Kempermann G; Gage FH. Running increases cell proliferation and neurogenesis in the adult mouse dentate gyrus. *Nat. Neurosci.*, 1999, 2, 266-270.

[46]   Farmer J; Zhao X; van Praag H; Wodtke K; Gage FH; Christie BR. Effects of voluntary exercise on synaptic plasticity and gene expression in the dentate gyrus of adult male Sprague-Dawley rats in vivo. *Neuroscience,* 2004, 124, 71-79.

[47]   Bramham CR; Messaoudi E. BDNF function in adult synaptic plasticity: the synaptic consolidation hypothesis. *Prog. Neurobiol.*, 2005, 76, 99-125.

[48]   Kirschenbaum B; Goldman SA. Brain-derived neurotrophic factor promotes the survival of neurons arising from the adult rat forebrain subependymal zone. *Proc. Natl. Acad. Sci. USA,* 1995, 92, 210–214.

[49]   Pencea P; Bingaman KD; Wiegand SJ; Luskin MB. Infusion of brainderived neurotrophic factor into lateral ventricle of the adult rat leads to new neuron in the parenchyma of the striatum, septum, thalamus, and hypothalamus. *J. Neurosci.,* 2001, 21, 6706–6717.

[50]   Lee J; Duan W; Mattson MP. Evidence that brain-derived neurotrophic factor is required for basal neurogenesis and mediates, in part, the enhancement of neurogenesis by dietary restriction in the hippocampus of adult mice. *J. Neurochem.*, 2002, 82, 1367-1375.

[51]   Carro E; Nuñez A; Busiguina S; Torres-Aleman I. Circulating insulin-like growth factor I mediates effects of exercise on the brain. *J. Neurosci.*, 2000, 20, 2926-2933.

[52]   Werther GA; Abate M; Hogg A; Cheesman H; Oldfield B; Hards D; Hudson P; Power B; Freed K; Herington AC. Localization of insulin-like growth factor-I mRNA in rat brain by in situ hybridization--relationship to IGF-I receptors.*Mol. Endocrinol.*, 1990, 4, 773-778.

[53]   Trejo JL; Carro E; Torres-Aleman I. Circulating insulin-like growth factor I mediates exercise-induced increases in the number of new neurons in the adult hippocampus.*J. Neurosci.*, 2001, 21, 1628-1634.

[54]   O'Kusky JR; Ye P; D'Ercole AJ. Insulin-like growth factor-I promotes neurogenesis and synaptogenesis in the hippocampal dentate gyrus during postnatal development. *J. Neurosci.*, 2000, 20, 8435-8442.

[55]   Storkebaum E; Carmeliet P. VEGF: a critical player in neurodegeneration. *J. Clin. Invest.*, 2004, 113, 14-18.

[56]   Neufeld G; Cohen T; Gengrinovitch S; Poltorak Z. Vascular endothelial growth factor (VEGF) and its receptors. *FASEB J.*, 1999, 13, 9-22.

[57]   Hong DL; Zhang YZ; Piacibello W; Aglietta M. Vascular Endothelial Growth Factor and Its Receptor KDR/flk-1 Play Important Roles in Hematopoiesis. Zhongguo Shi Yan Xue Ye Xue Za Zhi, 2001, 9, 268-272.

[58]   Jin K; Zhu Y; Sun Y; Mao XO; Xie L; Greenberg DA. Vascular endothelial growth factor (VEGF) stimulates neurogenesis in vitro and in vivo. *Proc. Natl. Acad. Sci. U S A,* 2002, 99, 11946-11950.

[59]   Nacher J; Crespo C; McEwen BS. Doublecortin expression in the adult rat telencephalon. Eur J Neurosci, 2001, 14, 629-644.

[60]   Seki T. Hippocampal adult neurogenesis occurs in a microenvironment provided by PSA-NCAM-expressing immature neurons. *J. Neurosci. Res.*, 2002, 69, 772-783.

[61]   Seki T. Microenvironmental elements supporting adult hippocampal neurogenesis. *Anat. Sci. Int.*, 2003, 78, 69-78.

[62]   Pereira AC; Huddleston DE; Brickman AM; Sosunov AA; Hen R; McKhann GM; Sloan R; Gage FH, Brown TR, Small SA. An in vivo correlate of exercise-induced neurogenesis in the adult dentate gyrus. *Proc. Natl. Acad. Sci. U S A*, 2007, 27, 104, 5638-5643.

[63]   Fabel K; Fabel K; Tam B; Kaufer D; Baiker A; Simmons N; Kuo CJ; Palmer TD. VEGF is necessary for exercise-induced adult hippocampal neurogenesis. Eur J Neurosci, 2003, 18, 2803-2312.

[64]   [64] Warren RS; Yuan H; Matli MR; Ferrara N; Donner DB. Induction of vascular endothelial growth factor by insulin-like growth factor 1 in colorectal carcinoma. *J. Biol. Chem.*, 1996, 271, 29483-2948.

[65]   Miele C; Rochford JJ; Filippa N; Giorgetti-Peraldi S; Van Obberghen E. Insulin and insulin-like growth factor-I induce vascular endothelial growth factor mRNA expression via different signaling pathways. *J. Biol. Chem.*, 2000, 275, 21695-21702.

[66]   Bennett EL; Rosenzweig MR; Diamond MC. Rat brain: effects of environmental enrichment on wet and dry weights. *Science*, 1969, 163, 825-826.

[67]   La Torre JC. Effect of differential environmental enrichment on brain weight and on acetylcholinesterase and cholinesterase activities in mice. *Exp. Neurol.*, 1968, 22, 493-503.

[68]   Kempermann G; Kuhn HG; Gage FH. More hippocampal neurons in adult mice living in an enriched environment. *Nature,* 1997, 386, 493-495.

[69]   Olson AK; Eadie BD; Ernst C; Christie BR. Environmental enrichment and voluntary exercise massively increase neurogenesis in the adult hippocampus via dissociable pathways. *Hippocampus*, 2006,16, 250-60.

[70]   Rossi C; Angelucci A; Costantin L; Braschi C; Mazzantini M; Babbini F; Fabbri ME; Tessarollo L; Maffei L; Berardi N; Caleo M. Brain-derived neurotrophic factor (BDNF) is required for the enhancement of hippocampal neurogenesis following environmental enrichment. *Eur. J. Neurosci.*, 2006, 24, 1850-1856.

[71]   orasdotter M; Metsis M; Henriksson BG; Winblad B; Mohammed AH.Environmental enrichment results in higher levels of nerve growth factor mRNA in the rat visual cortex and hippocampus. *Behav. Brain Res.*, 1998, 93, 83-90.

[72]   Torasdotter M; Metsis M; Henriksson BG; Winblad B; Mohammed AH. Expression of neurotrophin-3 mRNA in the rat visual cortex and hippocampus is influenced by environmental conditions. *Neurosci. Lett.*, 1996, 218, 107-110.

[73]   Refetoff S; Weiss RE; Usala SJ. The syndromes of resistance to thyroid hormone. *Endocr. Rev.*, 1993, 14, 348–399.

[74]   Nicholson JL; Altman J. Synaptogenesis in the rat cerebellum: effects of early hypo- and hyperthyroidism. *Science,* 1972, 176, 530–532.

[75]   Nicholson JL; Altman J. The effects of early hypo- and hyperthyroidism on the development of the rat cerebellar cortex II.Synaptogenesis in the molecular layer. *Brain. Res.*, 1972, 44, 25–36.

[76]   Oppenheimer JH; Schwartz HL. Molecular basis of thyroid hormone dependent brain development. *Endocr. Rev.*, 1997, 18, 462–475.

[77]   Rami A; Patel AJ; Rabie A. Thyroid hormone and development of the rat hippocampus: morphological alterations in granule and pyramidal cells. *Neuroscience,* 1986, 19, 1217-1226.

[78]   Gould E; Allan MD; McEwen BS. Dendritic spine density of adult hippocampal pyramidal cells is sensitive to thyroid hormone. *Brain Res.,* 1990, 525, 327-329.

[79]   Montero-Pedrazuela A; Venero C; Lavado-Autric R; Fernandez-Lamo I; Garcia-Verdugo JM; Bernal J; Guadano-Ferraz A. Modulation of adult hippocampal neurogenesis by thyroid hormones: implications in depressive-like behavior. *Mol. Psychiatry*, 2006,11, 361-371.

[80]   Uchida K; Yonezawa M; Nakamura S; Kobayashi T; Machida T. Impaired neurogenesis in the growth-retarded mouse is reversed by T3 treatment. *Neuroreport,* 2005,16,103-6.

[81]   Giordano T; Pan JB; Casuto D; Watanabe S; Arneric SP. Thyroid hormone regulation of NGF, NT-3 and BDNF RNA in the adult rat brain. B*rain Res. Mol. Brain. Res.*, 1992, 16, 239-245.

[82]   Alvarez-Dolado M; Iglesias T; Rodriguez-Pena A; Bernal J; Munoz A. Expression of neurotrophins and the trk family of neurotrophin receptors in normal and hypothyroid rat brain. *Brain Res. Mol. Brain Res.*, 1994, 27, 249-257.

[83]   Lindholm D. Role of neurotrophins in preventing glutamate induced neuronal cell death. *J. Neurol.*, 1994, 242, S16-18.

[84]   Tucker KL. Neurotrophins and the control of axonal outgrowth. *Panminerva Med.*, 2002, 44, 325-333.

[85]   Juurlink BH; Sweeney MI. Mechanisms that result in damage during and following cerebral ischemia. *Neurosci. Biobehav. Rev.*, 1997, 21, 121-128.

[86]   Kirino T. Delayed neuronal death in the gerbil hippocampus following ischemia. *Brain Res.*, 1982, 239, 57-69.

[87]   Liu J; Solway K; Messing RO; Sharp FR. Increased neurogenesis in the dentate gyrus after transient global ischemia in gerbils. *J. Neurosci.*, 1998, 18, 7768-7778.

[88]   Kee NJ; Preston E; Wojtowicz JM. Enhanced neurogenesis after transient global ischemia in the dentate gyrus of the rat. *Exp. Brain Res.*, 2001, 136, 313-320.

[89]   Jin K; Minami M; Lan JQ; Mao XO; Batteur S; Simon RP; Greenberg DA. Neurogenesis in dentate subgranular zone and rostral subventricular zone after focal cerebral ischemia in the rat. *Proc. Natl. Acad. Sci. U S A*, 2001, 98, 4710-4715.

[90]   Marti E; Ferrer I; Blasi J. Transient increase of synapsin-I immunoreactivity in the mossy fiber layer of the hippocampus after transient forebrain ischemia in the mongolian gerbil. *Brain Res.*, 1999, 824, 153-160.

[91]   Bernabeu R; Sharp FR. NMDA and AMPA/kainate glutamate receptors modulate dentate neurogenesis and CA3 synapsin-I in normal and ischemic hippocampus. *J. Cereb. Blood Flow Metab.*, 2000, 20, 1669-1680.

[92]   Arvidsson A; Collin T; Kirik D; Kokaia Z; Lindvall O. Neuronal replacement from endogenous precursors in the adult brain after stroke. *Nat. Med.*, 2002, 8, 963-970.

[93]   Nakatomi H; Kuriu T; Okabe S; Yamamoto S; Hatano O; Kawahara N; Tamura A; Kirino T; Nakafuku M. Regeneration of hippocampal pyramidal neurons after ischemic brain injury by recruitment of endogenous neural progenitors. *Cell*, 2002, 110, 429-441.

[94]   [94] Gould E; Woolley CS; McEwen BS. Adrenal steroids regulate postnatal development of the rat dentate gyrus: I. Effects of glucocorticoids on cell death. *J. Comp. Neurol.*, 1991, 313, 479-485.

[95]   Gould E; Woolley CS; Cameron HA; Daniels DC; McEwen BS. Adrenal steroids regulate postnatal development of the rat dentate gyrus: II. Effects of glucocorticoids and mineralocorticoids on cell birth. *J. Comp. Neurol.*, 1991, 313, 486-493.

[96]   [96] Gould E; Cameron HA; Daniels DC, Woolley CS, McEwen BS. Adrenal hormones suppress cell division in the adult rat dentate gyrus. *J. Neurosci.*, 1992, 12, 3642-3650.

[97]   Cameron HA; Gould E. Adult neurogenesis is regulated by adrenal steroids in the dentate gyrus. *Neuroscience*, 1994, 61, 203-209.

[98]   Gould E; McEwen BS; Tanapat P; Galea LA; Fuchs E. Neurogenesis in the dentate
        gyrus of the adult tree shrew is regulated by psychosocial stress and NMDA receptor
        activation. *J. Neurosci.,* 1997, 17, 2492-2498.

[99]   Tanapat P; Hastings NB; Rydel TA; Galea LA; Gould E. Exposure to fox odor
        inhibits cell proliferation in the hippocampus of adult rats via an adrenal hormone-
        dependent mechanism. *J. Comp. Neurol.,* 2001, 437, 496-504.

[100]   Alonso R; Griebel G; Pavone G; Stemmelin J; Le Fur G; Soubrie P. Blockade of
        CRF(1) or V(1b) receptors reverses stress-induced suppression of neurogenesis in a
        mouse model of depression. *Mol. Psychiatry,* 2004, 9, 278-286.

[101]   De Souza EB; Insel TR; Perrin MH; Rivier J; Vale WW; Kuhar MJ. Corticotropin-
        releasing factor receptors are widely distributed within the rat central nervous system:
        an autoradiographic study. *J. Neurosci.,* 1985, 5, 3189-3203.

[102]   Vaccari C; Lolait SJ; Ostrowski NL. Comparative distribution of vasopressin V1b
        and oxytocin receptor messenger ribonucleic acids in brain. *Endocrinology,* 1998,
        139, 5015-5033.

[103]   Malberg JE; Eisch AJ; Nestler EJ; Duman RS. Chronic antidepressant treatment
        increases neurogenesis in adult rat hippocampus. *J. Neurosci.,* 2000, 20, 9104-9110.

[104]   Duman RS; Nakagawa S; Malberg J. Regulation of adult neurogenesis by
        antidepressant treatment. *Neuropsychopharmacology,* 2001, 25, 836-844.

[105]   Thome J; Sakai N; Shin K; Steffen C; Zhang YJ; Impey S; Storm D; Duman RS.
        cAMP response element-mediated gene transcription is upregulated by chronic
        antidepressant treatment. *J. Neurosci.,* 2000, 20, 4030-4036.

[106]   Nibuya M; Nestler EJ; Duman RS. Chronic antidepressant administration increases
        the expression of cAMP response element binding protein (CREB) in rat
        hippocampus. *J. Neurosci.,* 1996, 16, 2365-2372.

In: Progress in Cell Growth Process Research
Editor: Takumi Hayashi, pp. 135-147

ISBN 978-1-60456-325-2
© 2008 Nova Science Publishers, Inc.

Chapter 5

VIRAL PROTEINS, HOST CELL PROTEINS, AND MANIPULATION OF THE CELL CYCLE BY VIRUSES

Kazuya Shirato[1] and Tetsuya Mizutani[23]
[1]Laboratory of Acute Respiratory Viral Diseases and Cytokines,
Department of Virology III,
[2]Department of Virology I, National Institute of Infectious Diseases, Gakuen 4-7-1,
Musashimurayama, Tokyo 208-0011 Japan

ABSTRACT

Manipulation of the cell cycle is an important strategy used by viruses to cope with the changing environments in virally infected cells. Viral infection may lead to inhibition or promotion of cell growth processes and may, in some cases, result in the arrest of the host cell cycle so as to promote viral replication. Cell growth may be slowed by inhibition of cellular DNA or RNA synthesis, inhibition of cell cycle progression by interaction with host cell proteins, and progression of apoptosis. These changes are thought to provide favorable conditions for the replication of viruses before elimination by the host immune system. After viral replication, apoptosis is often induced, resulting in lysis and the release of viruses. On the other hand, oncoproteins of DNA viruses are known to interact with proteins in the retinoblastoma family, which are tumor suppressors. These viruses have the potential to induce transformation of host cells. Such observations have led to experimental concepts regarding, for example, the culturing of cells from primary cells by expression of oncogenes. Signaling pathways, which may be activated or inactivated by viral infection, also play important roles in cell growth. In this review, we highlight molecular mechanisms of host cell growth regulation by the interactions of viral proteins and host proteins.

3 Corresponding author. Telephone +81-425-61-0771, Facsimile +81-425-65-3315, Email tmizutan@nih.go.jp.

ABSTRACT 2

A number of viruses are known to manipulate the cell cycles of their host cells to cope with changing cellular environments, and this change provides favorable conditions for the replication of viruses before elimination by the host immune system. Cell growth and division are strictly controlled by the cell cycle and the cell cycle consists of cycles of -G1-S-G2-M-. Transition from one phase to the next are regulated by different cyclins and cyclin-dependent kinases. For some type of virus infections, there have been numerous reports of the activities of cell cycle regulatory molecules being disturbed by viral proteins and the cell cycles of virus-infected cells being altered. Viruses manipulate the host cell cycle by using regulatory proteins to produce favorable environments for virus survival and replication.

ABBREVIATIONS

ADV:	denovirus
AcMNPV:	*utographa californica* multiple nucleopolyhedrovirus
bZIP:	asic leucine zipper
C:	core
CDK:	ifferent cyclin-dependent kinases
Cdc2:	ell division cycle 2 protein
EBV:	pstein-Barr virus
G:	ap stage
HBV:	he human hepatitis B virus
HCV:	uman hepatitis C virus
HIV-1:	uman immunodeficiency virus type 1
HTLV-1:	uman T-cell leukemia virus type I
IBV:	nfectious bronchitis virus
KSHV:	aposi's sarcoma-associated herpesvirus
LANA:	atency-associated nuclear antigen
M:	itosis phase
NS:	onstructural
ORF:	pen reading frame
S:	ynthesis stage
SV5:	imian parainfluenza virus 5
Rb:	etinoblastoma

INTRODUCTION

A number of viruses are known to manipulate the cell cycles of their host cells to cope with changing cellular environments. By selectively inhibiting or promoting host cell growth processes, viral replication can be favored. Host cell growth may be slowed by inhibition of cellular DNA or RNA synthesis, inhibition of cell cycle progression by the interaction of viral proteins with host cell proteins, and progression of apoptosis. These changes are thought to provide favorable conditions for the replication of viruses before elimination by the host immune system.

Cell growth and division are strictly controlled by the cell cycle. The cell cycle mainly divided into two periods, which are mitosis (M) phase and interphase. Besides, interphase are divided into three phases, which are post-mitosis gap stage (G_1), DNA synthesis stage (S), and pre-mitosis gap stage (G_2). Namely, cell cycle consists of cycles of -G1-S-G2-M-. The cell which is not in the cell division does not shift to S phase, the cell shifts into an arrest phase which is called a G_0 phase. Cyclin D/CDK4 or CDK6 complex promotes the progression from G_0 to G_1 by inhibiting the binding of the retinoblastoma (Rb) protein and E2F by phosphorylation of Rb. E2F up-regulates cyclin E expression and cyclin E/CDK2 complex promotes the transition from G_1 to the S phase. Cyclin A/or CDK2 or cell division cycle 2 protein (Cdc2) promotes the transition from the S phase to G_2, and cyclin B/Cdc2 is activated by Thr161 phosphorylation and initiates the M phase. The progression of the cell cycle is also checked and controlled at each stage by various CDK inhibitors and by guardian proteins, such as p53, and protein kinase ATM/ATR.

For some types of virus infections, there have been numerous reports of the activities of cell cycle regulatory molecules being disturbed by viral proteins and the cell cycles of virus-infected cells being altered. This chapter gives an overview of some common viruses that are able to affect either or both of the progression and the arrest of the cell cycle and discusses the advantages viruses may gain by influencing the cell cycles of their host cells.

REPRESENTATIVE VIRUSES KNOWN TO AFFECT PROGRESS OR ARREST OF THE CELL CYCLES OF THEIR HOST CELLS

1. Adenovirus Type 5

Adenovirus (ADV) type 5 is a DNA virus in the family *Adenoviridae*. The E1A polypeptides of adenoviruses are multifunctional proteins involved in many cellular processes, such as transcriptional activation and repression, immortalization, blockade of differentiation, and stimulation of DNA synthesis (Dyson and Harlow, 1992; Moran and Mathews, 1987). The E1A protein binds with coactivator p300/CREB-binding protein and retinoblastoma (Rb)-family proteins and inhibits the binding of Rb and transcriptional factor E2F, and expression of cyclin E are up-regulated, and then the cell cycle progression is up-regulated (Baluchamy *et al.*, 2007; Chellappan *et al.*, 1992; Eckner *et al.*, 1994; Howe *et al.*, 1990). The E1A protein shares a functional domain with simian virus 40 large T antigen and human papilloma virus E7 oncoprotein, and these proteins also bind Rb protein and therefore promote cell growth (Brehm *et al.*, 1999; Chellappan *et al.*, 1992; DeCaprio *et al.*, 1988).

2. Human T-Cell Leukemia Virus Type I

Human T-cell leukemia virus type I (HTLV-1) is in the family *Retroviridae* and is an etiological agent of adult T-cell leukemia (Hinuma *et al.*, 1981; Poiesz *et al.*, 1980). The Tax protein encoded in the HTLV-1 genome plays a critical role in cell transformation *in vitro* and *in vivo* (Grassmann *et al.*, 1989; Grossman *et al.*, 1995; Nerenberg *et al.*, 1987). The Tax protein was identified at first as a trans-acting transcriptional activator of the HTLV-1 promoter in the long terminal repeat (Felber *et al.*, 1985; Sodroski *et al.*, 1985). Tax protein directly up-regulates cell growth signaling, such as the transcriptional activator NF-κB signaling (Yoshida, 1995).

Tax protein induces cell cycle progression from the G_0/G_1 phase to the S and G_2/M phases. It has been reported that Tax protein up-regulates cell cycle regulatory molecules, such as cyclin D2, cyclin E, E2F1, CDK2, CDK4, and CDK6, through the NF-κB transcription pathway and down-regulates CDK inhibitors such as p16, p18, p19 and p27 (Huang *et al.*, 2001; Iwanaga *et al.*, 2001; Low *et al.*, 1997; Suzuki *et al.*, 1996; Suzuki *et al.*, 1999).

3. Herpesviruses

There have been many reports that viral proteins of viruses in the family *Herpesviridae* interact with cell cycle regulatory molecules and affect cell cycle progression. Kaposi's sarcoma-associated herpesvirus (KSHV), which is also called human herpesvirus 8, is in the subfamily *Gammaherpesvirinae,* as is the Epstein-Barr virus (EBV). Virus cyclin is a well-known cell cycle promoter of KSHV via direct interaction with CDK6 (Dittmer *et al.*, 1998; Kaldis *et al.*, 2001). In addition, the latency-associated nuclear antigen (LANA) of the KSHV can transform primary rat embryo fibroblasts by cooperating with the rat's oncogene and promoting cell growth with E2F activation by binding Rb, and moreover, LANA inhibits the p53 pathway and protects the cell against apoptosis (Friborg et al., 1999; Radkov, Kellam, and Boshoff, 2000). On the other hand, Zta is a basic leucine zipper (bZIP) transcription factor of EBV, and its KSHV homologue, K-bZIP, cause G_0/G_1 cell cycle arrest by down-regulating the cyclin E/CDK2 complex, and these bZIP transcription factors inhibit p53 induction and prevent cell apoptosis, prolonging the lives of infected cells (Cayrol and Flemington, 1996; Izumiya et al., 2003; Park et al., 2000a).

Other herpesviruses, such as the human cytomegalovirus, produce proteins, such as the UL69 protein, which block the cell cycle at G_1, even in the absence of virus replication, because UL69 is incorporated in the virion (Hayashi, Blankenship, and Shenk, 2000; Lu and Shenk, 1999), whereas human cytomegalovirus phosphoprotein 71 hastens cell cycle progression by inducing degradation of Rb family proteins in the proteasome pathway (Kalejta, Bechtel, and Shenk, 2003). In addition, it has been reported that the product of open reading frame (ORF) 68 of gammaherpesvirus induced cell-cycle arrest at G_2 by inhibiting the cyclin B/Cdc2 complex (Nascimento and Parkhouse, 2007).

4. Hepatitis B Virus

The human hepatitis B virus (HBV) is a member of the *Hepadnavirus* family and has a circular DNA consisting of a longer complete negative-sense strand, with a piece missing at a nick site, and an incomplete positive-sense strand. HBV causes acute and chronic hepatocyte injury and is associated with liver cancer (Beasley *et al.*, 1981). The HBV genome has four ORFs, and four gene products (surface, core, polymerase, and X) which are encoded in HBV. The HBV-X protein is a transcriptional activator and is also essential for viral infection (Spandau and Lee, 1988; Zoulim, Saputelli, and Seeger, 1994). HBV-X inhibits apoptosis (Gottlob *et al.*, 1998) and is able to induce liver cancer in HBV-X transgenic mice (Kim *et al.*, 1991; Koike *et al.*, 1994).

Benn and Schneider reported that HBV-X deregulated cell cycle checkpoint controls (Benn and Schneider, 1995). In brief, HBV-X activates the RAS-RAF-MAP kinase signal cascade and also activates the downstream transcriptional factors AP-1 and NF-κB and stimulates cell DNA synthesis. HBV-X stimulates cell cycle progression, hastening the emergence of cells from G_0 and entry into the S phase, and accelerating transit through checkpoint controls at G_0/G_1 and G_2/M. HBV-X can participate in the selection of cells that are genetically unstable, some of which may accumulate unrepaired transforming mutations (Benn and Schneider, 1995). On the other hand, Park et al, reported that HBV-X induced prolongation of G_1 to S phase in p53-mutant human hepatocellular carcinoma cells by increasing the expression of p21 and the binding of p21 and CDK2 (Park *et al.*, 2000b).

5. Hepatitis C Virus

Human hepatitis C virus (HCV) is in the family *Flaiviviridae* and causes acute, and in many cases chronic, hepatitis. Chronic hepatitis C is a major cause of liver cirrhosis and hepatic cancer (Erhardt *et al.*, 2002). It was reported that the core (C) protein of HCV can transform HCV-infected cells (Kato, 2001; Ray and Ray, 2001). The C protein of HCV activates extracellular signal-regulated kinase (ERK), c-Jun N-terminal kinase (JNK), and p38 mitogen-activated protein (MAP) kinase, induces MAP kinase phosphatase MKP-1 expression and increases cell proliferation (Erhardt *et al.*, 2002; Tsuchihara *et al.*, 1999). The C protein also protects cells from apoptosis induced by Fas or tumor necrosis factor-alpha by activating the NF-κB signaling pathway (Marusawa *et al.*, 1999).

In contrast, a nonstructural (NS) protein of HCV, NS5A, delays the cell cycle at G_2 by inducing the CDK inhibitor p21 which is dependent on p53 expression and by down-regulating cyclin/CDK1 activation (Arima *et al.*, 2001). The NS5B protein of HCV is also able to retard the cell cycle through the toll-like receptor 3 signaling pathway, which depends on interferon-beta induction, without replicating viral genomes (Naka *et al.*, 2006).

Infection by other flaviviruses, such as Japanese encephalitis virus and dengue virus type 2, activates the lipid kinase, phosphatidylinositol 3-kinase (PI3K) and its downstream target Akt signaling pathway, and protects cells from apoptosis in early stages of infection (Lee, Liao, and Lin, 2005).

6. Human Immunodeficiency Virus Type 1

Human immunodeficiency virus type 1 (HIV-1) is a single-stranded positive-sense RNA virus in the family *Retroviridae*, genus *Lentivirus*. HIV-1 has 9 genes, and they encode structural proteins (*gag, env*), polymerase (*pol*), transactivator (*rev, tat*), and accessory gene products (*vif, vpr, vpu,* and *nef*). The Vpr accessory protein is the one protein that is incorporated into the HIV-1 virion (Cohen *et al.*, 1990), affects the progression of the cell cycle, and has prevented the establishment of *in vitro* chronically infected HIV-1 producer cell lines (Rogel, Wu, and Emerman, 1995). The effects of the Vpr protein on the cell cycle are due to inhibiting the activation of the cyclin B/Cdc2 complex by preventing dephosphorylation of Cdc2 by binding Cdc25C phosphatase; Vpr causes HIV-1 infected cells to be in G_2 arrest (Goh, Manel, and Emerman, 2004; Goh et al., 1998; He et al., 1995; Re et al., 1995). In addition, the Vpr protein of HIV-1 induces cell-cycle arrest in G_1 in rodent cells and also induces apoptosis by increasing caspase-3 and caspase-9 activities by down-regulating caspase-3 and caspase-9 inhibitors (Azuma *et al.*, 2006).

7. Measles Virus

The measles virus is in the family *Paramyxoviridae*, genus *Morbillivirus*. It is lymphotropic and immunosuppressive during acute infection, and T and B lymphocytes and monocytes are infected (Joseph, Lampert, and Oldstone, 1975; Sullivan et al., 1975). Lymphocytes infected by measles virus are activated and permissive for efficient viral replication, but cells are nonresponsive to mitogens and are partially arrested at G_0/G_1 phase (McChesney, Altman, and Oldstone, 1988; McChesney et al., 1987). In lymphocytes infected with measles virus, expression of cyclin D3 and E are decreased, and high levels of p27 CDK inhibitor are maintained (Naniche, Reed, and Oldstone, 1999). Furthermore, cell cycle-related up-regulation of Rb protein synthesis does not occur in lymphocytes infected with measles virus (Naniche, Reed, and Oldstone, 1999).

Regarding other paramyxoviruses, it has for example been reported that simian parainfluenza virus 5 (SV5)-infected cells exhibit delayed transition from G_1 to the S phase and have prolonged progression through the S phase. The phosphorylation of Rb proteins is delayed in SV5-infected cells. The V protein of the SV5 virus is responsible for this delayed cell cycle (Lin and Lamb, 2000).

8. Coronaviruses

Cell cycle abnormalities and apoptosis have been observed in many host cells infected with coronaviruses. Infection by the avian coronavirus infectious bronchitis virus (IBV) causes cell cycle arrest at the G_2/M phase, which is characterized by the accumulation of hypophosphorylated Rb protein, and the replication of IBV increases during this cell cycle arrest period (Dove et al., 2006; Li, Tam, and Liu, 2007). In addition, apoptosis is induced only in a late stage of the IBV infection cycle.

Mouse hepatitis virus (MHV) infection also induces cell cycle arrest at G_0/G_1 phase (Chen and Makino, 2004). The NS protein of MHV p28 stabilizes p53, accumulated p53 causes up-regulation of CDK inhibitor p21, and increased p21 suppresses cyclin E/CDK 2 activity, inducing cell cycle arrest at G_0/G_1 phase (Chen et al., 2004).

In addition, infection of VeroE6 cells with severe acute respiratory syndrome coronavirus inhibits cell proliferation, and this inhibition is regulated by both the PI3K/Akt signaling pathway and by apoptosis in SARS-CoV infected VeroE6 cells (Mizutani et al., 2006).

9. Other Viruses

The effects of viral infection on host cell cycles have been reported for many other viruses in addition to those described above. The NS1 of the murine minute virus (MVM), in the family *Parvoviridae*, induces cell-cycle arrest at the G_1/S phase, depending on p53 activity, and also induces cell cycle arrest at G_2 by inducing CDK inhibitor p21 (Op De Beeck et al., 2001). In addition, Coxsackievirus group 3 (in the family *Picornaviridae*) induces cell cycle arrest in the G_1/S phase through an increase in ubiquitin-dependent proteolysis of cyclin D1 (Luo et al., 2003). Moreover, it has been reported that reovirus NSσ1s induces G_2/M cell cycle arrest (Cox and Shaw, 1974; Poggioli et al., 2000).

Interestingly, the relationship between viral infection and cell cycle arrest has also been reported for invertebrate cells. The *Autographa californica* multiple nucleopolyhedrovirus (AcMNPV) is in the *Baculoviridae* and is used as a virus vector. Braunagel et al., reported that AcMNPV infection of *Spodoptera frugiperda*-derived Sf9 cells resulted in cell cycle arrest at the G_2/M phase, and that this arrest may be due to a viral-encoded protein that has Cdc2-associated kinase activity (Braunagel et al., 1998).

ADVANTAGES FOR VIRUSES ABLE TO CONTROL THE HOST CELL CYCLE

Many viruses encode in their genomes functional proteins that can interact with cell cycle regulatory proteins to promote favorable conditions for viral replication by manipulating stages of host cell proliferation or arrest. The relationship between virus proteins and host cell cycle proteins are summarized in figure 1. Generally, the progression of the cell cycle is strictly controlled at checkpoints in G_1 or G_2 phase. When cells are stressed, such as when there are nutritional deficiencies, shortages of replication factors, genomic DNA damage, incomplete DNA replication, or during infection, the cell cycle may be arrested. Repair of genomic DNA is then started, and the cell cycle is not restarted until the problems are overcome. If the problems persist, the cell will die by apoptosis.

Some oncoviruses (such as ADV, HCV, HTLV, and KSHV) transform infected cells into immortalized phenotypes, progress the host cell cycle, and inhibit apoptosis by interfering with guardian mechanisms of the host cell, producing a prolonged infection and effective replication. Other viruses usually induce cell cycle arrest and stop host cell gene transcription and protein production in order to induce favorable conditions for viral protein synthesis and viral genomic replication. Some viruses also inhibit cell apoptosis so as to prolong infection.

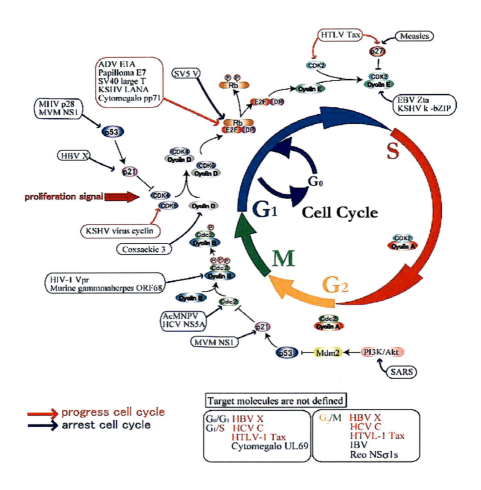

Figure 1. The relationship between virus proteins and host cell cycle proteins. The cell cycle and cell cycle regulatory molecules are shown. Red arrow indicates virus proteins which effect on cell proliferation, and blue arrow indicates cell cycle arrest.

In addition, induction of cell cycle arrest by viruses (such as the measles virus), in which the target cells are immunocells, leads to inhibition of immunocell cloning, and this inhibition leads to the suppression of the host immunosystem and is thus advantageous for virus survival. Among the viruses that can manipulate the cell cycle, some herpesviruses (cytomegalovirus, KSHV) and HCV simultaneously encode cell cycle promoter proteins and cell cycle delayer proteins. This suggests that they used different functional proteins in specific ways to induce a favorable environment for viral replication. Moreover, viral proteins (such as the UL69 protein of the human cytomegalovirus) that can interact with cell cycle regulators are incorporated in virions and can produce effects immediately after infection, even before viral replication occurs.

As described above, some viruses manipulate the host cell cycle by using regulatory proteins to produce favorable environments for virus survival and replication. Further studies of viral host cell cycle regulation promise to improve control of viral diseases and to improve understanding of the cell cycle.

REFERENCES

Arima, N., Kao, C. Y., Licht, T., Padmanabhan, R., Sasaguri, Y., and Padmanabhan, R. (2001). Modulation of cell growth by the hepatitis C virus nonstructural protein NS5A. *J. Biol. Chem.* 276(16), 12675-84.

Azuma, A., Matsuo, A., Suzuki, T., Kurosawa, T., Zhang, X., and Aida, Y. (2006). Human immunodeficiency virus type 1 Vpr induces cell cycle arrest at the G(1) phase and apoptosis via disruption of mitochondrial function in rodent cells. *Microbes Infect.* 8(3), 670-9.

Baluchamy, S., Sankar, N., Navaraj, A., Moran, E., and Thimmapaya, B. (2007). Relationship between E1A binding to cellular proteins, c-myc activation and S-phase induction. *Oncogene* 26(5), 781-7.

Beasley, R. P., Hwang, L. Y., Lin, C. C., and Chien, C. S. (1981). Hepatocellular carcinoma and hepatitis B virus. A prospective study of 22 707 men in Taiwan. *Lancet* 2(8256), 1129-33.

Benn, J., and Schneider, R. J. (1995). Hepatitis B virus HBx protein deregulates cell cycle checkpoint controls. *Proc. Natl. Acad. Sci. U S A* 92(24), 11215-9.

Braunagel, S. C., Parr, R., Belyavskyi, M., and Summers, M. D. (1998). Autographa californica nucleopolyhedrovirus infection results in Sf9 cell cycle arrest at G2/M phase. *Virology* 244(1), 195-211.

Brehm, A., Nielsen, S. J., Miska, E. A., McCance, D. J., Reid, J. L., Bannister, A. J., and Kouzarides, T. (1999). The E7 oncoprotein associates with Mi2 and histone deacetylase activity to promote cell growth. *Embo. J.* 18(9), 2449-58.

Cayrol, C., and Flemington, E. (1996). G0/G1 growth arrest mediated by a region encompassing the basic leucine zipper (bZIP) domain of the Epstein-Barr virus transactivator Zta. *J .Biol. Chem* .271(50), 31799-802.

Chellappan, S., Kraus, V. B., Kroger, B., Munger, K., Howley, P. M., Phelps, W. C., and Nevins, J. R. (1992). Adenovirus E1A, simian virus 40 tumor antigen, and human papillomavirus E7 protein share the capacity to disrupt the interaction between transcription factor E2F and the retinoblastoma gene product. *Proc. Natl. Acad. Sci. U S A* 89(10), 4549-53.

Chen, C. J., and Makino, S. (2004). Murine coronavirus replication induces cell cycle arrest in G0/G1 phase. *J. Virol.* 78(11), 5658-69.

Chen, C. J., Sugiyama, K., Kubo, H., Huang, C., and Makino, S. (2004). Murine coronavirus nonstructural protein p28 arrests cell cycle in G0/G1 phase. *J. Virol* .78(19), 10410-9.

Cohen, E. A., Dehni, G., Sodroski, J. G., and Haseltine, W. A. (1990). Human immunodeficiency virus vpr product is a virion-associated regulatory protein. *J. Virol.*64(6), 3097-9.

Cox, D. C., and Shaw, J. E. (1974). Inhibition of the initiation of cellular DNA synthesis after reovirus infection. *J. Virol.* 13(3), 760-1.

DeCaprio, J. A., Ludlow, J. W., Figge, J., Shew, J. Y., Huang, C. M., Lee, W. H., Marsilio, E., Paucha, E., and Livingston, D. M. (1988). SV40 large tumor antigen forms a specific complex with the product of the retinoblastoma susceptibility gene. *Cell* 54(2), 275-83.

Dittmer, D., Lagunoff, M., Renne, R., Staskus, K., Haase, A., and Ganem, D. (1998). A cluster of latently expressed genes in Kaposi's sarcoma-associated herpesvirus. *J. Virol.* 72(10), 8309-15.

Dove, B., Brooks, G., Bicknell, K., Wurm, T., and Hiscox, J. A. (2006). Cell cycle perturbations induced by infection with the coronavirus infectious bronchitis virus and their effect on virus replication. *J. Virol.* 80(8), 4147-56.

Dyson, N., and Harlow, E. (1992). Adenovirus E1A targets key regulators of cell proliferation. *Cancer Surv.* 12, 161-95.

Eckner, R., Ewen, M. E., Newsome, D., Gerdes, M., DeCaprio, J. A., Lawrence, J. B., and Livingston, D. M. (1994). Molecular cloning and functional analysis of the adenovirus E1A-associated 300-kD protein (p300) reveals a protein with properties of a transcriptional adaptor. *Genes Dev .*8(8), 869-84.

Erhardt, A., Hassan, M., Heintges, T., and Haussinger, D. (2002). Hepatitis C virus core protein induces cell proliferation and activates ERK, JNK, and p38 MAP kinases together with the MAP kinase phosphatase MKP-1 in a HepG2 Tet-Off cell line. *Virology* 292(2), 272-84.

Felber, B. K., Paskalis, H., Kleinman-Ewing, C., Wong-Staal, F., and Pavlakis, G. N. (1985). The pX protein of HTLV-I is a transcriptional activator of its long terminal repeats. *Science* 229(4714), 675-9.

Friborg, J., Jr., Kong, W., Hottiger, M. O., and Nabel, G. J. (1999). p53 inhibition by the LANA protein of KSHV protects against cell death. *Nature* 402(6764), 889-94.

Goh, W. C., Manel, N., and Emerman, M. (2004). The human immunodeficiency virus Vpr protein binds Cdc25C: implications for G2 arrest. *Virology* 318(1), 337-49.

Goh, W. C., Rogel, M. E., Kinsey, C. M., Michael, S. F., Fultz, P. N., Nowak, M. A., Hahn, B. H., and Emerman, M. (1998). HIV-1 Vpr increases viral expression by manipulation of the cell cycle: a mechanism for selection of Vpr in vivo. *Nat. Med.* 4(1), 65-71.

Gottlob, K., Fulco, M., Levrero, M., and Graessmann, A. (1998). The hepatitis B virus HBx protein inhibits caspase 3 activity. *J. Biol .Chem.*273(50), 33347-53.

Grassmann, R., Dengler, C., Muller-Fleckenstein, I., Fleckenstein, B., McGuire, K., Dokhelar, M. C., Sodroski, J. G., and Haseltine, W. A. (1989). Transformation to continuous growth of primary human T lymphocytes by human T-cell leukemia virus type I X-region genes transduced by a Herpesvirus saimiri vector. *Proc. Natl. Acad. Sci. U S A* 86(9), 3351-5.

Grossman, W. J., Kimata, J. T., Wong, F. H., Zutter, M., Ley, T. J., and Ratner, L. (1995). Development of leukemia in mice transgenic for the tax gene of human T-cell leukemia virus type I. *Proc. Natl. Acad. Sci. U S A* 92(4), 1057-61.

Hayashi, M. L., Blankenship, C., and Shenk, T. (2000). Human cytomegalovirus UL69 protein is required for efficient accumulation of infected cells in the G1 phase of the cell cycle. *Proc.Natl. Acad. Sci. U S A* 97(6), 2692-6.

He, J., Choe, S., Walker, R., Di Marzio, P., Morgan, D. O., and Landau, N. R. (1995). Human immunodeficiency virus type 1 viral protein R (Vpr) arrests cells in the G2 phase of the cell cycle by inhibiting p34cdc2 activity. *J.Virol.* 69(11), 6705-11.

Hinuma, Y., Nagata, K., Hanaoka, M., Nakai, M., Matsumoto, T., Kinoshita, K. I., Shirakawa, S., and Miyoshi, I. (1981). Adult T-cell leukemia: antigen in an ATL cell line and detection of antibodies to the antigen in human sera. *Proc. Natl. Acad. Sci. U S A* 78(10), 6476-80.

Howe, J. A., Mymryk, J. S., Egan, C., Branton, P. E., and Bayley, S. T. (1990). Retinoblastoma growth suppressor and a 300-kDa protein appear to regulate cellular DNA synthesis. *Proc. Natl. Acad. Sci. U S A* 87(15), 5883-7.

Huang, Y., Ohtani, K., Iwanaga, R., Matsumura, Y., and Nakamura, M. (2001). Direct trans-activation of the human cyclin D2 gene by the oncogene product Tax of human T-cell leukemia virus type I. *Oncogene* 20(9), 1094-102.

Iwanaga, R., Ohtani, K., Hayashi, T., and Nakamura, M. (2001). Molecular mechanism of cell cycle progression induced by the oncogene product Tax of human T-cell leukemia virus type I. *Oncogene* 20(17), 2055-67.

Izumiya, Y., Lin, S. F., Ellison, T. J., Levy, A. M., Mayeur, G. L., Izumiya, C., and Kung, H. J. (2003). Cell cycle regulation by Kaposi's sarcoma-associated herpesvirus K-bZIP: direct interaction with cyclin-CDK2 and induction of G1 growth arrest. *J. Virol.*77(17), 9652-61.

Joseph, B. S., Lampert, P. W., and Oldstone, M. B. (1975). Replication and persistence of measles virus in defined subpopulations of human leukocytes. *J. Virol.* 16(6), 1638-49.

Kaldis, P., Ojala, P. M., Tong, L., Makela, T. P., and Solomon, M. J. (2001). CAK-independent activation of CDK6 by a viral cyclin. *Mol. Biol. Cell* 12(12), 3987-99.

Kalejta, R. F., Bechtel, J. T., and Shenk, T. (2003). Human cytomegalovirus pp71 stimulates cell cycle progression by inducing the proteasome-dependent degradation of the retinoblastoma family of tumor suppressors. *Mol. Cell Biol.* 23(6), 1885-95.

Kato, N. (2001). Molecular virology of hepatitis C virus. *Acta Med Okayama* 55(3), 133-59.

Kim, C. M., Koike, K., Saito, I., Miyamura, T., and Jay, G. (1991). HBx gene of hepatitis B virus induces liver cancer in transgenic mice. *Nature* 351(6324), 317-20.

Koike, K., Moriya, K., Iino, S., Yotsuyanagi, H., Endo, Y., Miyamura, T., and Kurokawa, K. (1994). High-level expression of hepatitis B virus HBx gene and hepatocarcinogenesis in transgenic mice. *Hepatology* 19(4), 810-9.

Lee, C. J., Liao, C. L., and Lin, Y. L. (2005). Flavivirus activates phosphatidylinositol 3-kinase signaling to block caspase-dependent apoptotic cell death at the early stage of virus infection. *J. Virol.* 79(13), 8388-99.

Li, F. Q., Tam, J. P., and Liu, D. X. (2007). Cell cycle arrest and apoptosis induced by the coronavirus infectious bronchitis virus in the absence of p53. *Virology*.

Lin, G. Y., and Lamb, R. A. (2000). The paramyxovirus simian virus 5 V protein slows progression of the cell cycle. *J. Virol.* 74(19), 9152-66.

Low, K. G., Dorner, L. F., Fernando, D. B., Grossman, J., Jeang, K. T., and Comb, M. J. (1997). Human T-cell leukemia virus type 1 Tax releases cell cycle arrest induced by p16INK4a. *J. Virol.* 71(3), 1956-62.

Lu, M., and Shenk, T. (1999). Human cytomegalovirus UL69 protein induces cells to accumulate in G1 phase of the cell cycle. *J. Virol.* 73(1), 676-83.

Luo, H., Zhang, J., Dastvan, F., Yanagawa, B., Reidy, M. A., Zhang, H. M., Yang, D., Wilson, J. E., and McManus, B. M. (2003). Ubiquitin-dependent proteolysis of cyclin D1 is associated with coxsackievirus-induced cell growth arrest. *J. Virol.* 77(1), 1-9.

Marusawa, H., Hijikata, M., Chiba, T., and Shimotohno, K. (1999). Hepatitis C virus core protein inhibits Fas- and tumor necrosis factor alpha-mediated apoptosis via NF-kappaB activation. *J. Virol.* 73(6), 4713-20.

McChesney, M. B., Altman, A., and Oldstone, M. B. (1988). Suppression of T lymphocyte function by measles virus is due to cell cycle arrest in G1. *J. Immunol.* 140(4), 1269-73.

McChesney, M. B., Kehrl, J. H., Valsamakis, A., Fauci, A. S., and Oldstone, M. B. (1987). Measles virus infection of B lymphocytes permits cellular activation but blocks progression through the cell cycle. *J. Virol.* 61(11), 3441-7.

Mizutani, T., Fukushi, S., Iizuka, D., Inanami, O., Kuwabara, M., Takashima, H., Yanagawa, H., Saijo, M., Kurane, I., and Morikawa, S. (2006). Inhibition of cell proliferation by SARS-CoV infection in Vero E6 cells. *FEMS Immunol Med Microbiol* 46(2), 236-43.

Moran, E., and Mathews, M. B. (1987). Multiple functional domains in the adenovirus E1A gene. *Cell* 48(2), 177-8.

Naka, K., Dansako, H., Kobayashi, N., Ikeda, M., and Kato, N. (2006). Hepatitis C virus NS5B delays cell cycle progression by inducing interferon-beta via Toll-like receptor 3 signaling pathway without replicating viral genomes. *Virology* 346(2), 348-62.

Naniche, D., Reed, S. I., and Oldstone, M. B. (1999). Cell cycle arrest during measles virus infection: a G0-like block leads to suppression of retinoblastoma protein expression. *J. Virol.* 73(3), 1894-901.

Nascimento, R., and Parkhouse, R. M. (2007). Murine gammaherpesvirus 68 ORF20 induces cell-cycle arrest in G2 by inhibiting the Cdc2-cyclin B complex. *J. Gen. Virol.* 88(Pt 5), 1446-53.

Nerenberg, M., Hinrichs, S. H., Reynolds, R. K., Khoury, G., and Jay, G. (1987). The tat gene of human T-lymphotropic virus type 1 induces mesenchymal tumors in transgenic mice. *Science* 237(4820), 1324-9.

Op De Beeck, A., Sobczak-Thepot, J., Sirma, H., Bourgain, F., Brechot, C., and Caillet-Fauquet, P. (2001). NS1- and minute virus of mice-induced cell cycle arrest: involvement of p53 and p21(cip1). *J. Virol.* 75(22), 11071-8.

Park, J., Seo, T., Hwang, S., Lee, D., Gwack, Y., and Choe, J. (2000a). The K-bZIP protein from Kaposi's sarcoma-associated herpesvirus interacts with p53 and represses its transcriptional activity. *J. Virol.* 74(24), 11977-82.

Park, U. S., Park, S. K., Lee, Y. I., Park, J. G., and Lee, Y. I. (2000b). Hepatitis B virus-X protein upregulates the expression of p21waf1/cip1 and prolongs G1-->S transition via a p53-independent pathway in human hepatoma cells. *Oncogene* 19(30), 3384-94.

Poggioli, G. J., Keefer, C., Connolly, J. L., Dermody, T. S., and Tyler, K. L. (2000). Reovirus-induced G(2)/M cell cycle arrest requires sigma1s and occurs in the absence of apoptosis. *J. Virol.* 74(20), 9562-70.

Poiesz, B. J., Ruscetti, F. W., Gazdar, A. F., Bunn, P. A., Minna, J. D., and Gallo, R. C. (1980). Detection and isolation of type C retrovirus particles from fresh and cultured lymphocytes of a patient with cutaneous T-cell lymphoma. *Proc. Natl. Acad. Sci. U S A* 77(12), 7415-9.

Radkov, S. A., Kellam, P., and Boshoff, C. (2000). The latent nuclear antigen of Kaposi sarcoma-associated herpesvirus targets the retinoblastoma-E2F pathway and with the oncogene Hras transforms primary rat cells. *Nat. Med.* 6(10), 1121-7.

Ray, R. B., and Ray, R. (2001). Hepatitis C virus core protein: intriguing properties and functional relevance. *FEMS Microbiol. Lett.* 202(2), 149-56.

Re, F., Braaten, D., Franke, E. K., and Luban, J. (1995). Human immunodeficiency virus type 1 Vpr arrests the cell cycle in G2 by inhibiting the activation of p34cdc2-cyclin B. *J. Virol.* 69(11), 6859-64.

Rogel, M. E., Wu, L. I., and Emerman, M. (1995). The human immunodeficiency virus type 1 vpr gene prevents cell proliferation during chronic infection. *J. Virol.* 69(2), 882-8.

Sodroski, J., Rosen, C., Goh, W. C., and Haseltine, W. (1985). A transcriptional activator protein encoded by the x-lor region of the human T-cell leukemia virus. *Science* 228(4706), 1430-4.

Spandau, D. F., and Lee, C. H. (1988). trans-activation of viral enhancers by the hepatitis B virus X protein. *J. Virol* .62(2), 427-34.

Sullivan, J. L., Barry, D. W., Lucas, S. J., and Albrecht, P. (1975). Measles infection of human mononuclear cells. I. Acute infection of peripheral blood lymphocytes and monocytes. *J. Exp. Med.* 142(3), 773-84.

Suzuki, T., Kitao, S., Matsushime, H., and Yoshida, M. (1996). HTLV-1 Tax protein interacts with cyclin-dependent kinase inhibitor p16INK4A and counteracts its inhibitory activity towards CDK4. *Embo. J.* 15(7), 1607-14.

Suzuki, T., Narita, T., Uchida-Toita, M., and Yoshida, M. (1999). Down-regulation of the INK4 family of cyclin-dependent kinase inhibitors by tax protein of HTLV-1 through two distinct mechanisms. *Virology* 259(2), 384-91.

Tsuchihara, K., Hijikata, M., Fukuda, K., Kuroki, T., Yamamoto, N., and Shimotohno, K. (1999). Hepatitis C virus core protein regulates cell growth and signal transduction pathway transmitting growth stimuli. *Virology* 258(1), 100-7.

Yoshida, M. (1995). HTLV-1 oncoprotein Tax deregulates transcription of cellular genes through multiple mechanisms. *J Cancer Res Clin Oncol* 121(9-10), 521-8.

Zoulim, F., Saputelli, J., and Seeger, C. (1994). Woodchuck hepatitis virus X protein is required for viral infection in vivo. *J. Virol.* 68(3), 2026-30.

In: Progress in Cell Growth Process Research
Editor: Takumi Hayashi, pp. 149-165

ISBN 978-1-60456-325-2
© 2008 Nova Science Publishers, Inc.

Chapter 6

NICOTINE AND LUNG CANCER: MECHANISMS AND IMPLICATIONS FOR EARLY DETECTION AND TREATMENT

ShouWei Han[1, 4], Cherry Wongtrakool[1] and Jesse Roman[1, 2, 3]
[1]Division of Pulmonary, Allergy and Critical Care Medicine,
Department of Medicine, Emory University School of Medicine, Atlanta, GA, USA
[2]Atlanta Veterans Affairs Medical Center, Atlanta, GA, USA

ABSTRACT

Lung carcinoma is one of the most common malignant tumors in the world, and is the leading cause of carcinoma death in the United States. Despite recent advances in understanding the molecular biology of lung carcinoma and the introduction of multiple new chemotherapeutic agents for its treatment, its dismal 5-year survival rate (< 15%) has not changed substantially. It is well known that tobacco use is the most important risk factor for the development of lung carcinoma in the United States. In particular, non-small cell lung cancer (NSCLC), the most common lung malignancy, demonstrates a strong etiologic association with smoking. Smoking susceptibility is influenced by both genetic and environmental factors. Although nicotine, the major pharmacologically active substance in cigarette smoke, has been shown to be involved in lung cancer, the mechanisms by which this agent affects human lung cancer occurrence and progression remain incompletely elucidated. Recent work suggests that multiple factors and pro-oncogenic signaling pathways are involved in this process. In this review, we summarize the extensive network of co-mediators and cellular mechanisms that have implicated nicotine in lung tumorigenesis with the hope of improving understanding in this field. Our intention is to foster the development of new strategies to successfully break the

---

4 Address all correspondence and requests for reprints to: ShouWei Han, M.D., Ph.D. or Jesse Roman, M.D. Division of Pulmonary, Allergy and Critical Care Medicine Emory University School of Medicine Whitehead Bioresearch Building 615 Michael Street, Suite 205-M Atlanta, Georgia, 30322. E-mail: shan2@emory.edu or jroman@emory.edu, Tel: 404-712-2661 Fax: 404-712-2151.

cycle of nicotine-mediated lung carcinogenesis. Further work in this area is likely to lead to the identification of novel targets for early detection and treatment.

INTRODUCTION

Lung carcinoma is the leading cause of carcinoma death in the United States with a 5-year survival rate of less than 15% [21]. It is well known that tobacco use is one of the most important risk factors for the development of lung carcinoma in the United States and is associated with at least 87% of cancer deaths [45]. Both small cell lung cancer (SCLC) and non-small cell lung cancer (NSCLC) demonstrate a strong etiologic association with smoking. Unraveling the molecular basis of smoking-related lung cancer including mechanisms of activation and detoxification of various constituents of tobacco smoke and the genetic basis of smoking persistence, is the focus of many current epidemiologic studies and bench research.

Nicotine in tobacco smoke leads to tobacco addiction and therefore represents an important target of investigation. Although nicotine does not appear to be carcinogenic by itself, its metabolism leads to the generation of potent carcinogens [39]. Also, nicotine can stimulate cancer cell proliferation and angiogenesis, and suppress apoptosis induced by certain agents [71]. Evidence to date suggests that these effects of nicotine and its derivatives are mediated by nicotinic acetylcholine receptors (nAChRs) expressed on the surface of tumor cells, thereby contributing to tumor progression [16, 17, 38]. However, the molecular mechanisms underlying the role that nicotine plays in promoting lung cancer biology are unclear. This review describes pathways and networks involved in cancer cell growth and survival that are affected by nicotine, and the potential steps that could be targeted through the development of novel anti-cancer therapies.

NICOTINE METABOLISM AND NICOTINIC ACETYLCHOLINE RECEPTORS

Nicotine is the principal alkaloid in the leaves of commercially used tobacco (*Nicotiana tabacum and N. rustica*). Nicotine in tobacco leaves and in plant-derived preparations exists mostly in the (S)-nicotine isomeric form. However, tobacco smoke contains up to 10% (R)-nicotine, probably because of racemization during combustion [31]. Nicotine is the addictive compound in tobacco and is a commonly used psychoactive drug. It enters the body by systemic absorption through cigarette smoking, oral snuff, pipe tobacco, cigars, and chewing tobacco use [4, 32]. It can also enter in purified form as a medication. In cigarette smoke, nicotine is carried into the body on particulate matter where it is rapidly absorbed in the small airways and alveoli of the lung [52]. In this neutral pH environment, it is un-ionized and soluble, and can be transferred across cell membranes into the blood. It moves into the pulmonary venous circulation, to the left ventricle of the heart, and into the systemic arterial circulation [58]. It travels to the brain within seconds where it binds to nicotinic cholinergic receptors and activates the dopaminergic reward system [54]. Other forms of nicotine (such as nicotine gum, transdermal patch, inhaler, lozenges and sublingual tablets) are usually buffered at alkaline pH and quickly traverse cell membranes, but most reach the blood and brain more slowly. Consequently, they are less likely to cause addiction because of the delayed reward of nicotine [31].

In humans, the primary site of nicotine metabolism is the liver. There is little evidence in the literature for any extrahepatic metabolism, despite the presence of isoforms of nicotine metabolizing enzymes in other tissues [31]. Nicotine and its metabolites such as cotinine, desmethylcotinine, N-methylbutyramide, oxobutyric acid, and nicotine N-oxide are excreted in urine where they have been analyzed and quantitated [5, 44].

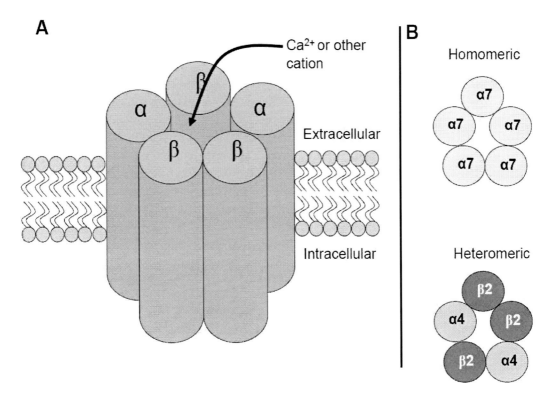

Figure 1. Organization and structure of nAChRs. (A) Schematic representation of the nAChR cation channel in the cell membrane. (B) Subunit arrangement in the homomeric α7 and heteromeric α4β2 subtypes.

Nicotine acts through nAChRs, which are widely distributed throughout the brain, neuromuscular junctions, and in a variety of non-neuronal tissues including the lung(10). NAChRs are a family of cationic channels consisting of different subunits, each having a specific pharmacological, physiological, and anatomical distribution in brain and ganglia. These receptors belong to the gene superfamily of ligand-gated ion channels (of which muscle AChRs are the prototype), which includes the gamma aminobutyric acid (GABA$_A$ and GABA$_C$) and glycine and 5-hydroxytryptamine (5-HT$_3$) receptors [47]. NAChRs have a pentameric structure consisting of the homomeric or heteromeric combination of 12 different subunits (α2–α10, β2–β4) (Figure 1)[23]. Genes encoding for individual nAChR subunits are named CHRNA1-10 for the α subunits and CHRNB1-4 for the β subunits. Neuronal nAChRs contain only two types of subunits: either a combination of α and β subunits or five copies of the same α subunits [63]. Both the α and β subunits are thought to contribute to the physiologic properties of nAChR, where the α subunit contains the principal sites for agonist binding, such as acetylcholine, and β subunits are believed to regulate the rate of binding and dissociation by agonists [53]. NAChRs contribute to a wide range of brain activities and influence a number of physiological functions. Dysfunction of nAChRs has been linked to a number of human diseases such as schizophrenia, Alzheimer's, and Parkinson's diseases, but the role of non neuronal nAChRs in disease states remains incompletely elucidated [48].

Expression of nAChR subunits has been observed in epithelial and endothelial cells [43, 72]. Human bronchial epithelial cells (BEC) and aortic endothelial cells (AEC) express the α7 subunit of nAChR, which forms functional homomeric nAChRs. The presence of α7 nAChR in BEC and AEC suggests that some toxic effects of tobacco smoke could be mediated through these nicotine-sensitive receptors [72]. Other nAChR subunits present in human airway cells include α3, α5, β2, and β4, as well as the other potentially homomeric receptors composed of α9 and α10[10] [56, 69]. α3, α5, α7, β2, and β4 subunits are not only found in pulmonary neuroendocrine cells, NSCLC, and SCLC cell lines, but also in skin keratinocytes, vascular tissues, airway-related vagal preganglionic neurons, human lymphocytes, and eosinophils [7, 11, 18, 38, 41, 49, 68]. High level expression of the α7 nAChR has been demonstrated in SCLC cell lines and in hamster pulmonary neuroendocrine cells, which serve as a model for the cell of origin of human SCLC [61]. The presence of nAChRs in lung is important because nicotine in cigarette smoke reaches lung cells at high concentrations and plays a role in stimulating the growth of tumor cells [23].

NAChRs are the target of natural ligands and toxins including nicotine, and its highly carcinogenic derivative 4 (methylnitrosamine)-1-(3-pyridyl)-1-butanone [23, 60]. However, although nicotine is most often considered to be an agonist or activator of nAChRs, it has several effects on receptor function that complicate this assignment and require attention in any experimental design that employs this compound. For example, unlike endogenous ligands such as acetylcholine or choline, which are either rapidly degraded or removed from the receptor vicinity, nicotine is not readily degraded or removed. On the contrary, it accumulates in certain tissues well beyond the concentration measured in serum because of its lipophilic property [19].

In addition, nicotine can stimulate the expression of its own receptors in lung and other tissues [37, 62]. For example, nicotine stimulates α7 nAChR expression in lung fibroblasts and human bronchial epithelial cells [57, 72]. Prenatal nicotine exposure has been shown to upregulate α7 nAChR expression in fetal monkey lungs [64]. Increased numbers of fetal pulmonary neuroendocrine cells seen in the offspring of maternal smokers are thought to result from upregulation of α7 nAChR, subsequent activation of MAP kinases extracellular signal regulated kinase 1 (ERK1) and extracellular signal regulated kinase 2 (ERK2), and stimulation of DNA synthesis (62). Recently, we showed that nicotine dramatically increases the expression of α7 nAChR in NSCLC cells [79].

Nicotine and nAChRs also interact during fetal lung development. It is well established that maternal smoking during pregnancy is a leading preventable cause of low birth weight and prematurity. Less appreciated is that maternal smoking during pregnancy is also associated with alterations in pulmonary function at birth and greater incidence of respiratory illnesses after birth [64]. Epidemiological studies have shown that offspring of women who smoke during pregnancy have abnormal lung function and show higher incidences of lower respiratory disorders [65]. A lower birth weight in children born at term is associated with a transiently increased risk of respiratory symptoms. This effect is enhanced by environmental tobacco smoke exposure [13]. Since nicotine traverses the placenta and nAChRs are expressed in fetal tissues, the direct interaction between nicotine and nAChR in fetal lung may underlie the postnatal pulmonary abnormalities seen in such infants [65, 66]. The expression of nAChRs in fetal lung tissues has not been extensively evaluated. Animal studies show that $\alpha 7$ nAChRs are present in the developing lung in airway epithelial cells, cells surrounding large airways and blood vessels, alveolar type II cells, free alveolar macrophages, and pulmonary neuroendocrine cells [64]. These findings demonstrate that nicotine can alter fetal lung development by crossing the placenta to interact directly with nicotinic receptors on non-neuronal cells in the developing lung, and that similar effects can occur in human infants whose mothers smoke during pregnancy. In mice, nicotine stimulates lung branching morphogenesis through $\alpha 7$ nAChR and may contribute to dysanaptic lung growth which, in turn, may predispose the host to airways disease in the postnatal period [75]. Thus, in a fetus exposed to maternal or passive smoking, nicotine might lead subtle alterations in lung development resulting in airway disfunction and a reduction in the complexity of the gas-exchange surface [64].

It should be emphasized that the endogenous ligand for nAChRs is not nicotine, but acetylcholine, which is produced by the synthetic enzyme choline acetyltransferase which uses acetyl coenzyme A and choline as substrates for the formation of acetylcholine. Dietary choline and phosphatidylcholine serve as the sources of free choline for acetylcholine synthesis. Upon release, acetylcholine is metabolized into choline and acetate by acetylcholinesterase, and other nonspecific esterases. It acts as a neurotransmitter in the central and peripheral nervous systems in humans. Acetylcholine release can be excitatory or inhibitory depending on the type of tissue and the nature of the receptor with which it interacts. Interestingly, acetylcholine is also found in non-neuronal cells such as in mesothelial, endothelial, glial, and circulating blood cells (platelets, mononuclear cells), as well as in alveolar macrophages [73].

NICOTINE IN TUMOR CELL PEROLIFERATION AND APOPTOSIS

While nicotine is not a carcinogen by itself, it has been shown to induce tumor cell proliferation and differentiation through nAChR [12, 38, 60]. The mitogenic effects of nicotine in NSCLC are analogous to those of growth factors, and involve activation of multiple signaling pathways [16, 17]. Nicotine has been shown to induce NSCLC proliferation by activation of the c-Src and c-Raf pathways, and phosphoinositide 3-kinase

(PI-3)/Akt dependent changes in cyclin D1 expression [17, 71]. Also, accelerated migration and invasion of human lung cancer cells has been associated with nicotine-induced phosphorylation of both mu- and m-calpains via activation of atypical protein kinase Ciota (PKCiota) [77].

NAChRs appear to play an important role in mediating the effects of nicotine on cell proliferation and survival. Activation of nAChRs may promote cell growth and proliferation by stimulating the epidermal growth factor receptor and c-Myc signaling pathways through mitogen activated protein kinase (MAPK) [35, 36]. We have reported that nicotine stimulates NSCLC proliferation through induction of fibronectin, a matrix glycoprotein highly expressed in acute and chronic forms of lung disease that has been implicated in the biology of lung cancer, and that these events are mediated through α7 nAChR-mediated signals that include ERK and PI3-K/mTOR pathways [79]. In addition, we found that Akt signaling and MAPK (p44/42) phosphorylation were downstream events to these pathways and could be inhibited by nAChR antagonists such as α-bungarotoxin [11]. It appears the MAPK pathway likely mediates the effect of nicotine through ERK1/2 and JNK, but not p38MAPK in HBECs exposed to nicotine (70). Nicotine-stimulated proliferation of SCLC cells is associated with increased expression of α7 nAChR, influx of Ca(2+), and activation of phosphoinositide-specific phospholipase C, Raf-1, ERK1/2, and c-Myc [61].

The metabolites of nicotine have also been found to have effects on cell proliferation and survival. Nitrosamine 4-(methylnitrosamino)-1-(3-pyridyl)-1-butanone (NNK) formed by nitrosation of nicotine has been identified as the most potent carcinogen contained in cigarette smoke which contributes to smoking-related lung cancer. Inhibition of binding of NNK and N'-Nitrosonornicotine (NNN), another metabolite of nicotine, to nAChRs in lung carcinoma cells abolishes tumor cell acquisition of anchorage-independent growth [2]. In SCLC cell lines, NNK induces expression of α7 nAChR and promotes cell survival and stimulates proliferation, in part, through phosphorylation of Raf-1 and ERK1/2, and c-myc activation [35, 62, 74]. NNK also stimulates normal human bronchial cell proliferation through activation of the nuclear transcription factor kappaB (NF-κB) which, in turn, up-regulates cyclin D1 expression [30]. Other studies show that NNK induces functional cooperation of Bcl2 and c-Myc in promoting cell survival and proliferation, and that this might contribute to the development of lung cancer and/or chemoresistance [34]. More recently, NNK was found to induce lung tumors in A/J mice in an mTOR-dependent manner. Rapamycin, an inhibitor of mTOR, markedly reduced the development and growth of NNK-induced lung tumors [24].

Inhibition of apoptosis is a hallmark in tumor progression and propels development of cancer. Nicotine can inhibit apoptosis in a nAChR-dependent fashion. In concentrations found in smokers, nicotine was found to block the induction of apoptosis in human lung cancer cells. This effect was reversed by nAChR antagonists. Several pathways appear important in the suppression of apoptosis by nicotine including PKC, nitric oxide, upregulation of NF-κB, and induction of X-linked inhibitor of apoptosis (XIAP) and survivin, a new member of the IAP family [42]. Nicotine inhibits nitric oxide (NO)-induced apoptosis in oral epithelial cells, which likely contributes to tobacco-induced oral carcinogenesis [3]. In NSCLC, nicotine prevents chemotherapy-induced apoptosis through blocking the inhibition of PKC and ERK2 activity by anti-cancer agents [25]. Nicotine also activates MAPK, specifically the ERK2 pathway, in lung cancer cells, resulting in increased expression of the Bcl-2 protein and further inhibition of apoptosis in these cells. Similarly, nicotine induces survival through multi-site phosphorylation of Bad, an anti-apoptotic factor, which may lead to development of human lung cancer and/or chemoresistance [34]. In mouse models of lung cancer, nicotine reduced the number of apoptotic cells after 24-hour exposure to hypoxia, and annexin V expression was decreased in the nicotine-treated cells. The anti-apoptotic effect of nicotine in these studies was blocked by hexamethonium, a specific antagonist of nAChR [29].

NICOTINE IN ANGIOGENESIS AND TUMOR VASCULARIZATION

Angiogenesis is required for lung cancer growth, which is mediated by various growth factors such as vascular endothelial growth factor (VEGF) [59]. Increases in VEGF and angiogenesis have been correlated with poor prognosis and survival in patients with lung cancer [20]. Several studies provide anatomic and functional evidence that nicotine induces angiogenesis and subsequently tumor growth [15, 16, 29, 75]. Nicotine increases the number of human umbilical-vein endothelial cells and human coronary artery endothelial cells in culture, particularly at concentrations seen in smokers [29]. In a mouse model of lung cancer, nicotine-stimulated-tumor growth correlated with increased vascularization of the tumor tissue [29]. In addition, the combination of nicotine and estradiol, a hormone that has been shown to promote angiogenesis, seems to play an important role in lung tumor initiation and progression. Estradiol and nicotine exposure enhanced the growth of bronchioloalveolar carcinoma xenografts in mice through the stimulation of cell proliferation, VEGF secretion, and angiogenesis. Furthermore, estradiol promoted VEGF secretion from various NSCLC cells, and this effect was enhanced by nicotine in a tumor xenograft model [33]. Thus, nicotine appears to have additive effects on the induction of angiogenesis through the stimulation of VEGF secretion during NSCLC progression. In other studies, Lewis lung cancer cells were injected subcutaneously into mice subsequently exposed to sidestream smoke or clean room air. Sidestream smoke significantly increased tumor size, weight, and capillary density in association with increased VEGF and monocyte chemoattractant protein-1 levels, and circulating endothelial progenitor cells. The effects of sidestream smoke were reduced when administered in combination with mecamylamine, a nAChR antagonist [80]. Another vascularization factor, hepatocyte growth factor, is induced by cigarette smoking and increased levels of this factor correlated with tumor staging in NSCLC [14].

Nicotine also induces hypoxia-inducible factor-1 (HIF-1) expression via nAChR-mediated signaling with activation of Ca(2+)/calmodulin, c-Src, protein kinase C, PI3-K, ERK1/2, and mTOR pathways [78]. HIF-1 plays an essential role in tumor angiogenesis and growth by regulating the transcription of several genes in response to hypoxic stress and changes in growth factors. This transcription factor mediates metabolic adaptation to hypoxia to activate tumor angiogenesis [9, 55]. As a master regulator of homeostasis, HIF-1 plays a pivotal role in hypoxia-induced angiogenesis through its regulation of VEGF [8]. This demonstrates a novel mechanism by which nicotine promotes tumor angiogenesis and metastasis, and provides further evidence that HIF-1α is a potential anti-cancer target in nicotine-associated lung cancer [50].

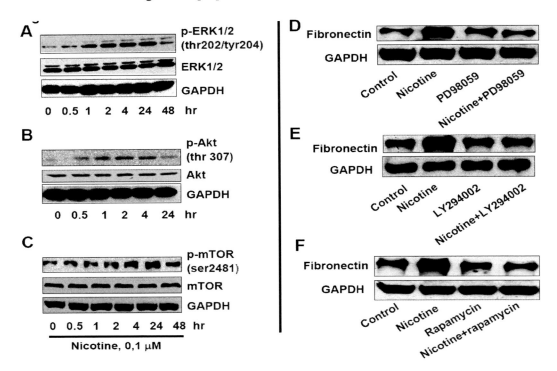

Figure 2. The effect of nicotine on the phosphorylation of ERK, Akt and mTOR, and the role of ERK and PI3-K/mTOR pathways in the induction of fibronectin by nicotine. A, Nicotine stimulates phosphorylation of ERK1/2 in a time-dependent fashion. Cellular protein (20 µg) was isolated from H460 cells treated with nicotine (0.1 µM) for the indicated period of time followed by Western blot analysis for phosphorylated-ERK1/2 (p-ERK1/2) and total ERK1/2 determinations. Blots were also incubated with an anti-GAPDH antibody to control for gel loading. B, Nicotine stimulates the phosphorylation of Akt in a time-dependent fashion. Cellular protein (30 µg) was isolated from H460 cells treated with nicotine (0.1 µM) for the indicated periods of time followed by Western blot analysis for phosphorylated-Akt (p-Akt) and total Akt determinations. Blots were also incubated with an anti-GAPDH antibody to control for gel loading. C, Nicotine stimulates the phosphorylation of mTOR in a time-dependent fashion. Cellular protein (20 µg) was isolated from H460 cells treated with nicotine (0.1 µM) for the indicated periods of time followed by Western blot analysis for phosphorylated-mTOR (p-mTOR) and total mTOR determinations. Blots were also incubated with an anti-GAPDH antibody to control for gel loading. D, Effect of an ERK1/2 inhibitor on nicotine-induced fibronectin protein expression. Cellular protein (5 µg) was isolated from H460 cells cultured for 1 hr in the presence or absence of PD98059 (25 µM) before exposure of cells to nicotine (0.1 µM) for an additional 48 hr, then subjected to Western blot analysis for fibronectin protein. E, Effect of PI3-K inhibitors on nicotine-induced fibronectin protein expression. Cellular protein (5 µg) was isolated from H460 cells cultured for 1 hr in the presence or absence of LY294002 (25 µM) before exposing the cells to nicotine (0.1 µM) for an additional 48 hr, followed by Western blot analysis for fibronectin protein. F, Effect of inhibitors of mTOR on nicotine-induced fibronectin protein expression. Cellular protein (5 µg) was isolated from H460 cells cultured for 1 hr in the presence or absence of rapamycin (10 nM) before exposure to nicotine (0.1 µM) for an additional 48 hr, then subjected to Western blot analysis for fibronectin protein.

NICOTINE AND TUMOR-STROMAL INTERACTIONS

Tumor growth and invasion are not only the result of malignant transformation, but also depend on environmental influences from their surrounding stroma, local growth factors, and systemic hormones. In particular, the composition of the extracellular matrix is believed to affect malignant behavior *in vivo*. One matrix glycoprotein implicated in lung cancer is fibronectin [40]. Nicotine induces lung fibroblasts to produce fibronectin by stimulating α7 nAChR-dependent signals that regulate the transcription of the fibronectin gene [57]. Expression of fibronectin is increased in lung carcinomas, especially in NSCLC [26, 46]. Several studies have suggested that excessive expression of fibronectin might create an extracellular environment that stimulates lung carcinoma proliferation. Consistent with this, we reported that nicotine binds to α7 nAChR thereby stimulating human lung carcinoma cell growth through activation of ERK1/2 and PI3-K/mTOR signaling pathways leading to fibronectin expression (Figure 2) [79]. Thus, tumor-derived fibronectin might be an important mediator of nicotine-induced tumor cell proliferation.

Data from our laboratory and that of others suggest that fibronectin, via its interaction with integrin α5β1 in tumor cells, affects lung carcinoma cell functions [1, 27, 28]. We also showed that silencing of α5 by α5 short hairpin RNA (shRNA) also inhibited cell growth induced by nicotine (Figure 3). These findings suggest a novel role for the integrin α5β1 in mediating the mitogenic effect of nicotine, and support the hypothesis that nicotine stimulates lung carcinoma cell growth, at least in part, through fibronectin-α5β1 interactions [79]. These results suggest that targeting these signals might aid in the development of novel agents with therapeutic potential for the prevention and treatment of human lung carcinoma related to tobacco exposure.

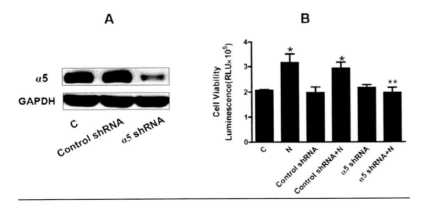

Figure 3. α5 shRNA inhibits cell growth induced by nicotine. A, α5 shRNA reduces α5 protein expression. Cellular protein (15 μg) was isolated from H460 cells, which were transfected by electroporation with α5 shRNA or control shRNA and incubated for 48 hr, and then subject to Western Blot analysis for the integrin α5. Blots were also incubated with an anti-GAPDH antibody for normalization purposes. B, α5 shRNA inhibits cell growth induced by nicotine. NSCLC H460 cells transfected with α5 shRNA or control shRNA by electroporation were added to 48 well tissue culture plates and incubated with 10^{-4} M nicotine for 5 days, then subjected to cell viability analysis. All data are depicted as mean $\pm$ SD. * indicates significant difference from control condition (P<0.05); **indicates significance of combination treatment as compared with nicotine alone. C, control.

IMPLICATIONS FOR PREVENTION AND THERAPY

The role of nicotine in the pathogenesis of lung cancer may identify novel targets for chemotherapeutics. Nicotine has been shown to activate growth-promoting pathways that facilitate the development of lung cancer and tumor growth. Some of these pathways are currently being exploited as potential chemotherapeutic targets such as the case with rapamycin, an mTOR inhibitor, and its derivatives CCI-779 and RAD001 [6, 67]. Delineation of the nAChR subtypes in lung cancer cells may accelerate the development of novel treatments. Future *in vivo* studies should establish the contribution of specific nAChR subtypes mediating the oncogenic action of tobacco-derived nitrosamines and also identify the receptor antagonists that can serve as chemopreventive agents [2]. Researchers can now profile these receptors, modify their function, and detect the presence or absence of specific receptors using imaging techniques *in vivo*. Several studies have demonstrated significant differences in nAChRs subunit expression patterns when comparing lung tumor and normal tissues, and also differences between lung adenocarcinomas depending on smoking or nicotine exposure [38]. These differences in nAChR subunit expression could potentially provide a biologic signature to guide therapy or even identify a lesion at risk for metastasis.

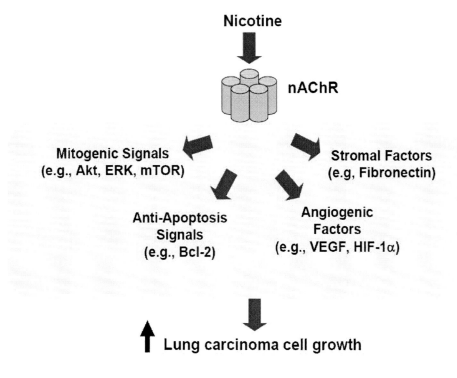

Figure 4. Nicotine promotes lung carcinoma growth and survival through AChRs. Nicotine acts on lung carcinoma cells through nAChRs that mediate signals involved in proliferation, inhibition of apoptosis, and the expression of angiogenic and stromal factors that promote tumor progression.

We recently found that rosiglitazone, one of the synthetic peroxisome proliferator-activated receptors gamma (PPARγ) ligands that are commonly used in diabetics, attenuated nicotine-induced NSCLC cell proliferation, at least, through activation of p38 mitogen activated protein kinase (p38MAPK) signaling pathway (Han et al, unpublished data). Even with new and potential chemotherapeutics, facilitating smoking cessation remains an important preventive step. Nicotinic AChRs have already been shown to play an important role in smoking cessation, most recently with the introduction of varenicline, a partial agonist of the $\alpha 4\beta 2$ nAChR [22].

Nicotine's effects on endogenous acetylcholine might also change the tumor biology and host response to tumorigenesis as well. Nicotine and its derivatives, by binding to nAChR on normal bronchial epithelial cells, can regulate cellular proliferation and apoptosis. Enzymes involved in endogenous acetylcholine metabolism (e.g., cholino-acetyltransferase, vesicular acetylcholine transporter and acetylcholinesterase) have been observed in NSCLC tumor biopsies and in NSCLC cell lines, and may be involved in cell growth regulation. A cholinesterase inhibitor, poly-APS, shows selective toxicity toward NSCLC cells while having no apparent toxicity towards normal cells and tissue *in vitro* and *in vivo* [51]. Acetylcholine is synthesized and secreted by the tumor cells and the released acetylcholine stimulates SCLC cell growth [68]. A chemotherapeutic agent targeting the endogenous acetylcholine pathways could potentially affect both tumor and host response in a complementary manner.

In summary, nicotine is an influential factor in the development of lung carcinoma in the setting of tobacco smoke exposure. Nicotine has proliferative and anti-apoptotic effects on lung carcinoma cells as well as normal lung cells. These effects are mediated through a number of nAChR-dependent pathways that can be potentially exploited for novel chemotherapeutic targets (Figure 4). Thus, nAChRs are emerging as important players in the biology of lung carcinoma and may play a future role in the design of therapeutic and preventive agents.

ACKNOWLEDGMENTS

This work was supported by an American Lung Association Grant RG-10215N (S.W.H), by American Thoracic Society/LunGevity Foundation Partnership Grant LC-06-004 (S.W.H), National Heart, Lung, and Blood Institute Grant HL080293 (C.W), Department of Defense Grant PR043305 (J.R), and by a Merit Review Grant from the Department of Veterans Affairs (J.R).

REFERENCES

[1]   Adachi, M., T. Taki, M. Higashiyama, N. Kohno, H. Inufusa, and M. Miyake. 2000. Significance of integrin alpha5 gene expression as a prognostic factor in node-negative non-small cell lung cancer. *Clin. Cancer Res.* 6:96-101.

[2]   Arredondo, J., A. I. Chernyavsky, and S. A. Grando. 2006. The nicotinic receptor antagonists abolish pathobiologic effects of tobacco-derived nitrosamines on BEP2D cells. *J. Cancer Res. Clin. Oncol.* 132:653-63.

[3]   Banerjee, A. G., V. K. Gopalakrishnan, and J. K. Vishwanatha. 2007. Inhibition of nitric oxide-induced apoptosis by nicotine in oral epithelial cells. Mol Cell Biochem.

[4]   Benowitz, N. L., and P. Jacob, 3rd. 1984. Daily intake of nicotine during cigarette smoking. *Clin. Pharmacol. Ther.* 35:499-504.

[5]   Benowitz, N. L., P. Jacob, 3rd, I. Fong, and S. Gupta. 1994. Nicotine metabolic profile in man: comparison of cigarette smoking and transdermal nicotine. *J. Pharmacol. Exp. Ther.* 268:296-303.

[6]   Bjelogrlic, S. K., T. Srdic, and S. Radulovic. 2006. Mammalian target of rapamycin is a promising target for novel therapeutic strategy against cancer. *J. Buon.* 11:267-76.

[7]   Blanchet, M. R., A. Langlois, E. Israel-Assayag, M. J. Beaulieu, C. Ferland, M. Laviolette, and Y. Cormier. 2007. Modulation of eosinophil activation in vitro by a nicotinic receptor agonist. *J. Leukoc. Biol.* 81:1245-51.

[8]   Bozova, S., and G. O. Elpek. 2007. Hypoxia-inducible factor-1alpha expression in experimental cirrhosis: correlation with vascular endothelial growth factor expression and angiogenesis. *Apmis.* 115:795-801.

[9]   Bruegge, K., W. Jelkmann, and E. Metzen. 2007. Hydroxylation of hypoxia-inducible transcription factors and chemical compounds targeting the HIF-alpha hydroxylases. *Curr .Med. Chem.* 14:1853-62.

[10]   Carlisle, D. L., T. M. Hopkins, A. Gaither-Davis, M. J. Silhanek, J. D. Luketich, N. A. Christie, and J. M. Siegfried. 2004. Nicotine signals through muscle-type and neuronal nicotinic acetylcholine receptors in both human bronchial epithelial cells and airway fibroblasts. *Respir. Res.* 5:27.

[11]   Carlisle, D. L., X. Liu, T. M. Hopkins, M. C. Swick, R. Dhir, and J. M. Siegfried. 2006. Nicotine activates cell-signaling pathways through muscle-type and neuronal nicotinic acetylcholine receptors in non-small cell lung cancer cells. *Pulm. Pharmacol. Ther.*

[12]   Cattaneo, M. G., A. Codignola, L. M. Vicentini, F. Clementi, and E. Sher. 1993. Nicotine stimulates a serotonergic autocrine loop in human small-cell lung carcinoma. *Cancer Res.* 53:5566-8.

[13]   Caudri, D., A. Wijga, U. Gehring, H. A. Smit, B. Brunekreef, M. Kerkhof, M. Hoekstra, J. Gerritsen, and J. C. de Jongste. 2007. Respiratory symptoms in the first 7 years of life and birth weight at term: the PIAMA Birth Cohort. *Am. J. Respir. Crit. Care Med.* 175:1078-85.

[14]   Chen, J. T., T. S. Lin, K. C. Chow, H. H. Huang, S. H. Chiou, S. F. Chiang, H. C. Chen, T. L. Chuang, T. Y. Lin, and C. Y. Chen. 2006. Cigarette smoking induces overexpression of hepatocyte growth factor in type II pneumocytes and lung cancer cells. *Am. J. Respir. Cell Mol. Biol.* 34:264-73.

[15]   Cooke, J. P. 2007. Angiogenesis and the role of the endothelial nicotinic acetylcholine receptor. *Life Sci.* 80:2347-51.

[16]   Dasgupta, P., and S. P. Chellappan. 2006. Nicotine-mediated cell proliferation and angiogenesis: new twists to an old story. *Cell Cycle* 5:2324-8.

[17]   Dasgupta, P., S. Rastogi, S. Pillai, D. Ordonez-Ercan, M. Morris, E. Haura, and S. Chellappan. 2006. Nicotine induces cell proliferation by beta-arrestin-mediated activation of Src and Rb-Raf-1 pathways. *J. Clin. Invest.* 116:2208-2217.

[18]   Dehkordi, O., P. Kc, K. V. Balan, and M. A. Haxhiu. 2006. Airway-related vagal preganglionic neurons express multiple nicotinic acetylcholine receptor subunits. *Auton. Neurosci.* 128:53-63.

[19]   Gahring, L. C., and S. W. Rogers. 2005. Neuronal nicotinic acetylcholine receptor expression and function on nonneuronal cells. *Aaps. J.* 7:E885-94.

[20]   Giaccone, G. 2007. The potential of antiangiogenic therapy in non-small cell lung cancer. *Clin. Cancer Res.* 13:1961-70.

[21]   Gilligan, D., M. Nicolson, I. Smith, H. Groen, O. Dalesio, P. Goldstraw, M. Hatton, P. Hopwood, C. Manegold, F. Schramel, H. Smit, J. van Meerbeeck, M. Nankivell, M. Parmar, C. Pugh, and R. Stephens. 2007. Preoperative chemotherapy in patients with resectable non-small cell lung cancer: results of the MRC LU22/NVALT 2/EORTC 08012 multicentre randomised trial and update of systematic review. *Lancet* 369:1929-37.

[22]   Glover, E. D., and J. M. Rath. 2007. Varenicline: progress in smoking cessation treatment. *Expert Opin. Pharmacother.* 8:1757-67.

[23]   Gotti, C., and F. Clementi. 2004. Neuronal nicotinic receptors: from structure to pathology. *Prog. Neurobiol.* 74:363-96.

[24]   Granville, C. A., N. Warfel, J. Tsurutani, M. C. Hollander, M. Robertson, S. D. Fox, T. D. Veenstra, H. J. Issaq, R. I. Linnoila, and P. A. Dennis. 2007. Identification of a highly effective rapamycin schedule that markedly reduces the size, multiplicity, and phenotypic progression of tobacco carcinogen-induced murine lung tumors. *Clin. Cancer Res.* 13:2281-9.

[25]   Grozio, A., A. Catassi, Z. Cavalieri, L. Paleari, A. Cesario, and P. Russo. 2007. Nicotine, lung and cancer. *Anticancer Agents Med. Chem .*7:461-6.

[26]   Han, J. Y., H. S. Kim, S. H. Lee, W. S. Park, J. Y. Lee, and N. J. Yoo. 2003. Immunohistochemical expression of integrins and extracellular matrix proteins in non-small cell lung cancer: correlation with lymph node metastasis. *Lung Cancer* 41:65-70.

[27]   Han, S., F. R. Khuri, and J. Roman. 2006. Fibronectin stimulates non-small cell lung carcinoma cell growth through activation of Akt/mammalian target of rapamycin/S6 kinase and inactivation of LKB1/AMP-activated protein kinase signal pathways. *Cancer* Res 66:315-23.

[28]   Han, S., N. Sidell, S. Roser-Page, and J. Roman. 2004. Fibronectin stimulates human lung carcinoma cell growth by inducing cyclooxygenase-2 (COX-2) expression. *Int. J. Cancer* 111:322-31.

[29]   Heeschen, C., J. J. Jang, M. Weis, A. Pathak, S. Kaji, R. S. Hu, P. S. Tsao, F. L. Johnson, and J. P. Cooke. 2001. Nicotine stimulates angiogenesis and promotes tumor growth and atherosclerosis. *Nat. Med.* 7:833-9.

[30]   Ho, Y. S., C. H. Chen, Y. J. Wang, R. G. Pestell, C. Albanese, R. J. Chen, M. C. Chang, J. H. Jeng, S. Y. Lin, Y. C. Liang, H. Tseng, W. S. Lee, J. K. Lin, J. S. Chu, L. C. Chen, C. H. Lee, W. L. Tso, Y. C. Lai, and C. H. Wu. 2005. Tobacco-specific carcinogen 4-(methylnitrosamino)-1-(3-pyridyl)-1-butanone (NNK) induces cell proliferation in normal human bronchial epithelial cells through NFkappaB activation and cyclin D1 up-regulation. *Toxicol. Appl. Pharmacol.* 205:133-48.

[31] Hukkanen, J., P. Jacob, 3rd, and N. L. Benowitz. 2005. Metabolism and disposition kinetics of nicotine. *Pharmacol. Rev.* 57:79-115.

[32] Jacob, P., 3rd, L. Yu, A. T. Shulgin, and N. L. Benowitz. 1999. Minor tobacco alkaloids as biomarkers for tobacco use: comparison of users of cigarettes, smokeless tobacco, cigars, and pipes. *Am. J. Public Health* 89:731-6.

[33] Jarzynka, M. J., P. Guo, I. Bar-Joseph, B. Hu, and S. Y. Cheng. 2006. Estradiol and nicotine exposure enhances A549 bronchioloalveolar carcinoma xenograft growth in mice through the stimulation of angiogenesis. *Int. J. Oncol.* 28:337-44.

[34] Jin, Z., F. Gao, T. Flagg, and X. Deng. 2004. Nicotine induces multi-site phosphorylation of Bad in association with suppression of apoptosis. *J. Biol. Chem.* 279:23837-44.

[35] Jull, B. A., H. K. Plummer, 3rd, and H. M. Schuller. 2001. Nicotinic receptor-mediated activation by the tobacco-specific nitrosamine NNK of a Raf-1/MAP kinase pathway, resulting in phosphorylation of c-myc in human small cell lung carcinoma cells and pulmonary neuroendocrine cells. *J. Cancer Res. Clin. Oncol.* 127:707-17.

[36] Kanda, Y., and Y. Watanabe. 2007. Nicotine-induced vascular endothelial growth factor release via the EGFR-ERK pathway in rat vascular smooth muscle cells. *Life Sci.* 80:1409-14.

[37] Katono, T., T. Kawato, N. Tanabe, N. Suzuki, K. Yamanaka, H. Oka, M. Motohashi, and M. Maeno. 2006. Nicotine treatment induces expression of matrix metalloproteinases in human osteoblastic Saos-2 cells. *Acta Biochim. Biophys. Sin.* (Shanghai) 38:874-82.

[38] Lam, D. C., L. Girard, R. Ramirez, W. S. Chau, W. S. Suen, S. Sheridan, V. P. Tin, L. P. Chung, M. P. Wong, J. W. Shay, A. F. Gazdar, W. K. Lam, and J. D. Minna. 2007. Expression of Nicotinic Acetylcholine Receptor Subunit Genes in Non-Small-Cell Lung Cancer Reveals Differences between Smokers and Nonsmokers. *Cancer Res.* 67:4638-47.

[39] Li, M. D. 2006. The genetics of nicotine dependence. Curr Psychiatry Rep 8:158-64.

[40] Limper, A. H., and J. Roman. 1992. Fibronectin. A versatile matrix protein with roles in thoracic development, repair and infection. *Chest* 101:1663-73.

[41] Macklin, K. D., A. D. Maus, E. F. Pereira, E. X. Albuquerque, and B. M. Conti-Fine. 1998. Human vascular endothelial cells express functional nicotinic acetylcholine receptors. *J. Pharmacol. Exp. Ther.* 287:435-9.

[42] Maneckjee, R., and J. D. Minna. 1994. Opioids induce while nicotine suppresses apoptosis in human lung cancer cells. *Cell Growth Differ.* 5:1033-40.

[43] Maus, A. D., E. F. Pereira, P. I. Karachunski, R. M. Horton, D. Navaneetham, K. Macklin, W. S. Cortes, E. X. Albuquerque, and B. M. Conti-Fine. 1998. Human and rodent bronchial epithelial cells express functional nicotinic acetylcholine receptors. *Mol. Pharmacol.* 54:779-88.

[44] Meger, M., I. Meger-Kossien, A. Schuler-Metz, D. Janket, and G. Scherer. 2002. Simultaneous determination of nicotine and eight nicotine metabolites in urine of smokers using liquid chromatography-tandem mass spectrometry. J Chromatogr B Analyt Technol *Biomed. Life Sci.* 778:251-61.

[45]   Meuwissen, R., and A. Berns. 2005. Mouse models for human lung cancer. *Genes Dev.* 19:643-64.

[46]   Nanki, N., J. Fujita, Y. Yang, S. Hojo, S. Bandoh, Y. Yamaji, and T. Ishida. 2001. Expression of oncofetal fibronectin and syndecan-1 mRNA in 18 human lung cancer cell lines. Tumour Biol 22:390-6.

[47]   Nashmi, R., and H. A. Lester. 2006. CNS localization of neuronal nicotinic receptors. *J. Mol. Neurosci.* 30:181-4.

[48]   Ng, H. J., E. R. Whittemore, M. B. Tran, D. J. Hogenkamp, R. S. Broide, T. B. Johnstone, L. Zheng, K. E. Stevens, and K. W. Gee. 2007. Nootropic alpha7 nicotinic receptor allosteric modulator derived from GABAA receptor modulators. *Proc. Natl. Acad. Sci. U S A* 104:8059-64.

[49]   Nguyen, V. T., A. I. Chernyavsky, J. Arredondo, D. Bercovich, A. Orr-Urtreger, D. E. Vetter, J. Wess, A. L. Beaudet, Y. Kitajima, and S. A. Grando. 2004. Synergistic control of keratinocyte adhesion through muscarinic and nicotinic acetylcholine receptor subtypes. *Exp. Cell Res.* 294:534-49.

[50]   Oh, S. H., J. K. Woo, Q. Jin, H. J. Kang, J. W. Jeong, K. W. Kim, W. K. Hong, and H. Y. Lee. 2007. Identification of novel antiangiogenic anticancer activities of deguelin targeting hypoxia-inducible factor-1 alpha. *Int. J. Cancer.*

[51]   Paleari, L., S. Trombino, C. Falugi, L. Gallus, S. Carlone, C. Angelini, K. Sepcic, T. Turk, M. Faimali, D. M. Noonan, and A. Albini. 2006. Marine sponge-derived polymeric alkylpyridinium salts as a novel tumor chemotherapeutic targeting the cholinergic system in lung tumors. *Int. J. Oncol.* 29:1381-8.

[52]   Pankow, J. F. 2001. A consideration of the role of gas/particle partitioning in the deposition of nicotine and other tobacco smoke compounds in the respiratory tract. *Chem. Res. Toxicol.* 14:1465-81.

[53]   Papke, R. L. 1993. The kinetic properties of neuronal nicotinic receptors: genetic basis of functional diversity. *Prog. Neurobiol.* 41:509-31.

[54]   Perry, D. C., M. I. Davila-Garcia, C. A. Stockmeier, and K. J. Kellar. 1999. Increased nicotinic receptors in brains from smokers: membrane binding and autoradiography studies. *J. Pharmacol. Exp. Ther.* 289:1545-52.

[55]   Post, D. E., E. M. Sandberg, M. M. Kyle, N. S. Devi, D. J. Brat, Z. Xu, M. Tighiouart, and E. G. Van Meir. 2007. Targeted cancer gene therapy using a hypoxia inducible factor dependent oncolytic adenovirus armed with interleukin-4. *Cancer Res.* 67:6872-81.

[56]   Proskocil, B. J., H. S. Sekhon, Y. Jia, V. Savchenko, R. D. Blakely, J. Lindstrom, and E. R. Spindel. 2004. Acetylcholine is an autocrine or paracrine hormone synthesized and secreted by airway bronchial epithelial cells. *Endocrinology* 145:2498-506.

[57]   Roman, J., J. D. Ritzenthaler, A. Gil-Acosta, H. N. Rivera, and S. Roser-Page. 2004. Nicotine and fibronectin expression in lung fibroblasts: implications for tobacco-related lung tissue remodeling. *Faseb. J.* 18:1436-8.

[58]   Rose, J. E., F. M. Behm, E. C. Westman, and R. E. Coleman. 1999. Arterial nicotine kinetics during cigarette smoking and intravenous nicotine administration: implications for addiction. *Drug Alcohol Depend.* 56:99-107.

[59]   Sandler, A. 2007. Bevacizumab in non small cell lung cancer. *Clin. Cancer Res.* 13:4613s-6s.

[60]   Schuller, H. M. 1989. Cell type specific, receptor-mediated modulation of growth kinetics in human lung cancer cell lines by nicotine and tobacco-related nitrosamines. *Biochem. Pharmacol.* 38:3439-42.

[61]   Schuller, H. M. 2007. Nitrosamines as nicotinic receptor ligands. *Life Sci.* 80:2274-80.

[62]   Schuller, H. M., B. A. Jull, B. J. Sheppard, and H. K. Plummer. 2000. Interaction of tobacco-specific toxicants with the neuronal alpha(7) nicotinic acetylcholine receptor and its associated mitogenic signal transduction pathway: potential role in lung carcinogenesis and pediatric lung disorders. *Eur. J. Pharmacol.* 393:265-77.

[63]   Schuller, H. M., and M. Orloff. 1998. Tobacco-specific carcinogenic nitrosamines. Ligands for nicotinic acetylcholine receptors in human lung cancer cells. *Biochem. Pharmacol.* 55:1377-84.

[64]   Sekhon, H. S., Y. Jia, R. Raab, A. Kuryatov, J. F. Pankow, J. A. Whitsett, J. Lindstrom, and E. R. Spindel. 1999. Prenatal nicotine increases pulmonary alpha7 nicotinic receptor expression and alters fetal lung development in monkeys. *J. Clin. Invest.* 103:637-47.

[65]   Sekhon, H. S., J. A. Keller, N. L. Benowitz, and E. R. Spindel. 2001. Prenatal nicotine exposure alters pulmonary function in newborn rhesus monkeys. *Am. J. Respir. Crit. Care Med.* 164:989-94.

[66]   Sekhon, H. S., P. Song, Y. Jia, J. Lindstrom, and E. R. Spindel. 2005. Expression of lynx1 in developing lung and its modulation by prenatal nicotine exposure. *Cell Tissue Res.* 320:287-97.

[67]   Shen, C., C. S. Lancaster, B. Shi, H. Guo, P. Thimmaiah, and M. A. Bjornsti. 2007. TOR Signaling is a Determinant of Cell Survival in Response to DNA Damage. *Mol. Cell Biol.*

[68]   Song, P., H. S. Sekhon, Y. Jia, J. A. Keller, J. K. Blusztajn, G. P. Mark, and E. R. Spindel. 2003. Acetylcholine is synthesized by and acts as an autocrine growth factor for small cell lung carcinoma. *Cancer Res.* 63:214-21.

[69]   Tournier, J. M., K. Maouche, C. Coraux, J. M. Zahm, I. Cloez-Tayarani, B. Nawrocki-Raby, A. Bonnomet, H. Burlet, F. Lebargy, M. Polette, and P. Birembaut. 2006. alpha3alpha5beta2-Nicotinic acetylcholine receptor contributes to the wound repair of the respiratory epithelium by modulating intracellular calcium in migrating cells. *Am. J. Pathol.* 168:55-68.

[70]   Tsai, J. R., I. W. Chong, C. C. Chen, S. R. Lin, C. C. Sheu, and J. J. Hwang. 2006. Mitogen-activated protein kinase pathway was significantly activated in human bronchial epithelial cells by nicotine. *DNA Cell. Biol.* 25:312-22.

[71]   Tsurutani, J., S. S. Castillo, J. Brognard, C. A. Granville, C. Zhang, J. J. Gills, J. Sayyah, and P. A. Dennis. 2005. Tobacco components stimulate Akt-dependent proliferation and NFkappaB-dependent survival in lung cancer cells. *Carcinogenesis* 26:1182-95.

[72]   Wang, Y., E. F. Pereira, A. D. Maus, N. S. Ostlie, D. Navaneetham, S. Lei, E. X. Albuquerque, and B. M. Conti-Fine. 2001. Human bronchial epithelial and

endothelial cells express alpha7 nicotinic acetylcholine receptors. *Mol. Pharmacol.* 60:1201-9.

[72] Wessler, I., C. J. Kirkpatrick, and K. Racke. 1998. Non-neuronal acetylcholine, a locally acting molecule, widely distributed in biological systems: expression and function in humans. *Pharmacol. Ther.* 77:59-79.

[74] West, K. A., J. Brognard, A. S. Clark, I. R. Linnoila, X. Yang, S. M. Swain, C. Harris, S. Belinsky, and P. A. Dennis. 2003. Rapid Akt activation by nicotine and a tobacco carcinogen modulates the phenotype of normal human airway epithelial cells. *J. Clin. Invest.* 111:81-90.

[75] Wong, H. P., L. Yu, E. K. Lam, E. K. Tai, W. K. Wu, and C. H. Cho. 2007. Nicotine promotes colon tumor growth and angiogenesis through beta-adrenergic activation. *Toxicol. Sci.* 97:279-87.

[76] Wongtrakool, C., S. Roser-Page, H. N. Rivera, and J. Roman. 2007. Nicotine alters lung branching morphogenesis through the {alpha}7 nicotinic acetylcholine receptor. *Am. J. Physiol. Lung Cell Mol. Physiol.*

[77] Xu, L., and X. Deng. 2006. Suppression of cancer cell migration and invasion by protein phosphatase 2A through dephosphorylation of mu- and m-calpains. *J. Biol. Chem.* 281:35567-75.

[73] Zhang, Q., X. Tang, Z. F. Zhang, R. Velikina, S. Shi, and A. D. Le. 2007. Nicotine Induces Hypoxia-Inducible Factor-1{alpha} Expression in Human Lung Cancer Cells via Nicotinic Acetylcholine Receptor Mediated Signaling Pathways. *Clin. Cancer Res.* 13:4686-94.

[79] Zheng, Y., J. D. Ritzenthaler, J. Roman, and S. Han. 2007. Nicotine Stimulates Human Lung Cancer Cell Growth by Inducing Fibronectin Expression. *Am. J Respir Cell. Mol. Biol.*

[80] Zhu, B. Q., C. Heeschen, R. E. Sievers, J. S. Karliner, W. W. Parmley, S. A. Glantz, and J. P. Cooke. 2003. Second hand smoke stimulates tumor angiogenesis and growth. *Cancer Cell* 4:191-6.

In: Progress in Cell Growth Process Research
Editor: Takumi Hayashi, pp. 167-185

ISBN 978-1-60456-325-2
© 2008 Nova Science Publishers, Inc.

Chapter 7

ELECTRICAL IMPEDANCE MONITORING OF CELL MONOLAYER GROWTH *IN VITRO*

Sungbo Cho[5] and Hagen Thielecke

Biohybrid Systems, Fraunhofer Institute for Biomedical Engineering
Ensheimerstr. 48 66386 St. Ingbert Germany

ABSTRACT

The monitoring of cell growth *in vitro* is used not only for the investigation of cultivation processes but also for medical diagnosis, cytotoxicity testing, and drug development. The *in vitro* characterization of cells without any labelling is required increasingly required to guarantee the cell culture environment during the experiments. As one of those non-invasive methods, electrical impedance spectroscopy has been investigated over the last decades. Impedance spectroscopy is a reliable and quantifiable technique to measure the ratio of alternating potential to current. Since the bi-lipid layer of cell membrane has low conductivity, the behaviour of cells (e.g. movement, adhesion, spreading, or detachment) affects current flow or potential distribution across the cell layer. The electrical properties of thin cell monolayer and even single cell related with morphological changes have been measured by micro systems with impedance spectroscopy. Under various environments (e.g. during the cell cultivation, toxification, or infection), the impedances dependent on the minute changes in the cell/substrate and cell/cell gap have been monitored. In this chapter, a technical and applicative review of impedance spectroscopy for *in vitro* monitoring of cell monolayer growth is presented.

1. INTRODUCTION

For the investigation of cell physiology or pathology, an *in vitro* cell-based system is increasingly utilized to non-invasively monitor the cell growth under various environments

(Mack *et al.* 2001). During the growth of most mammalian cells under the culture condition, they attach, spread, and proliferate on the surface of glass dishes releasing traces of material (Fuhr *et al.* 1998). Further, the cells migrate under biochemical stimulations or infectious/toxic conditions by using membrane protrusion adhered to the substrate for the transformation of cellular contraction forces (Kirfel *et al.* 2004). Therefore, the investigation of the cellular adhesion, the binding of a cell to another cell or to a surface, has a key role in understanding the responses of cells to specific conditions. Cells adhere to specific molecules on the opposing cell or surface by using the adhesion molecules of cell membranes termed "receptors". The receptors are linked to the intracellular cytoskeleton supporting the mechanical stability of cellular adhesion. The pathways regulating the cellular adhesion are determined not only by the extracellular proteins such as cytokines or growth factors but also the signalling molecules such as GTPases or Ca2+ -regulated proteins (Takai *et al.* 1995, 2001, Ridley 2002). These lead to cytoskeletal activity and changes in focal adhesion. Due to the presence of adhesive proteins, transport organelles, and the cellular receptors, there are nano-meter scaled adhesion clefts in the cell/cell or cell/substrate junction (Giebel *et al* 1999).

To characterize the properties within the adhesion clefts, several biophysical techniques such as electrical impedance spectroscopy, quartz crystal microscopy, and optical waveguide light-mode spectroscopy have been investigated (Hug 2003). These label-free essays provide their unique quantitative information about the cell-substrate interaction in real-time and have a potential for medical diagnosis and drug development. Among these methods, in this chapter, the electrical impedance spectroscopy for *in vitro* monitoring of cell growth is presented. For this, a theoretical background and technical review about the impedance measurement of cells is described. Further, the current state of art is outlined through a review of various applications using the electrical technique.

2. IMPEDANCE SPECTROSCOPY

Impedance spectroscopy (IS) is a non-invasive and reliable technique to measure the frequency dependent electrical properties of materials (Grimnes and Martinsen 2000). By using the weak alternating electric fields, the impedance of biological materials can be monitored during the physiological and morphological changes in them. The impedance is a ratio of alternating potential to current and a complex which consists of a real resistance and imaginary reactance and has a unit of ohms (Ω). Under linear conditions, when an alternating current (I) source with a certain frequency is applied to materials, the response can be an alternating voltage (V). In the presence of the dielectric properties of materials, the differences of phase and amplitude between the source and response signal are observed. When the alternating current is applied with the amplitude of I_m and phase of ϕ_I as the measured potential with the amplitude of V_m and phase of ϕ_V is

---

[5] http://www.ibmt.fhg.de, Tel. +49 6894 980 274, Fax +49 6894 980 400, E-mail: sungbo.cho@ibmt.fhg.de.

$$I = I_m e^{j(\omega t + \phi_I)}$$ (1)

$$V = V_m e^{j(\omega t + \phi_V)}$$ (2)

where $j = (-1)^{1/2}$, $\omega = 2\pi f$ with the frequency of f, and t is time.

Therefore, the ratio of V to I can be presented as the electrical impedance (Z) with the amplitude of Z_m and phase of θ as follows.

$$Z = \frac{V}{I} = \frac{V_m e^{j(\omega t + \phi_V)}}{I_m e^{j(\omega t + \phi_I)}} = \frac{V_m}{I_m} e^{j(\phi_V - \phi_I)} = Z_m e^{j\theta}$$ (3)

To measure the impedance, the electrodes for applying the source and measuring the response are required. According to the number and configuration of electrodes, the measurement can be called two- or four-electrode method. The setup of the two-electrode method is simpler than the four-electrode method; however the total impedance measured by the two-electrode method contains the electrode impedance. The electrode impedance is characterized by electrical double layers and diffusion on the electrode (Bard and Faulkner 2001). When a current flows from the electrode to electrolytes, an electrostatic interaction between the ions in the electrolyte and electrode surface occurrs (Langmuir 1929). The attracted ions make a charged layer on the electrode surface for neutralization, and therefore the electrical double layer forms on the electrode. In addition, the ions concentrating at the electrode result in the diffusion of ions near the electrode. As the electrode area decreases, or as the frequency is lower, the contribution of electrode impedance on total impedance increases. De Boer and van Osterom (1978) have modelled the frequency and area dependent electrode impedance as a constant phase element. This electrode impedance can be avoided theoretically from the impedance measurement by using the four-electrode method, which uses a pair of electrodes for recording the potential and another pair of electrodes for applying the current.

3. ELECTRICAL PROPERTIES OF CELLS

The cell has a membrane, ultra-thin layers surrounding the intra cellular fluid, the cytoplasm (Curtis and Barnes 1989). The cell membrane is composed of bi-layer lipids, proteins, transport organelles, and ionic channels for electrogenic pumps. The electrogenic current density in excitable animal cells is usually of the order of a few $\mu A/cm^2$. South and Grant (1973), and Takashima and Schwan (1974) have investigated the passive properties of the excitable cell membrane. By the sodium/potassium pumps of the active ionic channel, the interior potentials of excitable and non-excitable cells are about -70 mV and -10 mV to -20 mV with respect to the extra cellular liquid, respectively. The membrane of the cell breaks down when the potential difference through cells is increased more than 150 mV. The voltage dependence of the membrane capacitance was studied by Cole (1972) and Takashima and Yantorno (1977). Asami *et al.* (1990) have measured the impedance of HeLa and Myeloma membrane by using the micropipette technique, and found that the conductance and capacitance of the membrane are about 100 μScm^{-2} and $1.0 \sim 1.9 \ \mu F/cm^2$ in the frequency range of 1 Hz to 1 kHz.

The cells/tissue can be regarded as an inhomogeneous, dielectric, and anisotropic material because the size and orientation of cells are uneven. The electrical properties of cells/tissue are dependent on the temperature and frequency strongly as well. When electric fields are applied externally to tissue, the dipoles are formed with bound ions, and the tissue is polarized (Malmivuo and Plonsey 1995). If the frequency of electric fields is low enough so that all charges in the tissue are allowed to change their position, the polarization is maximal (Grimnes and Martinsen 2000). To characterize this time dependence, Maxwell (1873) first introduced the concept of relaxation. Later Debye (1929) used this relaxation theory to explain the time required for dipolar molecules to orient themselves. The frequency domain concept corresponding to relaxation is dispersion. Schwan (1957) roughly divided the dispersions of cells/tissue into three groups with the terms of α, β, and γ. In the first dispersion region (α), the relative permittivity ε_r decreases between 1 Hz and 10 kHz. In this frequency range, the current flows through the extra cellular space, and therefore the impedance of tissues is strongly determined by the extra cellular conditions (e.g. volume or conductivity). This α dispersion is caused by ionic diffusion and surface ionic conduction at the boundaries of cell membrane. The second dispersion region (β) is observed from about 100 kHz to 100 MHz and caused by the passive cell membrane capacitance short-circuiting the membrane resistance. The current flows through the extra and intra cellular space. The third dispersion region (γ) is appeared from about 100 MHz to 100 GHz and caused by the relaxation of the water molecules.

4. IMPEDANCE MEASUREMENT OF CELLS GROWTH

Giaever and Keese (1984) have pioneered the impedance measurement of cell layer on a planar electrode-based chip. They have measured the potential fluctuated caused by the movement of cells on planar electrodes during the cultivation by applying an alternating current at the frequency of 4 kHz (Giaever and Keese 1986, 1993). Since they configured a two-electrode system including small electrodes with the area of $3 \times 10^{-4} \ cm^2$ and a relatively large electrode of $2 \ cm^2$, the region of smaller electrode mainly contributed to the total measured impedance. When the cells were introduced in the electrode-based cell chip, the measured impedance began to increase and to fluctuate with cultivation time. The rise in impedance was observed as the cells spread and cover the surface of electrodes and as cell density increases. Afterwards, the impedance became relatively constant and the fluctuation was somewhat decreased since the locomotion of individual cells is reduced at enough high density of cells on the limited area of electrode surface. Further, Giaever and Keese (1991) derived an analytical solution for the frequency dependent impedance of cell monolayer on electrodes as Figure 1 with assumption that the cells are cylindrical shape with average radius of r_c and gap between the ventral surface of cell and substratum of h. From the estimation of potential and current distribution in the model, they deduced the whole specific impedance of cells on electrode Z_c (Ωcm^2) with parameters involved with cell/cell (R_b) and cell/substrate gap (α) as Eq. 4. In case of rectangularly shaped cells on electrode, the whole specific impedance of cell monolayer was derived by Lo and Ferrier (1998).

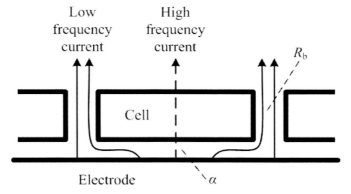

Figure 1. A schematic model of cell monolayer on electrode, R_b and α are parameters involved with cell/cell and cell/substrate gap, respectively.

$$\frac{1}{Z_c} = \frac{1}{Z_n} \left\{ \frac{Z_n}{Z_m + Z_n} + \frac{\dfrac{Z_m}{Z_m + Z_n}}{\dfrac{\gamma r_c}{2} \dfrac{I_0(\gamma r_c)}{I_1(\gamma r_c)} + R_b \left(\dfrac{1}{Z_m} + \dfrac{1}{Z_n} \right)} \right\}$$

$$\gamma r_c = r_c \sqrt{\frac{\rho}{h} \left(\frac{1}{Z_m} + \frac{1}{Z_n} \right)} = \alpha \sqrt{\frac{1}{Z_m} + \frac{1}{Z_n}} \tag{4}$$

where I_0 and I_1 are modified Bessel function of the first kind of order 0 and 1, respectively. Z_n, Z_m specific impedance of cell-free electrode and cell layer, ρ resistivity of medium, R_b junctional resistance between adjacent cells over a unit cell area, α parameter related with cell adhesion region.

Another electrical property of cell layer without considering the cell morphology was presented by a macro equivalent circuit of a resistance (R_{cl}) and a parallel-connected capacitance (C_{cl}) as Figure 2 (Wegener *et al.* 1996). For this model, it was premised that these parameters, resistance and capacitance of cell layer, are determined by the whole paracellular shunt, cells adhesion/spreading, and extra cellular matrix. By non-linear curve fitting the derived models on the measured impedance spectra, the parameters in the model were adjusted to minimize the sum of squared deviations between the model and measured data.

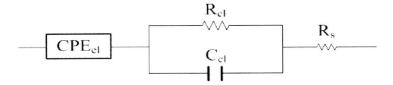

Figure 2. An equivalent circuit for cell on electrodes, R_{cl} and C_{cl} are the resistance and the capacitance of cell layer, respectively, CPE_{el} the constant phase element for electrode impedance R_s the resistance of medium.

As other systems for the impedance measurement of cell growth, Ehret *et al.* (1997, 1998) have developed an interdigitated electrode structure (IDES) and monitored the impedance of cellular behaviour on IDES. It was found that the capacitance of cell layer on IDES shows decreasing patterns during the cell cultivation. A field effect transistor (FET) was used to measure the extracellular resistance of single cells between the ventral cell membrane and silicon dioxide substrate (Kiessling *et al.* 2000, Braun and Fromherz 2004). Hagedorn *et al.* (1995) have fabricated a thin insulated silicon membrane with micro pores and measured the impedance related with cell mobility on the holes. Cho and Thielecke (2007) have fabricated a micro hole-based chip and measured the impedance of single cells on a micro hole during the cultivation or toxification.

5. ELECTRODE-BASED CHIP FOR MONITORING OF CELLS

Here, it was shown to utilize the impedance monitoring of cells as cytotoxicity test or diagnosis of virus infection by using a fabricated electrode-based chip. The fabrication process in semiconductor technology for the electrode-based chip was briefly described below. First, silicon nitride layer was deposited on a silicon wafer by plasma enhanced chemical vapour deposition (PE-CVD). Afterwards, circular gold electrodes and interconnection lines were deposited and patterned on the silicon nitride layer. As insulation layer, a second silicon nitride layer was deposited on the whole substrate by PE-CVD. The electrode sites and connecting pads were opened by reactive ion etching. The radius of exposed electrode was 250 μm (area ≈ 1.96×10^{-3} cm^2). The electrode substrate was packaged with a ceramic chip carrier. The pads of chip were connected with the individual conductive lines of chip carrier by wire-bonding. Then, the conductive lines, pads, and wires were insulated by using the silicon resin. A cylindrical glass dish conserving the cell culture medium was integrated with the electrode structure. The inner radius and height of the dish was 3 cm and 1 cm, respectively. For the impedance measurement, the chip was electrically connected to an impedance analyzer Solartron 1260 (Solartron Analytical, Farnborough, UK) by the combination of chip with chip adapter. A platinum wire was used as a counter electrode. Since the contact area of counter electrode was much larger than one of sensing gold electrode, the surface area of gold electrodes mostly contributed to the total measured impedance. A schematic of impedance measurement of cells on electrodes was shown in Figure 3. During the cultivation of cells on electrodes at 7.5% CO_2 and 37 °C in an incubator Heraeus BB 6220 (Heraeus-Christ, Hanau, Germany), the impedance of cell chip was measured from 100 Hz to 1 MHz by the impedance analyser. The applied input potential was 10 mV. By using a multiplexer integrated with the impedance analyser and programming of experimental schedule, it was enable to do computer-controlled impedance monitoring of cell layer during the long-term cultivation.

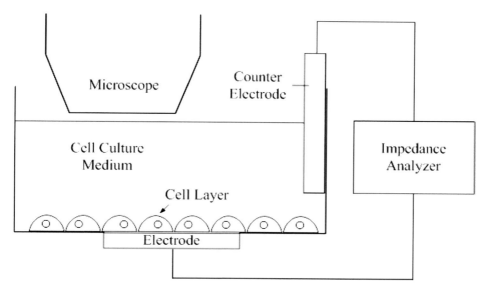

Figure 3. Schematic of impedance measurement of cells on electrodes, not scaled.

5.1. L-929 Fibroblasts and Cytotoxic Test

For the experiments, L-929 fibroblasts (3.6×10^6 / ml) and 3 ml of culture medium (RPMI 1640, 10 % fetal calf serum, 0.5 % penicillin / streptavidin) were applied into the chip. The culture medium in the cell chip was refreshed every day during the cultivation. For a cytotoxic test, 10 μl of RPMI culture medium containing 5% of the cell toxic substance dimethylsulfoxide (DMSO) was prepared. It was found that DMSO is polar and easily diffused through the cell membrane where it can replace water molecules associated with cellular constituents (Tokuhiro *et al.* 1974). It causes the dehydration of the lipid bilayer and the morphological changes of cell (Vessey *et al.* 1991, Gordeliy *et al.* 1998). While the medium with 5% DMSO was applied to L-929 cells cultivated on the electrode for one day, the impedance was recorded at 40 kHz in real time.

Figure 4 showed the micrograph of L-929 cells on electrode when applied (0 h) or after cultivation for 3 days (72 h). When L-929 fibroblasts were applied on the electrode, the measured impedance spectrum was not different from one of no cells on the electrode. In the low frequency range of measured spectra in Figure 4(c), the impedance presented the electrode impedance and decreased with increasing frequency. At enough high frequency, the value became a constant of spreading resistance (Newman 1966). More densely populated cells on the sensing electrode resulted in higher impedance magnitude in the frequency range. By fitting the measured spectra with an equivalent circuit based on Figure 2, it was shown that the specific R_{cl} increases but C_{cl} decreases according to the cultivation time (Figure 4(d)). In a confluent layer of L-929 fibroblasts, C_{cl} was about 0.9 µF/cm^2.

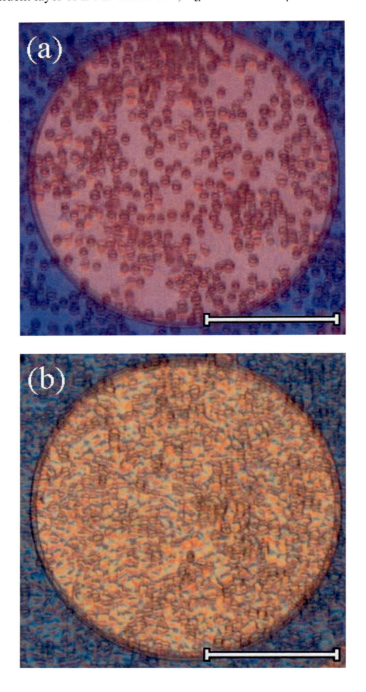

Figure 4. (Continued)

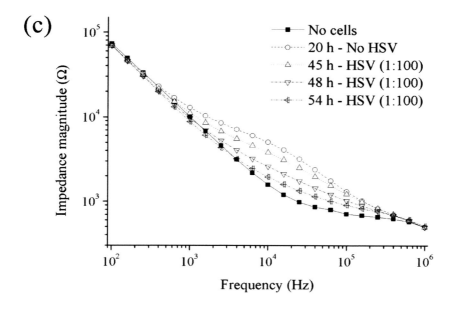

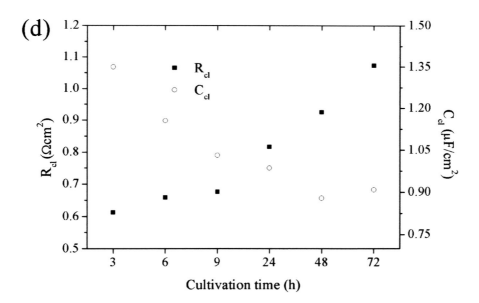

Figure 4. Monitoring of L-929 fibroblasts cultivation, micrograph of L-929 cells on electrode (a) when applying the cells (0 h) and (b) after cultivation for 3 days (72 h), scale bar: 200 μm, (c) measured and fitted spectra at 0 h and 72 h, (d) R_{cl} and C_{cl} (resistance and capacitance of cells, respectively) determined by fitting the measured spectra with an equivalent circuit based on Figure 2 versus the cultivation time.

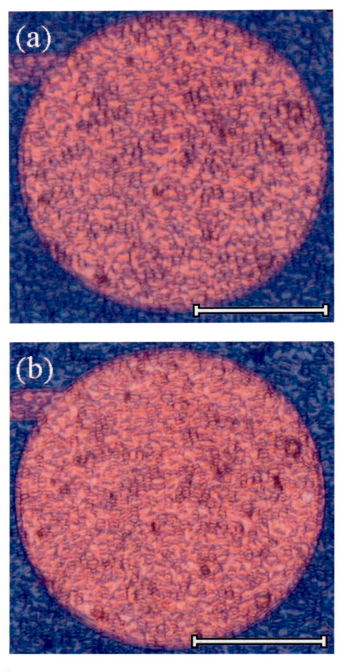

Figure 5. Continued

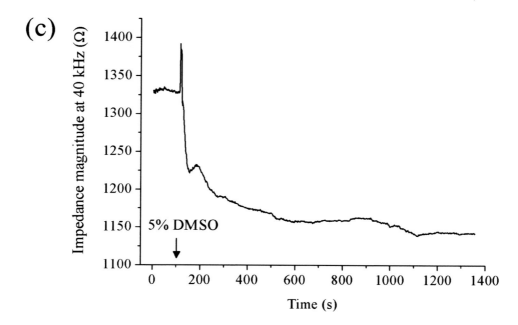

Figure 5. Effect of DMSO on the impedance of L-929 cells cultured for 24 h, micrograph of L-929 cells on electrode (a) before applying 5% DMSO and (b) after 30 minutes from applying 5% DMSO in the L-929 cell chip, scale bar: 200 μm, (c) impedance magnitude recorded at 40 kHz.

The cytotoxic effect of DMSO on L-929 cells cultured for a day was characterized by impedance as Figure 5. Figure 5(a) and (b) showed the micrograph of L-929 cells on the electrode before applying 5% DMSO and after 30 minutes from applying 5% DMSO, respectively. In the micrographs, no significant detachment or morphological change of cells was observed after applying the DMSO. However, the impedance magnitude at 40 kHz gradually decreased according to time after that (Figure 5(c)).

5.2. Vero Cells and Diagnosis of Virus Infection

Isolation of Herpes simplex virus (HSV) in Vero cell culture have provided the most reliable and specific method and been considered as the "Gold Standard" in the laboratory diagnosis (Athmananthan *et al.* 2002, El-Aal *et al.* 2006). Here, the diagnosis of HSV infection was characterized by impedance spectroscopy with electrode-based chip. For the impedance monitoring of cells during the virus infection, Vero cells and HSV were prepared. Vero cells (8×10^4) with 3 ml culture medium (D-MEM, 10% fetal bovine serum, 0.5 % penicillin / streptomycin) were applied in the electrode-based chip. After the cultivation of cells on electrode for one day, HSV with different concentration (dilution 1:20 and 1:100 of a standard HSV stock with TCID50 of 10^7 to 10^8 infection-unit) were injected in the cell chips separately.

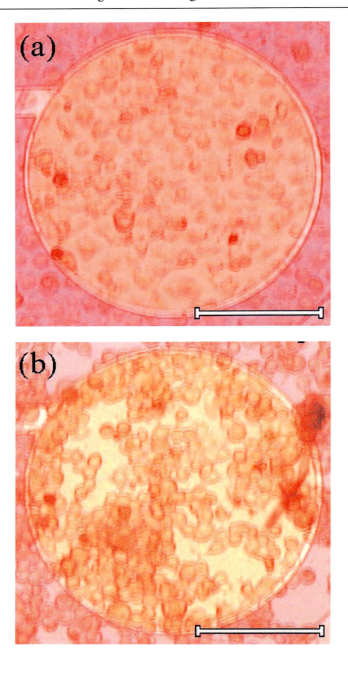

Figure 6. (Continued)

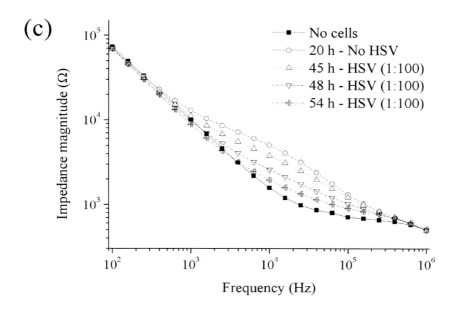

Figure 6. Continued

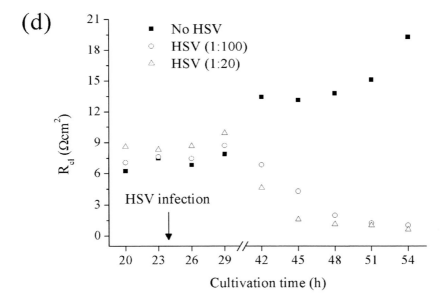

Figure 6. Effect of Herpes simplex virus (HSV) infection on Vero cells, micrograph of Vero cells on electrode (a) before (20 h) and (b) after HSV (1:100) infection (54 h), During HSV infection (c) measured spectra of Vero cells, (d) R_{cl} determined by fitting the measured spectra with an equivalent circuit based on Figure. 2.

Figure 6 showed the micrograph of Vero cells on electrode before and after 43 h from HSV (1:100) infection. The infected Vero cells were detached from the electrode after a certain period. During the cultivation of Vero cells, the measured impedance was increased in the frequency range of 500 Hz to 300 kHz as Figure 6(c). The largest change in the impedance magnitude was found in the frequency of 5 kHz to 15 kHz. After Vero cells were infected with HSV (1:100), the impedance magnitude was decreased gradually. The detachment of infected cells resulted in the increase of exposed electrode area and therefore the decrease of impedance magnitude. Finally, the impedance spectrum at 70 h became similar to one of no cells on electrode. Figure 6(d) showed R_{cl} determined by the fitting during Vero cells cultivation or infection with HSV. R_{cl} increased during the cultivation without infection (No HSV), however it decreased depending on the concentration of HSV.

5.3. Other Applications

Besides the examples described above, the adhesion and spreading of different cells onto electrodes were characterized electrically during the cultivation (Mitra et al. 1991, Lo et al. 1995, Takahashi et al. 1999, Wegener et al. 2000, Luong et al. 2001, Xiao et al. 2002a). For the cytotoxicity tests, the impedance of cells on the electrode was measured in real time while applying test substances (Xiao et al. 2002b, Xiao and Luong 2003, 2005). The morphological changes as the responses of cells to chemical and physical stimulations were investigated by using the electrical method (Lo et al. 1994, Smith et al. 1994, Wang et al. 1995, Ochoa et al. 1997, Patil et al. 1997, Noiri et al. 2001, De Blasio et al. 2004). During the apoptosis or chemotaxis, the impedance changes related with cell shape and migration were monitored (English et al. 1999, Hadjout et al. 2001, Arndt et al. 2004, Lee et al. 2006). The cell pathology was investigated by the electrode-based cell chip with impedance spectroscopy for the development of therapies or drugs (Sharma et al. 2001, Thielecke et al. 2001a, 2001b, Lundien et al. 2002, Kilani et al. 2004, McCoy et al. 2005, Cho et al. 2007).

6. CONCLUSION

Due to the guarantee of the cell's environment, the label-free test is increasingly required for the monitoring of cell growth, cytotoxicity tests, diagnosis of diseases, or development of therapies and drugs. Impedance spectroscopy has been used as a non-invasive and fast monitoring technique of cell behaviours in vitro. As a response of cell layers to various culture environments, the cellular adhesion and morphological changes of cells have been characterized by impedance spectroscopy with electrode-based chips. In this chapter, the theoretical background and applicative reviews of the electrical method were presented. Further, it was shown to utilize the electrode-based chip with impedance measurement to characterize the cytotoxic effect of dimethylsulfoxide on cells and the influence of herpes simplex virus infection on cell morphology.

REFEERNCES

Arndt, S., Seebach, J., Psathaki, K., Galla, H. J. and Wegener, J. (2004). Bioelectrical impedance assay to monitor changes in cell shape during apoptosis. *Biosensors and Bioelectronics* 19, 583-594.

Asami, K., Takahashi, Y. and Takashima, S. (1990). Frequency domain analysis of membrane capacitance of cultured cells (HeLa and myeloma) using the micropipette technique. *Biophysical Journal* 58, 143-148.

Athmananthan, S., Reddy, S. B., Nutheti, R. and Rao, G. N. (2002). Comparison of an immobilized human corneal epithelial cell line with Vero cells in the isolation of Herpes simplex virus-1 for the laboratory diagnosis of Herpes simplex keratitis. *BMC Ophthalmology* 2:3.

Bard, A. J. and Faulkner, L. R. (2001). Electrochemical Methods, Fundamentals and Applications. New York, Wiley.

Braun, D. and Fromherz, P. (2004). Imaging neuronal seal resistance on silicon chip using fluorescent voltage-sensitive dye. *Biophysical Journal* 87, 1351–1359.

Cho, S. and Thielecke, H. (2007). Micro hole based cell chip with impedance spectroscopy. *Biosensors and Bioelectronics* 22, 1764-1768.

Cho, S., Becker, S., von Briesen, H. and Thielecke, H. (2007). Impedance monitoring of herpes simplex virus-induced cytopathic effect in Vero cells. *Sensors and Actuators B: Chemical,* 123, 978–982.

Cole, K. S. (1972). Membranes, ions and impulses. Berkeley, University of California Press.

Curtis, H. and Barnes, N. S. (1989). Biology. New York, Worth Publishers.

De Blasio, B. F., Rottingen, J. A., Sand, K. L., Giaever, I. and Iversen, J. G. (2004). Global synchronous oscillations in cytosolic calcium and adherence in bradykinin-stimulated Madin-Darby canine kidney cells. *Acta Physiologica Scandinavica* 180, 335-346.

De Boer R. W. and van Osterom, A. (1978). Electrical properties of platinum electrodes: impedance measurements and time-domain analysis. *Medical and Biological Engineering and Computing* 16, 1-10.

Debye, P. (1929). Polar molecules. New York, Dover.

Ehret, R., Baumann, W., Brischwein, M., Schwinde, A., Stegbauer, K. and Wolf, B. (1997). Monitoring of cellular behaviour by impedance measurements on interdigitated electrode structures. *Biosensors and Bioelectronics* 12, 29-41.

Ehret, R., Baumann, W., Brischwein, M., Schwinde, A. and Wolf, B. (1998). On-line control of cellular adhesion with impedance measurements using interdigitated electrode structures. *Medical and Biological Engineering and Computing* 36, 365-370.

El-Aal, A. M., Sayed, M. E., Mohammed, E., Ahmed, M. and Fathy, M. (2006). Evaluation of herpes simplex detection in corneal scrapings by three molecular methods. *Current Microbiology* 52, 379-382.

English, D. A., Kovala, T., Welch, Z., Harvey, K. A., Siddiqui, R. A., Brindley, D. N. and Garcia, J. G. N. (1999). Induction of endothelial cell chemotaxis by sphingosine 1-phosphate and stabilization of endothelial monolayer barrier function by lysophosphatidic acid, potential mediators of hematopoietic angiogenesis. NCS Compendium 8, 627-634.

Fuhr, G. Richter, E., Zimmermann, H., Hitzler, H., Niehus, H. and Hagedorn, R. (1998). Cell traces-footprints of individual cells during locomotion and adhesion. *Biological Chemistry* 379, 1161-1173.

Giaever, I. and Keese, C. (1984). Monitoring fibroblast behavior in tissue culture with an applied electric field. *Proceedings of the National Academy of Sciences* 81, 3761–3764.

Giaever, I. and Keese, C. (1986). Use of electric fields to monitor the dynamical aspect of cell behavior in tissue culture. *IEEE Transactions on Biomedical Engineering* 33, 242 247.

Giaever, I. and Keese, C. R. (1991). Micromotion of mammalian cells measured electrically. Proceedings of the National Academy of Sciences 88, 7896-7900 (correction: (1993) *Proceedings of the National Academy of Sciences* 90, 1634).

Giaever, I. and Keese, C. R. (1993). A morphological biosensor for mammalian cells. *Nature* 366, 591-592.

Giebel, K. F., Bechinger, C., Herminghaus, S., Riedel, M., Leiderer, P., Weiland, U. and Bastmeyer, M. (1999). Imaging of cell/substrate contacts of living cells with surface plasmon resonance microscopy. *Biophysical Journal* 76, 509-516.

Gordeliy, V. I., Kiselev, M. A., Lesieur, P., Pole, A. V. and Teixeira, J. (1998). Lipid membrane structure and interactions in dimethylsulfoxide/water mixtures. *Biophysical Journal* 75, 2343-2351.

Grimnes, S. and Martinsen, Ø. G. (2000). Bioimpedance and bioelectricity basics. San Diego, Academic Press.

Hadjout, N., Laevsky, G., Knecht, D. A. and Lynes, M. A. (2001). Automated real-time measurement of chemotactic cell motility. *Biotechniques* 31, 1130-1138.

Hagedorn, R., Fuhr, G., Lichtwardt-Zinke, K., Richter, E., Hornung, J. and Voigt, A. (1995). Characterisation of cell movement by impedance measurement on fibroblasts grown on perforated Si-membranes. *Biochimica et Biophysica Acta* 1269, 221-232.

Hug, T. S. (2003). Biophysical methods for monitoring cell-substrate interactions in drug discovery. *Assay and Drug Development Technologies* 1, 479-488.

Kirfel, G., Rigort, A., Borm, B. and Herzog, V. (2004). Cell migration: mechanisms of rear detachment and the formation of migration tracks. *European Journal of Cell Biology* 83, 717-724.

Langmuir, I. (1929). The interaction of electron and positive ion space charges in cathode sheaths. *Physical Review* 33, 954-989.

Kiessling, V., Mueller, B. and Fromherz, P. (2000). Extracellular resistance in cell adhesion measured with a transistor probe. *Langmuir* 16, 3517-3521.

Kilani, M. M., Mohammed, K. A., Nasreen, N., Hardwick, J. A., Kaplan, M. H., Tepper, R. S. and Antony, V. B. (2004). Respiratory syncytial virus causes increased bronchial epithelial permeability. *Chest* 126, 186-191.

Lee, J. F., Zeng, Q., Ozaki, H., Wang, L., Hand, A. R., Hla, T., Wang, E. and Lee, M. J. (2006). Dual roles of tight junction-associated protein, zonula occludens-1, in sphingosine 1-phosphate-mediated endothelial chemotaxis and barrier integrity. *Journal of Biological Chemistry* 281, 29190-29200.

Lo, C. M., Keese, C. R. and Giaever, I. (1994). pH changes in pulsed CO2 incubators cause periodic changes in cell morphology. *Experimental Cell Research* 213, 391-397.

Lo, C. M., Keese, C. R. and Giaever, I. (1995). Impedance analysis of MDCK cells measured by electric cell-substrate impedance sensing. *Biophysical Journal* 69, 2800-2807.

Lo, C. M. and Ferrier, J. (1998). Impedance analysis of fibroblastic cell layers measured by electric cell-substrate impedance sensing. *Physical Review* E 57, 6982-6987.

Lundien, M. C., Mohammed, K. A., Nasreen, N., Tepper, R. S., Hardwick, J. A., Sanders, K. L., van Horn, R. D. and Antony, V. B. (2002). Induction of MCP-1 expression in airway epithelial cells: Role of CCR2 receptor in airway epithelial injury. *Journal of Clinical Immunology* 22, 144-152.

Luong, J. H. T., Habibi-Rezaei, M., Meghrous, J., Xiao, C., Male, K. B. and Kamen, A. (2001). Monitoring motility, spreading, and mortality of adherent insect cells using an impedance sensor. *Analytical Chemistry* 73, 1844-1848.

Mack, A., Thielecke, H. and Robitzki, A. (2001). 3D-biohybrid systems: Applications in drug screening. *TRENDS in Biotechnology* 20, 56-61.

McCoy, M. H. and Wang, E. (2005). Use of electric cell-substrate impedance sensing as a tool for quantifying cytopathic effect in influenza A virus infected MDCK cells in real-time. *Journal of Virological Methods* 130, 157-161.

Malmivuo, J. and Plonsey, R. (1995). Bioelectromagnetism: principles and application of bioelectric and biomagnetic fields. New York, Oxford University Press.

Maxwell, J. C. (1873). A treatise on electricity and magnetism. Oxford, Clarendon Press.

Mitra, P., Keese, C. and Giaever, I. (1991). Electric measurement can be used to monitor the attachment and spreading of cells in tissue culture. *BioTechniques* 4, 504-510.

Newman, J. (1966). Resistance for flow of current to a disk. *Journal of Electrochemical Society* 113, 501-502.

Noiri, E., Nakao, A., Uchida, K., Tsukahara, H., Ohno, M., Fujita, T., Brodsky, S. and Goligorsky, M. (2001). Oxidative and nitrosative stress in acute renal ischemia. *American Journal of Physiology-Renal Physiology* 281, F948-F957.

Ochoa, L., Waypa, G., Mahoney, J. R. Jr., Rodriguez, L. and Minnear, F. L. (1997). Contrasting effects of hypochlorous acid and hydrogen peroxide on endothelial permeability: prevention with cAMP drugs. *American Journal of Respiratory and Critical Care Medicine* 156, 1247-1255.

Patil, S., Kaplan, J. E. and Minnear, F. L. (1997). Protein, not adenosine or adenine nucleotides, mediates platelet decrease in endothelial permeability. *American Journal of Physiology* 273, H2304-H2311.

Ridley, A. J. (2002). Rho GTPases and cell migration. *Journal of Cell Science* 114, 2713-2722.

Schwan, H. P. (1957). Advances in biological and medical physics: Electrical properties of tissue and cell suspensions. New York, Academic Press.

Sharma, K. V., Koenigsberger, C., Brimijoin, S. and Bigbee, J. W. (2001). Direct evidence for an adhesive function in the noncholinergic role of acetylcholinesterase in neurite outgrowth. *Journal of Neuroscience Research* 63, 165-175.

Smith, T., Wang, H. S., Hogg, M. G., Henrikson, R. C., Keese, C. R. and Giaever, I. (1994). Prostaglandin E2 elicits a morphological change in cultured orbital fibroblasts from patients with graves ophthalmopathy. *Proceedings of the National Academy of Sciences* 91, 5094-5098.

South, G. P. and Grant, E. H. (1973). The contribution of proton fluctuation to dielectric relaxation in protein solutions. *Biopolymers* 12, 1937-1944.

Takahashi, N., Seko, Y., Noiri, E., Tobe, K., Kadowaki, T., Sabe, H. and Yazaki, Y. (1999). Vascular endothelial growth factor induces activation and subcellular translocation of focal adhesion kinase (p125FAK) in cultured rat cardiac myocytes. *Circulation Research* 84, 1194-1202.

Takai, Y., Sasaki, T., Tanaka, K. and Nakanishi, H. (1995). Rho as a regulator of the cytoskeleton. *Trends in Biochemical Sciences* 20, 227-231.

Takai, Y., Sasaki, T. and Matozaki, T. (2001). Small GTP-binding proteins. *Physiological Reviews* 81, 153-208.

Takashima, S. and Schwan, H. P. (1974). Passive electrical properties of the squid axon membrane. *Journal of Membrane Biology* 17, 51-68.

Takashima, S. and Yantorno, R. E. (1977). Investigation of the voltage dependent membrane capacity of squid axon. *Annals of the New York Academy of Sciences* 303, 306-321.

Thielecke, H., Mack, A. and Robitzki, A. (2001a). Biohybrid microarrays – Impedimetric biosensor with 3D in vitro tissues for toxicological and biomedical screening. Fresenius *Journal of Analytical Chemistry* 369, 23-29.

Thielecke, H., Mack, A. and Robitzki, A. (2001b). A multicellular spheroid-based sensor for anti-cancer therapeutics. *Biosensors and Bioelectronics* 16, 261-269.

Tokuhiro, T., Menafra, L. and Szmant, H. H. (1974). Contribution of relaxation and chemical shift results to the elucidation of the structure of the water-DMSO liquid system. *Journal of Chemical Physics* 61, 2275-2282.

Vessey, D. A., Cunningham, J. M., Selden, A. C., Woodman, A. C. and Hodgson, H. J. F. (1991). Dimethylsulphoxide induces a reduced growth rate, altered cell morphology and increased epidermal-growth-factor binding in Hep G2 cells. *Biochemical Journal* 277, 773-777.

Wang, H. S., Keese, C. R., Giaever, I. and Smith, T. (1995). Prostaglandin E2 alters human orbital fibroblast shape through a mechanism involving the generation of cyclic adenosine. *Journal of Clinical Endocrinology and Metabolism* 80, 3553-3560.

Wegener, J., Sieber, M. and Galla, H. J. (1996). Impedance analysis of epithelial and endothelial cell monolayers cultured on gold surfaces. *Journal of Biochemical and Biophysical Methods* 32, 151-170.

Wegener, J., Keese, C. R. and Giaever, I. (2000). Electric cell-substrate impedance sensing (ECIS) as a noninvasive means to monitor the kenetics of cell spreading to artificial surfaces. *Experimental Cell Research* 259, 158-166.

Xiao, C., Lachance, B., Sunahara, G. and Luong, J. H. T. (2002a). An in-depth analysis of electric cell-substrate impedance sensing to study the attachment and spreading mammalian cells. *Analytical Chemistry* 74, 1333-1339.

Xiao, C., Lachance, B., Sunahara, G. and Luong, J. (2002b). Assessment of cytotoxicity using electric cell-substrate impedance sensing: concentration and time response function approach. *Analytical Chemistry* 74, 5748-5753.

Xiao, C. and Luong, J. (2003). On-line monitoring of cell growth and cytotoxicity using electric cell-substrate impedance sensing (ECIS). *Biotechnology Progress* 19, 1000-1005.

Xiao, C. and Luong, J. H. T. (2005). Assessment of cytotoxicity by emerging impedance spectroscopy. *Toxicology and Applied Pharmacology* 206, 102-112.

In: Progress in Cell Growth Process Research
Editor: Takumi Hayashi, pp. 187-208

ISBN 978-1-60456-325-2
© 2008 Nova Science Publishers, Inc.

Chapter 8

LIPID PEROXIDATION END PRODUCT AS A MODULATOR OF CELL GROWTH

Suzana Borovic[16], Ivan Sunjic[2], Renate Wildburger[3], Martin Mittelbach[4], Georg Waeg[4] and Neven Zarkovic[1]

[1] Rudjer Boskovic Institute, Bijenicka 54, Zagreb, Croatia
[2] Pliva d.d., Baruna Filipovica 29, Zagreb, Croatia
[3] Medical University of Graz, Graz, Austia
[4] Karl Franzens University, Graz, Austria

ABSTRACT

Oxidative stress caused by reactive oxygen species (ROS) is capable of disturbing the integrity of cell membranes via peroxidation of membrane lipids and alteration of the structure and function of macromolecules. Reactive aldehydes, in particular 4-hydroxynonenal (HNE), are endogenous end products resulting from the lipid peroxidation of polyunsaturated fatty acids of membrane lipids. For a long time, HNE has been considered as a mainly toxic product of lipid peroxidation, implicated in the pathophysiology of several diseases such as neurodegenerative diseases, ischemia/reperfusion states, atherosclerosis, diabetes and cancer. However, HNE is permanently formed also under physiological conditions, and has signaling activities in regulation of cell cycle, proliferation, differentiation and apoptosis. A complex network of signal cascades involving HNE is intensively studied. Various signaling pathways are directly or indirectly affected by HNE, because HNE is able to react with a number of cellular elements. Due to the strong affinity to bind to bioactive macromolecules, in particular proteins and peptides, HNE could modify their structure and consequently their function. Formation of HNE-cell surface protein adducts could mimic ligand-cell surface receptor binding, and induce activation of receptor-triggered signal transduction. Thus, HNE is considered also as a growth regulating factor, interfering with the cytokine

---

6 Correspondence to: Tel: +385-1-4571213; Fax: +385-1-4561010; e-mail: borovic@irb.hr.

activities. Interaction of HNE with other growth factors and their influence on cell proliferation will be topic of this article.

Keywords: Lipid peroxidation, 4-Hydroxynonenal, growth factors, Cytokines, ^{3}H-Thymidine incorporation, cell proliferation, EGF, IGF-1, bFGF.

INTRODUCTION

Oxidative stress happens when reactive oxygen species (ROS) are formed in excess and the steady-state between formation and elimination of ROS is disturbed [1]. It could cause various acute as well as chronic diseases in almost every organic system and makes the pathological base for very difficult diseases such as cardiovascular [2] and neurodegenerative diseases [3], as well as the most severe diseases of the modern mankind, malignant tumors, which are also associated with oxidative stress [4].

When excessive amount of ROS is formed in the environment of cellular membranes, lipid peroxidation occurs and lipid components of cells are damaged. That has been particularly important, since lipids are essential constituents of the cell membranes being among the first molecules susceptible to the damage caused by ROS. Free radical reactions in tissues are accompanied by oxidative degradation of polyunsaturated fatty acids of membrane lipids [5]. This process results in the production of highly reactive aldehydes which are proposed to be "second toxic messengers" for the primary free radicals which initiated lipid peroxidation [6,7]. Unlike ROS, reactive aldehydes are relatively long-lived and therefore might diffuse from the side of their origin and attack distant targets intracellulary or extracellulary. Among the many different aldehydes, most intensively studied are malondialdehyde, acrolein and 4-hydroxyalkenals, in particular 4-hydroxynonenal (HNE). 4-Hydroxyalkenals are endogenous end products resulting from the lipid peroxidation of polyunsaturated fatty acids of membrane and lipoprotein phospholipids. HNE is the major lipid peroxidation product of ω-6 polyunsaturated fatty acids (linoleic and arachidonic acid) and also considered as major product of lipid peroxidation (Figure 1) [8,9,10].

HNE was discovered as a toxic product of lipid peroxidation and it was at first considered only as a toxic product of lipid peroxidation, especially when its connection with toxicity of oil samples obtained during investigations of the toxic-oil syndrome was discovered in Spain 1981. [11]. HNE concentrations usually referred as high, toxic concentrations are in the range from 10 μM to 1 mM. This range differs slightly depending on the experimental model used, as well as a type of cell while not all cells have the same sensitivity to HNE [12]. When used at these concentrations, the aldehyde is able to produce strong inhibitions of several cellular functions: mitochondrial respiration, synthesis of DNA and RNA. These effects are concentration-dependent [9,13].

The "grey" zone of effects falls into the range from 1 to 10 μM, and although usually not toxic in this range, HNE can have inhibitory effects on cellular processes. Addition of HNE to the cell cultures increases induction of apoptosis in cells of different origin, such as neural [14], blood vessels smooth muscle [15], leukemia [16], osteosarcoma and bone cells [12], etc. Inhibition of DNA and protein synthesis is also observed, probably due to the inhibition of

DNA-polymerase and altered cell cycle regulation [17,18]. Apoptosis induction in HeLa cells could be observed even if treated with low, 1 µM HNE [19].

When used, however, at concentration of 1 µM or lower, HNE displays a lot of activities regarding especially cell multiplication and differentiation. HNE inhibits proliferation and induces differentiation of MEL mice erythroleukemia cells [20], K562 erythroleukemia cells [21] and HL-60 human leukemia cell line [22]. As the concentrations indicated above are usually found in normal tissues, these effects may be considered as physiological.

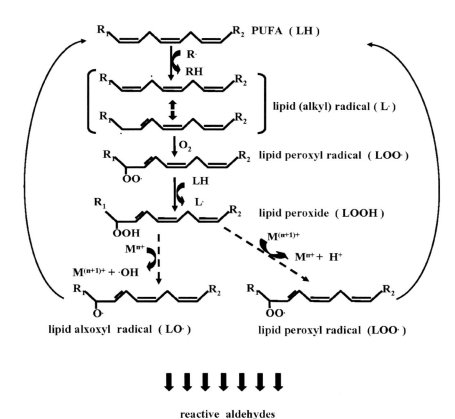

Figure 1. Schematic presentation of lipid peroxidation. Process of lipid peroxidation progress by a free radical chain reaction mechanism. It affects polyunsaturated fatty acids, because they contain multiple double bonds in between which lie methylene -CH$_2$- groups that posses especially reactive hydrogens. Free radical (R˙) abstracts hydrogen from the polyunsaturated fatty acid (PUFA) and creates radical. This radical reacts further with oxygen and another molecule of PUFA creating lipid peroxide. Reaction is further catalyzed by metal ions (M) resulting in alxoxyl and peroxyl radicals. These radicals can initiate process from the beginning starting chain reaction of lipid peroxidation. Upon disintegration, alxoxyl and peroxyl radicals generate reactive aldehydes, end products of lipid peroxidation.

Actually, HNE is found to be a physiological constituent of all tissues from animal and human origin studied [5,7,23]. However, the physiological role of HNE has not been clarified yet, but it seems that it could have an important role in cell growth control [13,22,24].

The importance of HNE has been considered in the pathophysiology of several diseases such as those involving chronic inflammation, many neurodegenerative diseases, ischemia/reperfusion, adult respiratory distress syndrome, atherogenesis and diabetes. More recently, it has been evidenced that HNE may act as a signaling molecule in pathological but also in physiological conditions [8,25]. As a low level of lipid peroxidation exists in normal tissues, the aldehyde displays signaling activities in normal cells. Among them, it is to consider the stimulation of neutrophil chemotaxis, activation of plasma membrane adenylate kinase, activation of membrane phospholipase C, inhibition of the oncogene c-myc expression, activation of the c-jun/jun kinases/AP-1 pathway, the effects on the cyclins and the activity of transcription factors [9,25].

Relatively high steady state concentrations of HNE in cell membranes were determined as the primary site of its origin (5–10 μM), [26] from where it can diffuse acting as a "second messenger" of free radicals [27]. Unlike free radicals or the other ROS, HNE has the unique feature to remain stable for some time and has high reactivity to bind to macromolecules; especially proteins, causing alteration of the structure and function of macromolecules. Such HNE-protein conjugates could be detected by the use of monoclonal antibodies [28,29]. HNE reacts mostly with SH groups of proteins and peptides, while such reaction with glutathione represents the most important mechanism for its detoxification [9, 30]. HNE can also react with amino groups, especially with amino acid side chains of proteins (mostly cysteine, lysine, arginine, proline and histidine), resulting in the generation of antigenic epitopes [9]. At certain extent, reactions of HNE are reversible, indicating that this is the way HNE could be carried to the distant places and released from proteins in convenient conditions, such as pH change, affecting biomolecules distant from the place of the HNE origin [9]. Such HNE-macromolecular conjugates might be even required for the biological activities of HNE [28,29]. Thus, in living systems biologically relevant interactions of HNE with macromolecules are complex. The simplest reaction is neutralization, where HNE is bound to macromolecules; hence the concentration of free aldehyde is decreased resulting in weaker toxicity of HNE. On the other hand, modification of cell growth in vitro in the presence of physiological concentrations of HNE (1μM) could depend on the presence of serum factors, but not serum albumin which is known to couple with HNE thus decreasing the effects of the aldehyde [19,31,32]. It is likely that interaction between serum growth factors and HNE could be not only direct, but on the signaling level as well.

MATERIAL AND METHODS

Preparation of Fresh HNE

HNE was obtained from Karl-Franzens University in Graz, Austria in the form of HNE-DMA (dimetilacetal) 1 mg/ml preserved in chloroform and kept at -20°C. Before use, it was activated according to the protocol: HNE-DMA was evaporated by nitrogen blow and 1 mM HCl was added to hydrolyze HNE for 1 h. HNE concentration was determined by spectrophotometer measuring the spectra from 200 to 350 nm and calculating value upon the absorption maximum at 223 nm. HNE concentration was calculated upon the formula:

$$c \text{ (mol/l)} = A \times d/13750$$

where is: c – concentration of HNE in mol/l; A – measured absorbance; d – sample dilution; 13750 – molar extinction coefficient of HNE in water (ε)[33].

Determination of HNE Stability in Water and in Cell Culture Media

Stability in water and in DMEM was measured because culture conditions require addition of HNE in cell culture medium. HNE was diluted to 100 μM and stability was followed by measuring absorbance at 223 nm every 10 minutes for 120 minutes. A HNE spectrum was measured from 200 to 350 nm. Measurement was done in quartz quvettes at UV-VIS spectrophotometer Biochrom 4060, LKB Pharmacia. HNE stability in DMEM was determined the same way as in water. Background of each solution (water or DMEM alone) was subtracted from respective solution.

Interaction of HNE with Proteins

Bovine serum albumin (BSA, Sigma) was taken as a model for interaction of HNE with proteins. It was dissolved in double distilled water and mixed with HNE to reach final concentrations of 0.1 mg/ml BSA and 100 μM HNE. Sample spectra from 200 to 350 nm were recorded every 10 minutes for 120 minutes at UV-VIS spectrophotometar Biochrom 4060, LKB Pharmacia).

Different concentrations of BSA were mixed with the same concentrations of HNE, reaching final concentrations ranging from 10^{-6} to 10 mg/ml BSA and 10 μM HNE. Solutions were left at room temperature for 30 minutes to ensure binding and were immediately analyzed by dot-blot method. The dot-blot method based on the affinity of proteins to bind to the nitrocellulose membrane was performed to determine saturation of BSA with HNE.

Determination of 4-Hydroxynonenal-Protein Adducts

The dot-blot method based on the affinity of proteins to bind to the nitrocellulose membrane was performed to determine saturation of BSA with HNE. Samples (400 μl) containing different amount of BSA but the same amount of HNE were applied to the nitrocellulose membrane. The primary monoclonal antibody against 4-hydroxynonenal-histidine conjugates (clone 1g4h7 TC) was applied for 3 hours at +4°C as described before [34]. Possible endogenous peroxidase activity of samples was blocked with 1.5% hydrogen peroxide, 0.1% (w/v) sodium azide (Kemika, Croatia) and 2% (w/v) bovine serum albumin (Sigma, USA) before secondary antibody addition. The detection of antibodies was conducted by measurement of peroxidase activity of enzyme-marked antibody applying DAB stain (Dako, Denmark), resulting in brown staining that indicated the presence of HNE.

HOS Cells

The human osteosarcoma cell line HOS was obtained from American Type Culture Collection (ATCC). Cells were mainteined in DMEM (Dulbecco's modified eagle's medium, Sigma, USA) with 10% (v/v) foetal calf serum (FCS, Sigma, USA) in an incubator (Heraeus, Germany) at 37°C, with a humid air atmosphere containing 5% CO_2. The cells were detached from semiconfluent cultures with a 0.25% (w/v) trypsin solution for 5 minutes. Viable cells (upon trypan blue exclusion) were counted on a Bürker-Türk hemocytometer and used for experiments.

Cell Proliferation Experiments

After counting, required cell number was taken and cells were washed twice with 5 ml of DMEM to remove excess of trypsin and FCS. The 1×10^4 cells were cultured in 96-well microtiter plates (Falcon, USA) in a final volume of 100 μl in the presence of 0.25% (v/v) FCS. After 24-96 hours of incubation, medium was changed for a 200 μl of fresh medium containing FCS, HNE or growth factors. All growth factors (insulin like growth factor 1 – IGF-1, epidermal growth factor – EGF, basic fibroblast growth factor – bFGF) were used in concentration of 10 mg/ml and were obtained from Sigma, USA. For neutralization protocols, growth factors were incubated with HNE for 30 minutes and then added to cell cultures. HNE was prepared immediately before use and added to cell cultures in less than 5 minutes. For each treatment fresh HNE was prepared.

^{3}H- Thymidine Incorporation Assay

The rate of radioactive ^{3}H-thymidine incorporation into DNA was used to estimate replicative activity of HOS cells. After 16 hours of incubation with compounds, radioactive ^{3}H-thymidine ([6-^{3}H] thymidine, 1 mCi/ml, Amersham Biosciences, USA) was added 0.1 μCi to each well and incubation was continued for following 8 hours. The cells were then harvested on glass filter in a cell harvester (Skatron, Norway) and ^{3}H-thymidine incorporation was measured using a liquid scintilation β-counter (Beckman 7400, USA).

Statistical Analysis

All assays were carried out in quadruplicates. The comparison of the mean values was done using Student's t-test considering values of $p < 0.05$ as significantly different.

RESULTS

HNE Stability in Solutions

Stability of 100 μM HNE in water and in DMEM was checked during a 120 min period, exposed to room temperature conditions, light and air to simulate working conditions with cell cultures. Whole UV-spectra of HNE was recorded, while results presented in Figure 2. show kinetic reaction with maximum absorbance measured at 223 nm. HNE gradually disintegrated both in DMEM solution, while in water this disintegration was very slow.

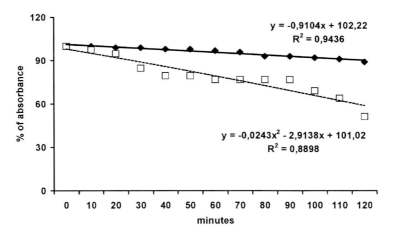

Figure 2. Stability of HNE in water and in DMEM. Absorbance of HNE was measured at 223 nm. HNE gradually disintegrated both in water and DMEM solution, but was much faster in DMEM.

Reaction of HNE with Proteins

Bovine serum albumin (BSA) was used as a model for reaction of HNE with proteins.

Changes in UV spectra of BSA were recorded in the presence of supraphysiological, 100 μM HNE and presented in Figure 3a. BSA had no particular absorbance maximum in the wavelength range from 200 to 350 nm, while HNE gave clear absorbance maximum at 223 nm. Interaction of BSA and HNE caused changes in BSA spectrum which resembled the summary spectrum of two compounds. Stability of this mixture was recorded for 120 minutes and presented at Figure 3b.

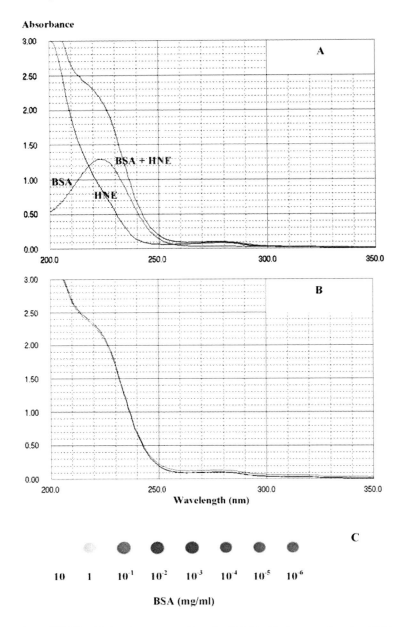

Figure 3. Reaction of HNE with bovine serum albumin (BSA). A) Spectra showing BSA, HNE and mixture of BSA and HNE are presented. Interaction of BSA and HNE caused changes in BSA spectrum which resembled the summary spectrum of two compounds. B) Spectra showing mixture of BSA and HNE. Stability of this mixture was recorded for 120 minutes (overlaid absorbencies).C) Immunochemical detection of HNE-protein conjugates. Different concentrations of BSA were mixed with the same amount of HNE (10 μM). Dot-blot immunochemical method for HNE detection was able to detect semi-quantitatively capacity of BSA to bind HNE.

Dot-blot immunochemical method for HNE detection was able to detect semi-quantitatively capacity of BSA to bind HNE (Figure 3c). Even such low amount of BSA as 1 ng/ml was able to bound detectable amount of HNE.

Cell Growth in the Presence of HNE and Serum

Human osteosarcoma cell line (HOS) cells were cultivated for different period of time in 0.25% FCS and then for 24 hours in serum-free conditions. The spontaneous incorporation of radioactive thymidine in cell cultures is presented in Figure 4. Cell proliferation was not blocked by cultivation in low serum conditions as the cells gradually increased ^{3}H-thymidine incorporation day by day (p<0.01).

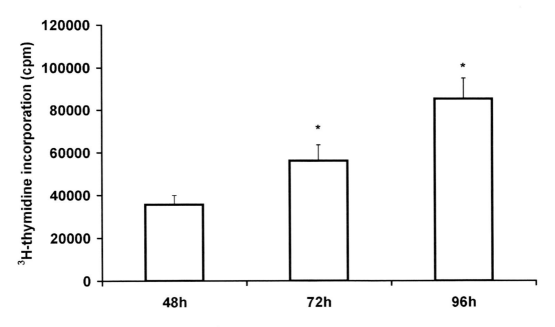

Figure 4. Spontaneous incorporation of ^{3}H-thymidine in HOS cell cultures. Cells were cultivated for different period of time in 0.25% FCS and then for 24 hours in serum-free conditions. ^{3}H-Thymidine was added for the last 8 hours of incubation. * Incorporation of ^{3}H-thymidine significantly different from previous time point, according to the Student's t-test (p<0.05).

Cellular response to growth-stimulating activity of serum was followed 48 hours after initial seeding of the cells in medium supplemented with only 0.25% FCS. Incorporation of ^{3}H-thymidine increased in the presence of FCS and was concentration-dependent as presented at Figure 5.

The same conditions were applied to check effects of HNE on ^{3}H-thymidine incorporation (Figure 6). Low, 1 and 2.5 μM HNE increased ^{3}H-thymidine incorporation (p<0.05); while 10 μM HNE decreased ^{3}H-thymidine incorporation (p<0.05).

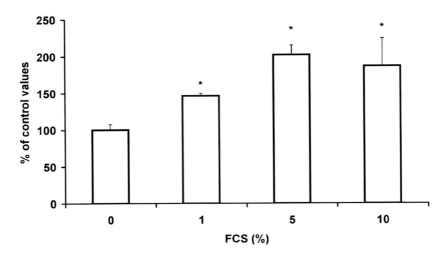

Figure 5. Serum-stimulated incorporation of ^{3}H-thymidine in HOS cell cultures. Cells were cultivated for 48 hours in 0.25% FCS and then for 24 hours in the presence of different concentrations of FCS. ^{3}H-Thymidine was added for the last 8 hours of incubation. * Incorporation of ^{3}H-thymidine significantly different from control cell culture (without FCS), according to the Student's t-test (p<0.05).

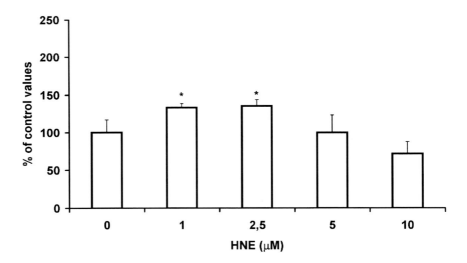

Figure 6. Incorporation of ^{3}H-thymidine in HOS cell cultures in the presence of HNE. Cells were cultivated for 48 hours in 0.25% FCS and then for 24 hours in the presence of different concentrations of HNE. ^{3}H-Thymidine was added for the last 8 hours of incubation. * Incorporation of ^{3}H-thymidine significantly different from control cell culture (without HNE), according to the Student's t-test (p<0.05).

Serum-stimulated incorporation of ^{3}H-thymidine in cell cultures after pretreatment with HNE is presented at Figure 7. HNE treatment attenuated incorporation of ^{3}H-thymidine in cell cultures after treatment with 1% FCS (p<0.05), while growth stimulation with 5% FCS was unaffected.

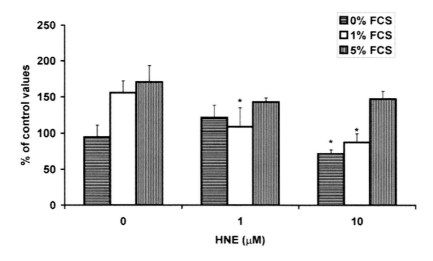

Figure 7. Incorporation of ^{3}H-thymidine in HOS cell cultures in the presence of HNE and FCS. Cells were cultivated for 48 hours in 0.25% FCS and then for 1 hour in the presence of HNE alone followed by addition of FCS for a total time of 24 hours. ^{3}H-Thymidine was added for the last 8 hours of incubation. * Incorporation of ^{3}H-thymidine significantly different from corresponding control cell culture, according to the Student's t-test ($p<0.05$).

Cell Growth in the Presence of HNE and Growth Factors

HOS cells were cultivated for 48 hours in 0.25% FCS and then for 24 hours in the presence of HNE alone or mixture of 10 μM HNE and 10 ng/ml growth factors. Results are presented at Figure 8. Incorporation of ^{3}H-thymidine decreased in the presence of HNE ($p<0.05$), while growth factors (EGF, IGF-1) partially blocked this effect of HNE ($p<0.05$).

Growth-factors stimulated incorporation of ^{3}H-thymidine in cell cultures after pretreatment with HNE as presented at Figures 9-11. All growth factors (IGF, bFGF, EGF) applied alone increased incorporation of radioactive thymidine in cell cultures ($p<0.05$). When pretreated with low, 1 μM HNE concentration, ^{3}H-thymidine incorporation in cell cultures incubated in the presence of growth factors was not affected by HNE-pretreatment; except for EGF which showed moderate increase ($p<0.05$). Higher, 10 μM HNE partially prevented increase in ^{3}H-thymidine incorporation caused by EGF ($p<0.05$) while increase in ^{3}H-thymidine incorporation in the presence of other growth factors was not affected.

DISCUSSION

When added into the cell culture, HNE should primarily affect cell membrane proteins including growth factor receptors rather than intracellular molecules. However, we cannot exclude possibility that low amounts of free HNE or the aldehyde bound to low molecular weight molecules could enter the cells, and be released afterwards under convenient conditions.

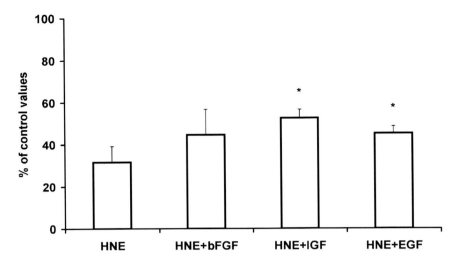

Figure 8. Incorporation of ^{3}H-thymidine in HOS cell cultures in the presence of mixtures of HNE and growth factors. Cells were cultivated for 48 hours in 0.25% FCS and then for 24 hours in the presence of mixtures of HNE and growth factors (preincubated for 30 minutes before addition to cell culture). ^{3}H-Thymidine was added for the last 8 hours of incubation. * Incorporation of ^{3}H-thymidine significantly different from corresponding control cell culture (treated with HNE alone), according to the Student's t-test (p<0.05).

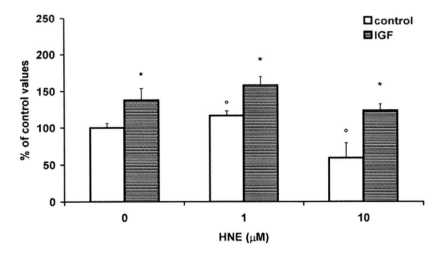

Figure 9. Incorporation of ^{3}H-thymidine in HOS cell cultures in the presence of HNE and IGF-1. Cells were cultivated for 48 hours in 0.25% FCS and then for 1 hour in the presence of HNE alone followed by addition of IGF-1 for a total time of 24 hours. ^{3}H-Thymidine was added for the last 8 hours of incubation. * Incorporation of ^{3}H-thymidine significantly different from corresponding HNE-treated cell culture, according to the Student's t-test (p<0.05).° Incorporation of ^{3}H-thymidine significantly different from corresponding control cell culture (with or without IGF-1), according to the Student's t-test (p<0.05).

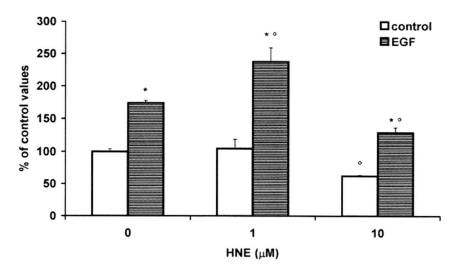

Figure 10. Incorporation of ^{3}H-thymidine in HOS cell cultures in the presence of HNE and EGF. Cells were cultivated for 48 hours in 0.25% FCS and then for 1 hour in the presence of HNE alone followed by addition of EGF for a total time of 24 hours. ^{3}H-Thymidine was added for the last 8 hours of incubation. * Incorporation of ^{3}H-thymidine significantly different from corresponding HNE-treated cell culture, according to the Student's t-test ($p < 0.05$).° Incorporation of ^{3}H-thymidine significantly different from corresponding control cell culture (with or without EGF), according to the Student's t-test ($p < 0.05$).

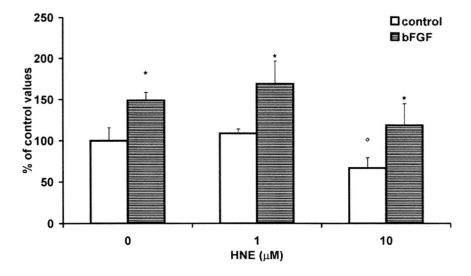

Figure 11. Incorporation of ^{3}H-thymidine in HOS cell cultures in the presence of HNE and bFGF. Cells were cultivated for 48 hours in 0.25% FCS and then for 1 hour in the presence of HNE alone followed by addition of bFGF for a total time of 24 hours. ^{3}H-Thymidine was added for the last 8 hours of incubation. * Incorporation of ^{3}H-thymidine significantly different from corresponding HNE-treated cell culture, according to the Student's t-test ($p < 0.05$).° Incorporation of ^{3}H-thymidine significantly different from corresponding control cell culture (with or without bFGF), according to the Student's t-test ($p < 0.05$).

The concentration of HNE added exogenously to the culture medium in most experiments may be much higher than endogenously formed in vivo. However, a wide range of concentrations of HNE, from potentially physiologically low (1-10 μM) to supra-physiologically high (10-100 μM), display a dose-dependent effect. The exogenous HNE should be eliminated rapidly reacting with proteins and amino acids in both the medium and cells before reacting with the target molecule, whereas endogenous HNE may be formed continuously at the site adjacent to membrane proteins and receptors. When HNE is applied together with serum, HNE-bounding to cell membranes is diminished due to reaction with serum proteins and growth suppressive activity of HNE decreased [19].

The dynamics of the local concentration of HNE surrounding the target molecules should be critical for the physiological effect. In the absence of biomolecules, HNE could be relatively stable, as we proved by incubation for 120 minutes in double distilled water that diminished HNE for only 10%. However, in cell culture medium free HNE disappeared faster; 50% of free HNE disappeared after 120 minutes. That was most likely due to the presence of HNE-bounding compounds with amino and thiol groups (amino acids) that bind HNE, reducing concentration of free aldehyde. However, we can not claim that such binding inactivated HNE; we can simply state that binding to components of cell culture medium influences groups responsible to absorbance of HNE at 223 nm. Interaction of HNE with proteins appears almost as immediate binding of the aldehyde [9], while interaction of BSA and HNE caused changes in their absorbance spectrum which resembled a summary spectrum of two compounds. Because chemical groups relevant for the specific absorbance of 223 nm wavelength by HNE are double bond and the aldehyde group, it seems that these groups were not affected by the HNE-BSA interaction, but it is also possible that new groups with similar spectroscopic features are formed. Reactions between gliceraldehid-phosphate dehydrogenase, aldolase, BSA, reduced BSA, reduced lactoalbumin, ovalbumin and 4-hydroxypentane [9] were studied, and the same mechanism of reaction was assumed for HNE also. Reaction between amino and thiol groups seems to be reversible at certain point and HNE could be removed by pH change, dialysis and with addition of SH donors [9]. Stable BSA-HNE spectra could suggest possible stabilization reaction of HNE in the presence of BSA, while in DMEM it probably disintegrated by loosing functional groups responsible for UV absorption of HNE.

Detoxification mechanisms of HNE are important to define the amount of cellular proteins modified by HNE. The most important intracellular molecule which protects cells from HNE is glutathione (GSH). Intracellular levels of GSH could determine the amount of HNE-modified proteins after treatment with HNE, which is determinal for cellular sensitivity to HNE toxicity [12]. Although GSH could act alone, reaction is much faster when GSH metabolizing enzymes are involved in this reaction. Majority of HNE is conjugated to GSH through the reaction catalyzed by glutathione S-transferases (GSTs) that form the GSH conjugate with the aldehyde (GS-HNE); while the rest of aldehyde can be reduced to alcohol by aldose reductase or oxidized to corresponding acids by aldehyde dehydrogenase [35]. Most of the major classes of GSTs present in mammalian tissues have some detectable activity towards HNE, but a subgroup of the α-class GST isozymes have higher catalytic efficiency for HNE [36]. Two GST isoenzymes, hGSTA4-4 and hGST5.8 belonging to this subgroup have been characterized in humans. GSTs discovered in rats (rGSTA4-4) and mice (π-GSTA4-4) are immunologically similar to human hGST5.8 [37]. After conjugation, GS-HNE is transported out of cells by ATP-dependent transporter RLIP76 (RALBP-1), a ral-binding GTPase activating protein [38]. Coordinated action of γ-GCL (responsible for GSH synthesis), GSTs and RLIP76 are important for regulated intracellular HNE concentration [39,40]. Concentrations of HNE in cells increase during oxidative stress, but limited information is available regarding the normal physiologic levels of HNE in cells. Nonetheless, HNE in varying amounts was found present in all cell lines and tissues analyzed [9]. Since the formation of HNE results from lipid peroxidation, an uncontrolled process depending on the redox status of cells, the intracellular levels of HNE should be controlled through its metabolism and subsequent transport of the metabolites as it was described above.

Role of HNE in signaling process is intriguing because its effects are concentration dependent and not well understood. Thus, the regulation of intracellular concentrations of HNE may be crucial for cell signaling. In earlier work we presented that sensitivity to HNE differs in cells of different origin; normal mesenchimal cells were less sensitive to apoptosis induction caused by HNE than malignant, and this depended on cellular GSH content [12]. In the current study we describe that HNE might induce proliferation of human osteosarcoma cells in concentration declared as "physiological" (1 μM). This was also noticed in previous work with HeLa cells [13]. Similarly, HNE also stimulates aortic smooth muscle cell growth at physiological concentrations of 1.0 and 2.5 μM. In these cells, treatment with HNE resulted in activation of extracellular signal-regulated protein kinases ERK1 and ERK2, induction of c-*fos* and c-*jun* protein expression, and an increase in transcription factor AP-1 DNA binding activity. In addition, HNE induces expression of platelet-derived growth factor (PDGF), while an anti–PDGF antibody specifically inhibits HNE-mediated DNA synthesis, suggesting that growth factor induction may play a role in HNE-induced vascular smooth muscle cell growth. The role of redox-sensitive mechanism in this process is further supported by the observation that HNE-induced DNA synthesis and AP-1 activation are inhibited by the antioxidants *N*-acetylcysteine and pyrrolidine dithiocarbamate [41].

These studies along with earlier observations that HNE induces various enzymes including phospholipase C [42], adenylate cyclase [43], caspase 3 [44], protein kinase C and other kinases involved in signal transduction cascades [45,46], strongly suggest a role of HNE in signaling cascades. This molecule is also able to influence cellular functions by regulating the genes encoding for other molecules, such as heat-shock genes [47], c-*myc* [18], c-*fos*, c-*jun* [43], c-*myb* [48], cyclins [18], p53 gene family [49], procollagen type I and TGF-β1 [50], etc.

The potentially unique pathways of intracellular signal transduction mediated by HNE and the primary molecular targets are still unknown. It seems that it is not necessary to have unique receptor for HNE to achieve growth regulating effect. A ligand-independent mechanism of epidermal growth factor receptor (EGFR) activation is achieved through direct binding of HNE with subsequent clustering of receptors [51,52]. HNE binds to EGFR and activates it, inducing phosphorylation of receptor tyrosine kinase, adaptor protein Shc and activating MAP kinase. In addition to the specific ligand EGF, a number of other agents such chemical agents, UV light and oxidized low density lipoproteins can also trigger phosphorylation of EGFR [54], probably also through HNE-mediated signaling mechanisms.

These results may help us to a further understanding of the molecular pathogenesis of oxidative stress-associated changes in cell growth regulation [53].

HNE also modulate the process of hepatic stellate cells (HSCs) activation, a process of early stages of liver injury associated with fibrogenesis [54]. Platelet-derived growth factor (PDGF) has been identified as the most potent mitogen for HSCs. By using non-cytotoxic, 1 µM concentrations of HNE, a inhibition of PDGF-dependent DNA synthesis was observed, together with activation of phosphatidylinositol-3-kinase (PI3K) and extracellular regulated kinases 1/2 (ERK1/2). Inhibition of DNA synthesis was reversible and recovery of PDGF-mediated mitogenic signaling occurred with upregulation of PDGFR gene expression. HNE inhibited tyrosine kinase activity associated with the PDGF receptor, but binding of PDGF to its receptor was unaffected.

We checked ability of HNE to interfere with growth-stimulating activity of serum, as a model of complex cellular growth-stimulating environment. When added before serum, 1 µM HNE was able to partially block growth-stimulating activity of serum, although HNE alone had mild growth-stimulating effect. This effect was present only when cell growth was stimulated with low, 1% serum concentrations, while 5% serum abolished effect of HNE. It is important to notice that treatments with serum or growth factors (IGF, EGF and bFGF) were performed 1h after HNE-treatment of the cells. Supraphysiological, 10 µM concentration of HNE partially blocked growth stimulating efficiency of growth factors, while growth factors diminished growth suppressive activity of high amount of HNE (10 µM) suggesting mutual dependence of the growth stimulating effects of the growth factors and inhibiting effect of HNE. On the contrary, low, 1 µM concentration of HNE showed additional stimulating affect but only when combined with growth promoting effects of EGF. Diminishing effect of growth factors on HNE-caused cytotoxicity is noticed earlier, when primary culture of hepatocytes sublethally damaged by HNE and recovered if exposed to soluble factors excreted by splenocytes activated by HNE-treated hepatocytes [55]. Due to the instability of HNE in cell culture medium and presence of cellular proteins in the medium we assume that direct interaction between HNE and growth factors can be excluded as mechanism of interactions of HNE and growth factors in experiments presented above. More likely, that this interaction was on signaling level. Nevertheless, direct interactions between growth factors and HNE could also be possible, however due to the low concentrations of the growth factors used to stimulate the growth of the cells this is neglectable.

CONCLUSION

Role of HNE in signaling process is intriguing because its effects are concentration dependent and unique pathways and the primary molecular targets of intracellular signal transduction mediated by HNE are still unknown. As it seems that unique receptor is not necessary for HNE to achieve growth regulating effect, complexity of possible interactions with signal-transduction pathways increased enormously. Possible mechanisms of interaction of HNE with growth factors signaling pathways are summarized at Figure 12. Our results support findings of HNE as a growth regulating mediator of oxidative stress which interacts with humoral growth factors. All growth factors used modulated effects of HNE on cell proliferation. However, we would like to point out at EGF, which seems to be the most important cytokine interfering with signaling activities of HNE under physiological conditions.

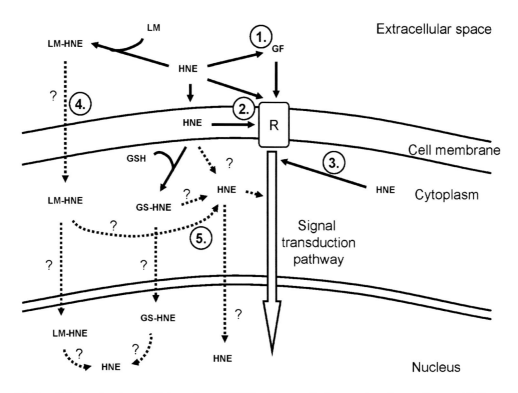

Figure 12. Possible mechanisms of interaction of HNE with growth factors signaling pathways. Full lines present known mechanisms by which HNE could interfere with signaling pathways, while dashed lines with question mark present hypothetic mechanisms which are not proved. HNE-protein conjugates are found in nucleus, demonstrating that free or bound HNE is transported into nucleus. HNE could interfere with signal transductions by different mechanisms: (**1.**) direct binding to growth factors (GF), which could change conformation and prevent binding to receptor; (**2.**) direct binding to growth factor receptor (R), which could affect active site of receptor and prevent growth factor binding or it could cause activation of receptor in the absence of growth factor; (**3.**) in the case that HNE is produced intracellulary direct binding to intracellular part of growth factor receptor (R), or interference with signal transduction pathway are possible; (**4.**) low molecular weight compounds (LM) extracellulary will bind HNE and (hypothetically) such conjugates will be transported into cell where it could be released and interfere with signal transduction pathways; (**5.**) HNE which enters the cell will be bound to GSH and (hypothetically) could be released and interferes with signal transduction pathways.

ACKNOWLEDGMENTS

The support of Croatian Ministry of Science, Education and Sport, by the Austrian National Bank Jubileums Fund and by COST Action B35 is gratefully acknowledged. The authors wish to express gratitude to Mrs Nevenka Hirsl for excellent technical assistance.

REFERENCES

[1]   Halliwell, B; Gutteridge, JMC. The chemistry of oxygen radicals and other oxygen-derived species. In: Halliwell B, Gutteridge JMC, editors. *Free Radicals in Biology and Medicine*, Oxford: Clarendon Press, 1989; 29-32.

[2]   Ignarro, LJ; Balestrieri, ML; Napoli C. Nutrition, physical activity, and cardiovascular disease: An update. *Cardiovascular Research*. 2007, 73, 326-340.

[3]   Emerit, J; Edeas, M; Bricaire, F. Neurodegenerative diseases and oxidative stress. *Biomedicine and Pharmacotherapy,* 2004, 58, 39–46.

[4]   Dreher, D; Junod, AF. Role of oxygen free radicals in cancer development. *European Journal of Cancer*, 1996, 32A, 30-38.

[5]   [5] Esterbauer, H; Zollner, H; Schaur, RJ. Aldehydes formed by lipid peroxidation: mechanisms of formation, occurence, and determination. In: Vigo-Pelfrey, C., editor. *Membrane Lipid Oxidation, Vol. I.* Boca Raton, Florida: CRC Press, Inc; 1990; 239-268.

[6]   Schauenstein, E; Esterbauer, H; Zollner, H. Aldehydes in biological systems; their natural occurence and biological activities. London: Pion Ltd; 1977.

[7]   Esterbauer, H; Weger, W. Über die wirkungen von aldehyden auf gesunde und maligne zellen; synthese von homologen 4-hydroxy-2-alkenalen. *Chemical Monthly,* 1967, 98, 1884-1891.

[8]   Zarkovic, N. 4-Hydroxynonenal as a bioactive marker of pathopysiological processes. *Molecular Aspects of Medicine*, 2003, 24, 281-291.

[9]   Esterbauer, H; Schaur, RJ; Zollner, H. Chemistry and biochemistry of 4-hydroxynonenal, malonaldehyde and related aldehydes. *Free Radicals Biology and Medicine*, 1991, 11, 81-128.

[10]   Schaur, RJ. Basic aspects of the biochemical reactivity of 4-hydroxynonenal. *Molecular Aspects of Medicine*, 2003, 24, 149-159.

[11]   Turner, WE; Hill RH; Hannon, WH; Bernert, JT; Kilbourne, EM; Bayse, DD. Bioassay Screening for Toxicants in Oil Samples from the Toxic-Oil Syndrome Outbreak in Spain. *Archives of Environmental Contamination and Toxicology*. 1985, 14, 261-271.

[12]   Borovic, S; Cipak, A; Meinitzer, A; Kejla, Z; Perovic, D; Waeg, G; Zarkovic, N. Differential sensitivity to 4-hydroxynonenal for normal and malignant mesenchymal cells. *Redox Report,* 2007, 12, 50-54.

[13]   Zarkovic, N; Ilic, Z; Jurin, M; Scahur, RJ; Puhl, H; Esterbauer, H. Stimulation of HeLa cell growth by physiological concentrations of 4-hydroxynonenal. *Cell Biochemistry and Function*, 1993, 11, 279-286.

[14]   Kruman, II; Mattson, MP. Pivotal role of mitochondrial calcium uptake in neural cell apoptosis and necrosis. *Journal of Neurochemistry*, 1999, 72, 529-540.

[15]   Ruef, T; Moser, M; Bode, C; Kubler, W; Runge, MS. 4-Hydroxynonenal induces apoptosis, NF-kappa B-activation and formation of 8-isoprostane in vascular smooth muscle cells. *Basic Research in Cardiology*, 2001, 96, 143-150.

[16]   Zhang, W; He, Q; Chan, LL; Zhou, F; El Naghy, M; Thompson, EB; Ansari, NH. Involvement of caspases in 4-hydroxy-alkenal-induced apoptosis in human leukemic cells. *Free Radical Biology and Medicine*, 2001, 30, 699-706.

[17]   Wonisch, W; Kohlwein, SD; Schaur, RJ; Tatzber, F; Guttenberger, H; Zarkovic, N; Winkler, R; Esterbauer, H. Treatment of the budding yeast saccharomyces cerevisiae with the lipid peroxidation product 4-HNE provokes a temporary cell cycle arrest in G1 phase. *Free Radical Biology and Medicine*. 1998, 25, 682-687.

[18]   Barrera, G; Pizzimenti, S; Laurora, S; Briatore, F; Toaldo, C; Dianzani, MU. 4-Hydroxynonenal and cell cycle. *BioFactors*, 2005, 24, 151-157.

[19]   Sovic, A; Borovic, S; Loncaric, I; Kreuzer, T; Zarkovic, K; Vukovic, T; Waeg, G; Hrascan, R; Wintersteiger, R; Klinger, R; Zurak, N; Schaur, RJ; Zarkovic, N. The carcinostatic and proapoptotic potential of 4-hydroxynonenal in HeLa cells is associated with its conjugation to cellular proteins. *Anticancer Research*, 2001, 21, 1997-2004.

[20]   [20] Rinaldi, M; Barrera, G; Aquino, A; Spinsanti, P; Pizzimenti, S; Farace, MG; Dianzani, MU; Fazio, VM. 4-hydroxynonenal-induced MEL cell differentiation involves PKC activity translocation. *Biochemical Biophysical Research Communications*, 2000, 272, 75-80.

[21]   Cheng, JZ; Singhal, SS; Saini, M; Singhal, J; Piper, JT; Van Kuijk, FJGM; Zimniak, P; Awasthi, YC; Awasthi, S. Effects of mGST A4 transfection on 4-hydroxynonenal-mediated apoptosis and differentiation of K562 human erythroleukemia cells. *Archives of Biochemistry and Biophysics,* 1999, 372, 29-36.

[22]   Barrera, G; Di Mauro, C; Muraca, R; Ferrero, D; Cavalli, G; Fazio, VM; Paradisi, L; Dianzani, MU. Induction of differentiation in human HL-60 cells by 4-hydroxynonenal, a product of lipid peroxidation. *Experimental Cell Research*, 1991, 197, 148-152.

[23]   Poli, G; Schaur, RJ. 4-Hydroxynonenal in the pathomechanisms of oxidative stress. *IUBMB Life,* 2000, 50, 315-21.

[24]   Kreuzer, T; Grube, R; Zarkovic, N; Schaur RJ. 4-Hydroxynonenal modifies the effects of serum growth factors on the expression of the c-fos proto-oncogene and the proliferation of HeLa carcinoma cells. *Free Radical Biology and Medicine*, 1998, 25, 42-49.

[25]   Dianzani, MU. 4-Hydroxy-2,3-nonenal from pathology to physiology. *Molecular Aspects of Medicine*, 2003, 24, 263-272.

[26]   Poli, G. Dianzani, MU; Cheeseman, KH. Separation and characterization of the aldehydic products of lipid peroxidation stimulated by carbon tetrachloride or ADP-iron in isolated rat hepatocytes and rat liver microsomal suspensions. *Biochemical Journal*, 1985, 227, 629-638.

[27]   Uchida, K; Shiraishi, M; Naito, Y; Torii, Y; Nakamura, Y; Osawa, T. Activation of stress signaling pathways by the end product of lipid peroxidation: 4-hydroxy-2-nonenal is a potential inducer of intracellular peroxide production. *Journal of Biological Chemistry*, 1999, 274, 2234-2242.

[28]   Zarkovic, K; Zarkovic, N; Schlag, G; Redl, H; Waeg, G. Histological aspects of sepsis-induced brain changes in a baboon model. In: Schlag, G, Redl, H, Traber, DL, editors. *Shock, Sepsis and Organ Failure, 5th Wiggers Bernard Conference.* Heidelberg: Springer-Verlag; 1997; 146-160.

[29]   Zarkovic, N; Zarkovic, K; Schaur, RJ; Stolc, S; Schlag, G; Redl, H; Waeg, G; Borovic, S; Loncaric, I; Juric, G; Hlavka, V. 4-Hydroxynonenal as a second messenger of free radicals and growth modifying factor. *Life Science*, 1999, 65, 1901-1904.

[30]   Schaur, RJ. Basic aspects of the biochemical reactivity of 4-hydroxynonenal. *Molecular Aspects of Medicine*, 2003, 24, 149-159.

[31]   Zarkovic, N; Schaur, R.J; Puhl, H; Jurin, M; Esterbauer, H. Mutual dependence of growth modifying effects of 4-hydroxy-nonenal and fetal calf serum in vitro. *Free Radical Biology and Medicine*, 1994, 16, 877-884.

[32]   Kreuzer, T; Zarkovic, N; Grube, R; Schaur, RJ. Inhibition of HeLa cell proliferation by 4-Hydroxynonenal is associated with enhanced expression of the c-fos oncogene. *Cancer Biotherapy Radiopharmaceuticals*, 1997, 12, 131-136.

[33]   Esterbauer, H; Weger, W. Über die Wirkungen von Aldehyden auf Gesunde und maligne Zellen. 3. Mitt. *Monatshefte für Chemie*, 1967, 98, 1994-2000.

[34]   Borovic, S; Tirzitis, G; Tirzite, D; Cipak, A; Khoschsorur, GA; Waeg, G; Tatzber, F; Scukanec-Spoljar, M; Zarkovic, N. Bioactive 1,4-dihydroisonicotinic acid derivatives prevent oxidative damage of liver cells. *European Journal of Pharmacology*, 2006, 537, 12-19.

[35]   Siems, W; Grune, T. Intracellular metabolism of 4-hydroxynonenal. *Molecular Aspects of Medicine*, 2003, 24, 167-175.

[36]   Zimniak, P; Eckles, MA, Saxena, M; Awasthi, YC. A subgroup of class alpha glutathione S-transferases. Cloning of cDNA for mouse lung glutathione S-transferase GST 5.7. *FEBS Letters*, 1992, 313, 173–176.

[37]   Cheng, JZ; Yang, Y; Singh, SP; Singhal, SS; Awasthi, S; Pan, S; Singh, SV; Zimniak, P; Awasthi, YC. Two distinct 4-hydroxynonenal metabolizing glutathione S-transferase isozymes are differentially expressed in human tissues. *Biochemical and Biophysical Research Communications*, 2001, 282, 1268-1274.

[38]   Sharma, R; Awasthi, S; Zimniak, P; Awasthi, YC. Transport of glutathione-conjugates in human erythrocytes. *Acta Biochimica Polonica,* 2000, 47, 751-762.

[39]   Forman, HJ; Dickinson, DA; Iles, KE. HNE-signaling pathways leading to its elimination. *Molecular Aspects of Medicine*, 2003, 24, 189-194.

[40]   Awasthi, S; Cheng, J; Singhal, SS; Saini, MK; Pandya, U; Pikula, S; Bandorowicz-Pikula, J; Singh, SV; Zimniak, P; Awasthi, YC. Novel function of human RLIP76: ATP-dependent transport of glutathione conjugates and doxorubicin. *Biochemistry*, 2000, 39, 9327-9334.

[41]   Ruef, J; Rao, GN; Li, F; Bode, C; Patterson, C; Bhatnagar, A; Runge, MS. Induction of rat aortic smooth muscle cell growth by the lipid peroxidation product 4-hydroxy-2-nonenal. *Circulation,* 1998, 97, 1071-1078.

[42]   [Rossi, MA; Fidale, F; Garramone, A; Esterbauer, H; Dianzani, MU. Effect of 4-hydroxyalkenals on hepatic phosphatidylinositol-4,5-bisphosphate-phospholipase C. *Biochemical Pharmacology,* 1990, 39, 1715-1719.

[43]   Paradisi, L; Panagini, C; Parola, M. Effects of 4-hydroxynonenal on adenylate cyclase and 5'-nucleotidase activities in rat liver plasma membranes. *Chemico-Biological Interactions*, 1985, 53, 209-217.

[44]   De Villiers, WJ; Song, Z; Nasser, MS; Deaciuc, IV; McClain, CJ. 4-Hydroxynonenal-induced apoptosis in rat hepatic stellate cells: Mechanistic approach. *Journal of Gastroenterology and Hepatology*, 2007, 22, 414-422.

[45]   Rinaldi, M; Barrera, G; Aquino, A; Spinsanti, P; Pizzimenti, S; Farace, MG; Dianzani, MU; Fazio, VM. 4-Hydroxynonenal-induced MEL cell differentiation involves PKC activity translocation. *Biochemical and Biophysical Research Communications,* 2000, 272, 75–80.

[46]   Leonarduzzi, G; Robbesyn, F; Poli, G. Signaling kinases modulated by 4-hydroxynonenal. *FreeRradical Biology and Medicine*, 2004, 37, 1694-1702.

[47]   Allevi, P; Anastasia, M; Cajone, F; Ciuffreda, P; Sanvito, AM. Structural requirements of aldehydes produced in LPO for the activation of the heat-shock genes in HeLa cells. *Free Radical Biology and Medicine*, 1995, 18, 107-116.

[48]   Barrera, G; Pizzimenti, S; Serra, A; Ferretti, C; Fazio, VM; Saglio, G; Dianzani, MU. 4-Hydroxynonenal specifically inhibits c-myb but does not affect c-fos expressions in HL-60 cells. *Biochemical and Biophysical Research Communications*, 1996, 227, 589-593.

[49]   Laurora, S; Tamagno, E; Briatore, F; Bardini, P; Pizzimenti, S; Toaldo, C; Reffo, P; Costelli, P; Dianzani, MU; Danni, O; Barrera, G. 4-Hydroxynonenal modulation of p53 family gene expression in the SK-N-BE neuroblastoma cell line. *Free Radical Biology and Medicine*, 2005, 38, 215– 225.

[50]   Poli, G; Parola, M. Oxidative damage and fibrogenesis. *Free Radical Biology and Medicine*, 1997, 22, 287-305.

[51]   Suc, I; Meilhac, O; Lajoie-Mazenc, I; Vandaele, J; Jurgens, G; Salvayre, R; Negre-Salvayre, A. Activation of EGF receptor by oxidized LDL. *FASEB Journal,* 1998, 12, 665–671.

[52]   Negre-Salvayre, A; Vieira, O; Escargueil-Blanc, I; Salvayre, R. Oxidized LDL and 4-hydroxynonenal modulate tyrosine kinase receptor activity. *Molecular Aspects of Medicine*, 2003, 24, 251–261.

[53]   Liu, W; Akhand, AA; Kato, Masashi; Yokoyama, I; Miyata, T; Kurokawa, K; Uchida, K; Nakashima, I. 4-Hydroxynonenal triggers an epidermal growth factor receptor-linked signal pathway for growth inhibition. *Journal of Cell Science*, 1999, 112, 2409-2417.

[54]   Robino, G; Parola, M; Marra, F; Caligiuri, A; De Franco, RMS; Zamara, E; Bellomo, G; Gentilini, P; Pinzani, M; Dianzani, MU. Interaction between 4-hydroxy2,3alkenals and the PDGF-beta receptor. Reduced tyrosine phosphorylation and downstream signaling in hepatic stellate cells. *Journal of Biological Chemistry,* 2000, 22, 40561–40567.

[55]   Cipak, A; Borovic, S; Scukanec-Spoljar, M; Kirac, I; Zarkovic, N. Possible involvement of 4-hydroxynonenal in splenocyte regulated liver regeneration. *Biofactors*, 2005, 24, 141-148.

In: Progress in Cell Growth Process Research
Editor: Takumi Hayashi, pp. 209-219

ISBN 978-1-60456-325-2
© 2008 Nova Science Publishers, Inc.

Chapter 9

EFFECTS OF PERIPHERAL GLUTAMATE RECEPTORS ON TUMOR CELL GROWTH – HOW NEUROTRANSMITTERS CAN AFFECT THE BODY

Helga Susanne Haas[7]

Department of Pathophysiology, Center of Molecular Medicine,
Medical University Graz, Heinrichstrasse 31A, 8010 Graz, Austria

ABSTRACT

Glutamate is not only the major excitatory neurotransmitter in the central nervous system (CNS); glutamate receptors have also been found in peripheral non-excitable cells. In addition to eliciting excitatory currents, glutamate can also regulate a broad range of other biological responses. Of particular interest is the discovery that peripheral glutamatergic signalling differentially modifies the proliferation of tumor cells, depending on ingredients in the external milieu (e.g. the external glutamate content). Furthermore, glutamate antagonists effectively suppress cancer growth, inhibit cell division and migration, enhance cell death, and alter the morphology of tumor cells. Our results indicate that glutamate, the receptor agonists kainate and AMPA (alpha-amino-3-hydroxy-5-methyl-4-isoxsazolepropionic acid), but also the antagonist CNQX (6-cyano-7-nitroquinoxaline-2,3-dione) significantly modified the proliferation of human promonocytic lymphoma (U937) cells. Furthermore, we could show that CPCCOEt (7-hydroxyiminocyclopropan[b]chromen-1a-carboxylic acid ethyl ester), a subtype-specific, non-competitive metabotropic glutamate receptor-1 antagonist, significantly, dose-dependently, and reversibly attenuated cell proliferation of both HBMC (human Bowes melanoma) and n15006 melanoma cells. In addition, we observed a synergistic effect of CPCCOEt and docetaxel, a commonly used cytostatic agent. Recent data now indicate that the same glutamate receptor antagonist can also inhibit the growth of multidrug resistant medullary thyroid carcinoma (MTC) cells. In conclusion, these data supply

---

7 Correspondence to: Helga Susanne Haas, Department of Pathophysiology, Center of Molecular Medicine, Medical University Graz, Heinrichstrasse 31A, 8010 Graz, Austria, E-mail: helga.haas@meduni-graz.at .

evidence that glutamate is far more than an excitatory neurotransmitter; glutamate has an important impact on cell growth as well, and glutamate receptor antagonists may augment existing cancer therapies either alone or through synergies with other chemotherapeutic drugs.

INTRODUCTION

In the last 30 years it has become apparent that there are intricate communication circuits between different physiological systems within the body, which account for the age-old notion that the mind can influence the body and in turn, susceptibility to disease, the course of disease and hence the length of human life. In this period, the field of "psychoneuroimmunology" has evolved, which investigates the multidirectional interactions between the nervous - , the immune - , and the neuroendocrine systems, proposing the use of a common chemical language for intra- and intercellular communication between the systems. The scientific background for this is that each of the systems can (i) express receptors of the other, (ii) produce as well as release hormones, cytokines and/or neurotransmitters that regulate cellular activity via these receptors, and (iii) that the systems share similar signal transduction pathways enabling autocrine as well as paracrine communication from cell to cell (Haas and Schauenstein, 1997; Haas and Schauenstein, 2001; Steinman, 2004; Besedovsky and del Rey, 2007; Blalock and Smith, 2007; Heijnen, 2007; Ziemssen and Kern, 2007).

Glutamate is the major excitatory neurotransmitter in the central nervous system (CNS) and acts through more than 20 receptors, which are divided into ionotropic (ligand-gated ion channels) and metabotropic (G-protein coupled) glutamate receptors (Ozawa et al., 1998; Bennett and Balcar, 1999; Pin and Acher et al., 2002; Kew and Kemp, 2005). In view of intersystem communications it is not surprising that glutamate receptors have also been found in peripheral non-excitable cells (e.g. taste buds, retina, intestine, heart, lung, spleen, thymus, pancreas, adrenal gland, kidney, skin, bone, bone marrow, hepatocytes, megakaryocytes, platelets and lymphocytes) (Lucas and Newhouse, 1957; Storto et al., 2000; Lombardi et al., 2001; Skerry and Genever, 2001; Leung et al., 2002; Nedergaard et al., 2002; Hinoi et al., 2004; Kalariti et al., 2005; Gill and Pulido, 2005). From the above discoveries, a burgeoning new field of science emerged and it became apparent that glutamate, in addition to eliciting excitatory currents, can regulate a broad range of other biological responses as well. Perhaps one of the most interesting aspects is the discovery that excessive glutamate release promotes tumor growth, and glutamate antagonists are capable to suppress cancer growth (Rzeski et al., 2001; Cavalheiro and Olney, 2001; Rothstein and Brem, 2001; Takano et al., 2001; Ishiuchi et al., 2002; Kalariti et al., 2005; Stepulak et al., 2005, Haas et al, 2005, 2007; Namkoong et al., 2007).

EFFECTS OF PERIPHERAL GLUTAMATE RECEPTORS ON TUMOR CELL GROWTH

It is well established that glutamate signalling has trophic functions in the developing brain (Ikonomidou et al., 1999; Behar et al., 1999; Luján et al., 2005; de Rivero Vaccari et al., 2006); consequently, first reports predominantly deal with brain tumors. In gliomas glutamate appears to play a dual role. During the process of invasion it serves to stimulate cell motility, whereas during tumor expansion it causes excitotoxic cell death (Sontheimer, 2003). Similar to what had been observed in the periphery (see below), AMPA (alpha-amino-3-hydroxy-5-methyl-4-isoxsazolepropionic acid) receptor agonists facilitated cell proliferation of human glioma cells in low-serum medium containing 0.5% fetal calf serum (FCS), whereas no effect was observed in serum-rich medium containing 10% FCS (Yoshida et al., 2006). Recent data indicate that Ca^{2+} signalling mediated by AMPA receptors regulates the growth and motility of human glioblastoma cells through activation of the protein serine-threonine kinase Akt (also called protein kinase B) (Ishiuchi et al., 2007). Blockade of Ca^{2+}-permeable AMPA receptors suppressed migration as well as proliferation, induced apoptosis, and inhibited phosphorylation of Akt in human glioblastoma cells (Ishiuchi et al., 2002, 2007). Furthermore, treatment with the NMDA (N-methyl-D-aspartate) receptor antagonist MK-801 ((±)-5-methyl-10,11-dihydro-5H-dibenzo(a,d)cyclohepten-5,10-imine/dizocilpine) or meman-ine significantly attenuated the growth of glutamate-secreting gliomas, *in situ* (Takano et al., 2001). Besides ionotropic glutamate receptors, metabotropic receptors also differentially modulate tumor cell proliferation. Pharmacological blockade of metabotropic glutamate receptors 2 and 3 (mGluR2/3) reduced the growth of human glioma cells in primary cell cultures as well as *in vivo* (D'Onofrio et al., 2003; Arcella et al., 2005). In contrast, pharmacological activation of mGluR4 can also inhibit the proliferation of medulloblastoma cells (Iacovelli et al., 2006), indicating that the different glutamate receptors act in a selective, subtype-specific manner.

First evidence for the effect of peripheral glutamate receptor signalling on tumor cell proliferation came from Rzeski et al. (2001). Glutamate stimulated the growth of lung carcinoma in serum-deprived medium or medium supplemented with serum-replacement medium, but did not affect proliferation of lung carcinoma or rhabdomyosarcoma/ medullo-blastoma cells in a medium containing 10% serum. These results indicate that peripheral glutamatergic signalling also differentially modifies the proliferation of tumor cells, depending on ingredients in the external milieu. This is partly in line with our findings, which describe the influence of ionotropic glutamate receptor reactive agents on the growth of human promonocytic lymphoma (U937) cells in a serum-glutamate-containing, but glutamine-free medium compared to serum- and glutamate-free conditions (Haas et al., 2005). When U937 cells were cultivated in serum- and glutamate-free conditions, the treatment with glutamate as well as with the receptor agonists kainate and AMPA resulted in increased cell growth, whereas the AMPA/KA receptor antagonist CNQX (6-cyano-7-nitroquinoxaline-2,3-dione) did not affect cell proliferation. In contrast, the same agonists, but also the antagonist CNQX significantly decreased the proliferation of U937 cells cultured in a serum- and glutamate-containing, but glutamine-free, medium (Haas et al., 2005). Furthermore, electron microscopy revealed that U937 cells exposed to the antagonist CNQX displayed enlarged mitochondria, which possibly may indicate changes in mitochondrial membrane depolarization (Haas et al., 2005). The work of Rzeski et al. (2001) also also demonstrated that different ionotropic glutamate receptor antagonists inhibit division and migration, enhance cell death, and alter the morphology of tumor cells *in vitro*. In these experiments, eight different tumor cell lines (SKNAS, human neuroblastoma; TE671, human rhabdomyosarcoma/medulloblastoma; MOGGCCM, human brain astrocytoma; FTC238, human thyroid carcinoma; A549, human Caucasian lung carcinoma; LS180, human Caucasian colon adenocarcinoma; T47D, human breast carcinoma; HT29, human colon adenocarcinoma) were tested and shown to be differentially sensitive to the cytostatic effects of the different glutamate receptor reagents. Furthermore, light microscopy revealed that the NMDA receptor antagonist dizocilpine induced rounded cell appearance with prominent vacuoles in the cytoplasm, whereas exposure to the AMPA receptor antagonist GYKI52466 (1-(4-aminophenyl)-4-methyl-7,8-methylenedioxy-5H-2,3-benzodiazepine) induced less prominent vacuoles and shrinkage of the cells (Rzeski et al., 2001). Electron microscopy showed that tumor cells exposed to glutamate receptor antagonists displayed a more noninvasive phenotype with fewer pseudopodial protrusions (Rzeski et al., 2001). An additional, clinically relevant finding of Rzeski and colleagues was the synergistic effect of NMDA and AMPA receptor antagonists and common cytostatic agents (cyclophosphamide, thiotepa, vinblastin, cisplatin) used in cancer therapy, whereby the enhancement of the antiproliferative effects was due to enhanced tumor cell death on the one hand, and decreased cell division on the other. Stepulak et al. (2005) determined that dizocilpine inhibits the extracellular-regulated kinases 1 and 2 (ERK 1/2) signalling pathway in human lung carcinoma A549 cells, reduces the phosphorylation of CREB (cAMP-responsive element binding protein), suppresses the expression of *cyclin D1, c-fos, c-jun* and *bcl-2*, and upregulated the cell cycle regulators and tumor suppressor proteins *p21* and *p53*. All these changes resulted in the slowing of cell cycle progression and proliferation of tumor cells *in vitro* and also achieved an anticancer effect in mice *in vivo* (Stepulak et al., 2005). The NMDA receptor subtype 2B (NMDAR2B) was shown to have a high frequency of methylation in primary human esophageal squamous cell carcinoma (ESCC) and strong apoptotic activity in ESCC cell lines, suggesting that this receptor subtype can suppress tumor growth (Kim et al., 2006). Similarly, recent data indicate that NMDAR2B methylation is also an important factor in human gastric cancer progression (Liu et al., in press). Overexpression of the glutamate receptor subunit NMDAR1 significantly correlated with tumor size, lymph node metastasis and cancer stage of oral squamous cell carcinoma (Choi et al., 2004). NMDA receptor expression has also been shown in human prostate cancer and the NMDA receptor antagonist memantine was found to inhibit the *in vitro* growth of human prostate cancer cell lines (Abdul and Hoosein, 2005). Peripheral glutamate receptors may also affect benign tumors. The AMPA receptor subunit GluR2, for example, is up-regulated in uterine leiomyomata relative to myometrium by 15- to 30-fold at the protein and mRNA level and is localized in endothelial cells (Tsibris et al., 2003).

As to G-protein coupled receptors (a receptor family also including mGluRs), recent microarray data revealed that overexpression occurs in several neoplasms (Li et al., 2005). mGluR4 expression was frequently identified in colorectal carcinoma, followed by malignant melanoma, and overexpression was associated with recurrence and poor disease-free survival

(Chang et al., 2005). Furthermore, pharmacological blockade of mGluR4 inhibited the proliferation of human colon cancer cell lines (Yoo et al., 2004). Keeping in mind the observation of Iacovelli et al. (2006, see also above) that activation of mGluR4 can inhibit the proliferation of medulloblastoma cells, it is reasonable to assume that central and peripheral glutamate receptor signalling differs in its mode of action. mGluR5 expression was evaluated in samples of oral squamous cell carcinoma patients and a mGluR5 agonist was shown to increase tumor cell migration, invasion as well as adhesion in oral tongue cancer cells (HSC3), which could be reversed by a mGluR5 antagonist (Park et al., 2007). mGluR1 mRNA expression was found in human MG-63 osteoblast-like osteosarcoma cells (Kalariti et al., 2004), as well as in Jurkat T cells (Pacheco et al., 2004), and upregulation of mGluR1 was detected in metastatic melanoma (Li et al., 2005). Compelling evidence for the importance of metabotropic glutamate receptor-1 signalling in melanocytic neoplasia is also provided by a study by Pamela M. Pollock et al. (2003). In these experiments, ectopic expression of mGluR1 was detected in a number of human melanoma cell lines as well as melanoma samples obtained from patients (Pollock et al., 2003). Furthermore, studies in a transgenic mouse melanoma model revealed that ectopic expression of mGluR1 in melanocytes is sufficient to induce the onset of melanoma (Pollock et al., 2003). In continuation of these experiments in mouse melanoma cell lines, Marín et al. (2006) showed that stimulation of mGluR1 with L-quisqualate results in inositol triphosphate (IP_3) accumulation and ERK 1/2 activation, both of which could be inhibited by pretreatment of the tumor cells with a mGluR1 subtype specific competitive antagonist LY367385. Recently, the group around Chen (Namkoong et al., 2007) reported that human melanoma cells released elevated levels of glutamate, implying a possible autocrine loop. Treatment of mGluR1 expressing human melanoma cells with subtype specific mGluR1 antagonists (LY367385, BAY36-7620) leads to a suppression of tumor cell proliferation (Namkoong et al., 2007), which is in line with our results with the non-competitive mGluR1 antagonist, CPCCOEt (7-hydroxyiminocyclopropan[b]chromen-1a-carboxylic acid ethyl ester) (Haas et al., 2007, see also below). Administration of the glutamate release inhibitor riluzole also resulted in an inhibition of melanoma cell growth and induced cell cycle arrest leading to apoptosis (Namkoong et al., 2007). In addition, treatment of human melanoma cell xenografts (nude mice) with riluzole leads to inhibition of tumor cell growth by 50% compared to controls (Namkoong et al., 2007). In our own studies we examined the effect of the subtype-specific, non-competitive metabotropic glutamate receptor-1 antagonist CPCCOEt on growth and morphology of two mGluR1 expressing human melanoma cell lines (human Bowes melanoma, HBMC; n15006 melanoma) (Haas et al., 2007). We show that CPCCOEt significantly, dose-dependently, and reversibly attenuated cell proliferation of both HBMC and n15006 melanoma cells. In these experiments, however, the effects were independent of the external glutamate content. Furthermore, we did not find an influence on apoptotic cell death. Interestingly, the competitive mGluR1 antagonist (RS)-1-aminoindan-1,5-dicarboxylic acid (AIDA), as well as the agonists (1S,3R-)1-aminocyclopentane- 1,3-dicarboxylic acid (ACPD) and glutamate per se did not affect cell proliferation of both cell lines (Haas et al., 2007). Scanning electron microscopy revealed that HBMC as well as n15006 melanoma cells appeared to be more spindle-shaped after treatment with CPCCOEt, which may indicate a loss of adherence (Haas et al., 2007). Furthermore, HBMC melanoma cells were subjected to treatment with either CPCCOEt, the chemotherapeutic drug docetaxel, or CPCCOEt in combination with docetaxel. CPCCOEt as well as docetaxel similarly inhibited cell proliferation. However, this antiproliferative effect was clearly enhanced in cells treated with both CPCCOEt and docetaxel (Haas et al., 2007). These findings indicate a synergistic effect of the metabotropic glutamate receptor antagonist and a commonly used chemotherapeutic drug, similar to observations by Rzeski et al. (2001).

These studies altogether show that, besides neurotransmission, glutamate receptor signalling involves fundamental processes of cell biology, such as cell proliferation and survival. Furthermore, mGluRs reactive drugs may represent novel targets for the treatment of different malignant tumors (Nicoletti et al., 2007).

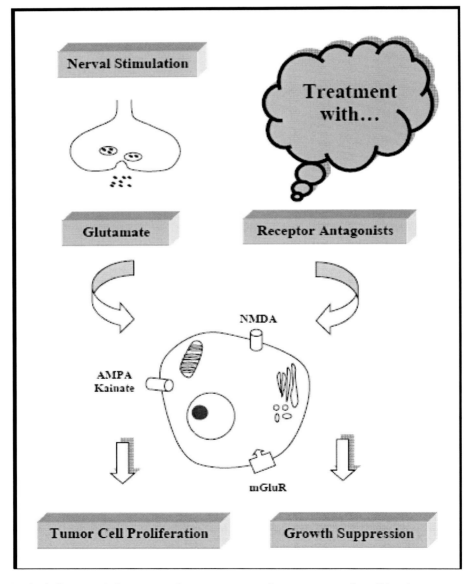

Figure 1. The influence of glutamate and receptor antagonists on tumor cell proliferation.

In particular, metabotropic glutamate receptor allosteric modulators, which exert their effects on the receptor through a binding site that is topographically distinct from the binding site of the endogenous ligand, have been described as promising novel therapeutic agents and have attracted increasing attention within the pharmaceutical industry (Kew, 2004; Ritzén et al., 2005). In view of this, we recently examined whether the subtype-specific, non-competitive metabotropic glutamate receptor-1 antagonist CPCCOEt exerts a similar antiproliferative effect on the growth of multi-drug resistant medullary thyroid carcinoma (MTC-SK) cells. MTC cells are derived from parafollicular C-cells of the thyroid and belong to the MEN2 (multiple endocrine neoplasia) symptom complex, which involves medullary thyroid carcinoma (MTC) in combination with parathyroid hyperplasia/adenoma and phaeochromocytoma (Monson, 2000; Thakker, 2001; Carling, 2005). Presently, nothing is known about glutamate receptor expression on these cells. Interestingly, CPCCOEt also significantly decreased the cell growth of MTC-SK cells in the same concentration as observed in melanoma cells (Haas et al., unpublished results). This may indicate a broader anticancer potential of allosteric mGluR antagonists than initially thought.

CONCLUSION

Recently, it was hypothesized that stimulation of neuronal as well as non-neuronal excitatory receptors may be a significant causative and pathogenic factor of cancer (Hoang et al., 2007). In agreement with data obtained in the developing brain (see above), there is increasing evidence that glutamate receptor signalling not only includes excitotoxicity, but also the activation of differential survival signalling pathways (Nicoletti et al., 1999; Vincent and Maiese, 2000; Hetman and Kharebava, 2006). The present report clearly indicates that a better understanding of the trophic functions of glutamate may provide a basis for new strategies to attack cancer (Figure 1). In addition, these data shall provide new challenges for cancer researchers and broaden our view of an integrative medicine – how neurotransmitters can affect the body.

ACKNOWLEDGMENTS

This research was supported by the by the Austrian National Bank Project Nr. 9365, Austrian Cancer Aid/Styria (Project-Nr. 06/2004), and Austrian National Bank Project Nr. 12598.

REFERENCES

Abdul, M; Hoosein, N. N-methyl-D-aspartate receptor in human prostate cancer. *J. Membr. Biol.*, 2005, 205, 125-128.

Arcella, A; Carpinelli, G; Battaglia, G; D'Onofrio, M; Santoro, F; Ngomba, RT; Bruno, V; Casolini, P; Giangaspero, F; Nicoletti, F. Pharmacological blockade of group II metabotropic glutamate receptors reduces the growth of glioma cells in vivo. *Neuro Oncol.*, 2005, 7, 236-245.

Behar, TN; Scott, CA; Greene, CL; Wen, X; Smith, SV; Maric, D; Liu, QY; Colton, CA; Barker, JL. Glutamate acting at NMDA receptors stimulates embryonic cortical neuronal migration. *J. Neurosci.*, 1999, 19, 4449-4461.

Bennett, MR; Balcar, VJ. Forty years of amino acid transmission in the brain. *Neurochem. Int.*, 1999, 35, 269-280.

Besedovsky, HO; del Rey, A. Physiology of psychoneuroimmunology: a personal view. *Brain Behav. Immun.*, 2007, 21, 34-44.

Blalock, JE; Smith, EM. Conceptual development of the immune system as a sixth sense. *Brain Behav. Immun.*, 2007, 21, 23-33.

Carling, T. Multiple endocrine neoplasia syndrome: genetic basis for clinical management. *Curr. Opin. Oncol.*, 2005, 17, 7-12.

Cavalheiro, EA; Olney, JW. Glutamate antagonists: deadly liaisons with cancer. *Proc. Natl. Acad. Sci. USA*, 2001, 98, 5947-5948.

Chang, HJ; Yoo, BC; Lim, S-B; Jeong, S-Y; Kim, WH; Park, J-G. Metabotropic glutamate receptor 4 expression in colorectal carcinoma and its prognostic significance. *Clin. Cancer Res.*, 2005, 11, 3288-3295.

Choi SW, Park SY, Hong SP, Pai H, Choi JY, Kim SG. The expression of NMDA receptor 1 is associated with clinicopathological parameters and prognosis in the oral squamous cell carcinoma. *J. Oral. Pathol. Med.*, 2004, 33, 533-537.

de Rivero Vaccari, JC; Casey, GP; Aleem, S; Park, WM; Corriveau, RA. NMDA receptors promote survival in somatosensory relay nuclei by inhibiting Bax-dependent developmental cell death. *Proc. Natl. Acad. Sci. U S A*, 2006, 103, 16971-16976.

D'Onofrio, M; Arcella, A; Bruno, V; Ngomba, RT; Battaglia, G; Lombari, V; Ragona, G; Calogero, A; Nicoletti, F. Pharmacological blockade of mGlu2/3 metabotropic glutamate receptors reduces cell proliferation in cultured human glioma cells. *J. Neurochem.*, 2003, 84, 1288-1295.

Gill, S; Pulido, O. Glutamate receptors in peripheral tissue. 1. Edition. New York: Kluwer Academic/Plenum Publishers; 2005.

Haas, HS; Schauenstein, K. Neuroimmunomodulation via limbic structures--the neuroanatomy of psychoimmunology. *Prog. Neurobiol.*, 1997, 5, 195-222.

Haas, HS; Schauenstein, K. Immunity, hormones, and the brain. *Allergy,* 2001, 5, 470-477.

Haas, HS; Pfragner, R; Siegl, V; Ingolic, E; Heintz, E; Schauenstein, K. Glutamate receptor-mediated effects on growth and morphology of human histiocytic lymphoma cells. *Int. J. Oncol.*, 2005, 27, 867-74.

Haas, HS; Pfragner, R; Siegl, V; Ingolic, E; Heintz, E; Schraml, E; Schauenstein, K. The non-competitive metabotropic glutamate receptor-1 antagonist CPCCOEt inhibits the *in vitro* growth of human melanoma. *Int. J. Oncol.*, 2007, 17, 1399-1404.

Heijnen, CJ. Receptor regulation in neuroendocrine-immune communication: current knowledge and future perspectives. *Brain Behav. Immun.*, 2007, 21, 1-8.

Hetman, M; Kharebava G. Survival signaling pathways activated by NMDA receptors. *Curr. Top Med. Chem.*, 2006, 6, 787-799.

Hinoi, E; Takarada, T; Ueshima, T; Tsuchihashi, Y; Yoneda, Y. Glutamate signaling in peripheral tissues. *Eur. J. Biochem.*, 2004, 271, 1-13.

Hoang, BX; Levine, SA; Pham, P; Shaw, DG. Hypothesis of the cause and development of neoplasms. *Eur. J. Cancer Prev.*, 2007, 16, 55-61.

Iacovelli, L; Arcella, A; Battaglia, G; Pazzaglia, S; Aronica, E; Spinsanti, P; Caruso, A; De Smaele, E; Saran, A; Gulino, A; D'Onofrio, M; Giangaspero, F; Nicoletti, F. Pharmacological activation of mGlu4 metabotropic glutamate receptors inhibits the growth of medulloblastomas. *J. Neurosci.*, 2006, 26, 8388-8397.

Ikonomidou, C; Bosch, F; Miksa, M; Bittigau, P; Vockler, J; Dikranian, K; Tenkova, TI; Stefovska, V; Turski, L; Olney, JW. Blockade of NMDA receptors and apoptotic neurodegeneration in the developing brain. *Science*, 1999, 283, 70-74.

Ishiuchi, S; Tsuzuki, K; Yoshida, Y; Yamada, N; Hagimura, N; Okado, H; Miwa, A; Kurihara, H; Nakazato, Y; Tamura, M; Sasaki, T; Ozawa, S. Blockage of Ca^{2+}-permeable AMPA receptors suppresses migration and induces apoptosis in human glioblastoma cells. *Nat. Med.*, 2002, 8, 971-978.

Ishiuchi, S; Yoshida, Y; Sugawara, K; Aihara, M; Ohtani, T; Watanabe, T; Saito, N; Tsuzuki, K; Okado, H; Miwa, A; Nakazato, Y; Ozawa, S. Ca2+-permeable AMPA receptors regulate growth of human glioblastoma via Akt activation. *J. Neurosci.*, 2007, 27, 7987-8001.

Kalariti, N; Lembessis, P; Koutsilieris, M. Characterization of the glutametergic system in MG-63 osteoblast-like osteosarcoma cells. *Anticancer Res.*, 2004, 24, 3923-2929.

Kalariti, N; Pissimissis, N; Koutsilieris, M. The glutamatergic system outside the CNS and in cancer biology. *Expert Opin Investig Drugs*, 2005, 14, 1487-1496.

Kew, JNC. Positive and negative allosteric modulation of metabotropic glutamate receptors: emerging therapeutic potential. *Pharmacol. Ther.*, 2004, 104, 233-244.

Kew, JNC; Kemp, JA. Ionotropic and metabotropic glutamate receptor structure and pharmacology. *Psychopharmacology*, 2005, 179, 4-29.

Kim, MS; Yamashita, K; Baek, JH; Park, HL; Carvalho, AL; Osada, M; Hoque, MO; Upadhyay, S; Mori, M; Moon, C; Sidransky, D. N-methyl-D-aspartate receptor type 2B is epigenetically inactivated and exhibits tumor-suppressive activity in human esophageal cancer. *Cancer Res.*, 2006, 66, 3409-3418.

Leung, JC; Travis, BR; Verlander, JW; Sandhu, SK; Yang, SG; Zea, AH; Weiner, ID; Silverstein, DM. Expression and developmental regulation of the NMDA receptor subunits in the kidney and cardiovascular system. *Am. J. Physiol. Regul. Integr. Comp. Physiol.*, 2002, 283, R964-R971.

Li, S; Huang, S; Peng, S-B. Overexpression of G protein-coupled receptors in cancer cells: involvement in tumor progression. *Int. J. Oncol.*, 2005, 27, 1329-1339.

Liu, JW; Kim, MS; Nagpal, J; Yamashita, K; Poeta, L; Chang, X; Lee, J; Park, HL; Jeronimo, C; Westra, WH; Mori, M; Moon, C; Trink, B; Sidransky D. Quantitative hypermethylation of NMDAR2B in human gastric cancer. *Int. J. Cancer*, 2007, in press.

Lombardi, G; Dianzani, C; Miglio, G; Canonico, PL; Fantozzi, R. Characterization of ionotropic glutamate receptors in human lymphocytes. *Br. J. Pharmacol.*, 2001, 133, 936-944.

Lucas, DR; Newhouse, JP. The toxic effect of sodium L-glutamate on the inner layers of the retina. *AMA Arch. Ophthalmol.*, 1957, 58, 193-201

Luján, R; Shigemoto, R; López-Bendito, G. Glutamate and GABA receptor signalling in the developing brain. *Neuroscience*, 2005, 130, 567-580.

Marín, YE; Namkoong, J; Cohen-Solal, K; Shin, S-S; Martino, JJ; Oka, M; Chen, S. Stimulation of oncogenic metabotropic glutamate receptor 1 in melanoma cells activates ERK1/2 via PKCepsilon. *Cell Signal*, 2006, 18, 1279-1286.

Monson, JP. The epidemiology of endocrine tumors. *Endocr Rel Cancer*, 2000, 7, 29-36.

Namkoong, J; Shin, SS; Lee, HJ; Marin, YE; Wall, BA; Goydos, JS; Chen, S. Metabotropic glutamate receptor 1 and glutamate signaling in human melanoma. *Cancer Res.*, 2007, 67, 2298-2305.

Nedergaard, M; Takano, T; Hansen AJ. Beyond the role of glutamate as a neurotransmitter. *Nat. Rev. Neurosci.*, 2002, 3, 748-755.

Nicoletti, F; Bruno, V; Catania, MV; Battaglia, G; Copani, A; Barbagallo, G; Cena, V; Sanchez-Prieto, J; Spano, PF; Pizzi, M. Group-I metabotropic glutamate receptors: hypotheses to explain their dual role in neurotoxicity and neuroprotection. *Neuropharmacology*, 1999, 38, 1477-1484.

Nicoletti, F; Arcella, A; Iacovelli, L; Battaglia, G; Giangaspero, F; Melchiorri, D. Metabotropic glutamate receptors: new targets for the control of tumor growth? *Trends Pharmacol. Sci.*, 2007, 28, 206-213.

Ozawa, S; Kamiya, H; Tsuzuki, K. Glutamate receptors in the mammalian central nervous system. *Prog Neurobiol*, 1998, 54, 581-618.

Pacheco, R; Ciruela, F; Casadó, V; Mallol, J; Gallart, T; Lluis, C; Franco, R. Group I metabotropic glutamate receptors mediate a dual role of glutamate in T cell activation. *J. Biol. Chem.*, 2004, 279, 33352-33358.

Park, SY; Lee, SA; Han, IH; Yoo, BC; Lee, SH; Park, JY, Cha, IH; Kim, J; Choi, SW. Clinical significance of metabotropic glutamate receptor 5 expression in oral squamous cell carcinoma. *Oncol. Rep.*, 2007, 17, 81-87.

Pin, JP; Acher, F. The metabotropic glutamate receptors: structure, activation mechanism and pharmacology. *Curr. Drug. Targets CNS Neurol. Disord.*, 2002, 1, 297-317.

Pollock, PM; Cohen-Solal, K; Sood, R; Namkoong, J; Martino, JJ; Koganti, A; Zhu, H; Robbins, C; Makalowska, I; Shin, SS; Marin, Y; Roberts, KG; Yudt, LM; Chen, A; Cheng, J; Incao, A; Pinkett, HW; Graham, CL; Dunn, K; Crespo-Carbone, SM; Mackason, KR; Ryan, KB; Sinsimer, D; Goydos, J; Reuhl, KR; Eckhaus, M; Meltzer, PS; Pavan, WJ; Trent, JM; Chen, S. Melanoma mouse model implicates metabotropic glutamate signaling in melanocytic neoplasia. *Nat. Genet.*, 2003, 34, 108-112.

Ritzén, A; Mathiesen, JM; Thomsen, C. Molecular pharmacology and therapeutic prospects of metabotropic glutamate receptor allosteric modulators. *Basic Clin. Pharmacol. Toxicol.*, 2005, 97, 202-213.

Rothstein, JD; Brem, H. Excitotoxic destruction facilitates brain tumor growth. *Nat. Med.*, 2001, 7, 994-995.

Rzeski, W; Turski, L; Ikonomidou, C. Glutamate antagonists limit tumor growth. *Proc. Natl. Acad. Sci. USA*, 2001, 98, 6372-6377.

Skerry, TM; Genever, PG. Glutamate signalling in non-neuronal tissues. *Trends Pharmacol. Sci.*, 2001, 22, 174-181.

Sontheimer, H. Malignant gliomas: perverting glutamate and ion homeostasis for selective advantage. *Trends Neurosci.*, 2003, 26, 543-549.

Steinman, L. Elaborate interactions between the immune and nervous systems. *Nat. Immunol.*, 2004, 5, 575-581.

Stepulak, A; Sifringer, M; Rzeski, W; Endesfelder, S; Gratopp, A; Pohl, EE; Bittigau, P; Felderhoff-Mueser, U; Kaindl, AM; Buhrer, C; Hansen, HH; Stryjecka-Zimmer, M; Turski, L; Ikonomidou, C. NMDA antagonist inhibits the extracellular signal-regulated kinase pathway and suppresses cancer growth. *Proc Natl Acad Sci U S A*, 2005, 102, 15605-15610.

Storto, M; de Grazia, U; Battaglia, G; Felli, MP; Maroder, M; Gulino, A; Ragona, G; Nicoletti, F; Screpanti, I; Frati, L; Calogero; A. Expression of metabotropic glutamate receptors in murine thymocytes and thymic stromal cells. *J. Neuroimmunol.*, 2000, 109, 112-120.

Takano, T; Lin, JH-C; Arcuino, G; Gao, Q; Yang, J; Nedergaard, M. Glutamate release promotes growth of malignant tumors. *Nat. Med.*, 2001, 7, 1010-1015.

Thakker, RV. Multiple endocrine neoplasia. *Horm. Res.*, 2001, 56, 67-72.

Tsibris, JC; Maas, S; Segars, JH; Nicosia, SV; Enkemann, SA; O'Brien, WF; Spellacy, WN. New potential regulators of uterine leiomyomata from DNA arrays: the ionotropic glutamate receptor GluR2. *Biochem Biophys Res Commun.*, 2003, 312, 249-254.

Vincent, AM; Maiese K. The metabotropic glutamate system promotes neuronal survival through distinct pathways of programmed cell death. *Exp Neurol*, 2000, 166, 65-82.

Yoo, BC; Jeon, E; Hong, SH; Shin, YK; Chang, HJ; Park JG. Metabotropic glutamate receptor 4-mediated 5-Fluorouracil resistance in a human colon cancer cell line. *Clin. Cancer Res.*, 2004, 10, 4176-4184.

Yoshida, Y; Tsuzuki, K; Ishiuchi, S; Ozawa, S. Serum-dependence of AMPA receptor-mediated proliferation in glioma cells. *Pathol. Int.*, 2006, 56, 262-271.

Ziemssen, T; Kern, S. Psychoneuroimmunology - Cross-talk between the immune and nervous systems. *J. Neurol.*, 2007, 254 Suppl 2, II8-II11.

INDEX

C

F

G

H

I

M

S

T

X

Y

Z

W